Treatise on
Heart Disease in Indians

Treatise on Heart Disease in Indians

Enas A Enas
MD FACC
Founder President and CEO
Coronary Artery Disease among Asian Indians (CADI)
Research Foundation and Advanced Heart Lipid Clinic
Downers Grove, Illinois, USA
President, Association of Kerala Medical Graduates (AKMG) (1985–1988)
Chair, Board of Trustees, AAPI (1991–1992)

Basil Varkey
MD FRCP FCCP
Professor Emeritus
Department of Medicine
Elected Member (Alpha Omega Alpha Honor Medical Society)
Teaching Scholar (Society of Teaching Scholars)
Distinguished Service Awardee
Medical College of Wisconsin, USA

Foreword
Salim Yusuf

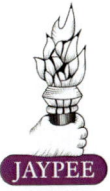

JAYPEE BROTHERS MEDICAL PUBLISHERS
The Health Sciences Publisher
New Delhi | London

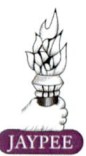

Jaypee Brothers Medical Publishers (P) Ltd

Headquarters
EMCA House, 23/23-B
Ansari Road, Daryaganj
New Delhi 110 002, India
Landline: +91-11-23272143, +91-11-23272703
+91-11-23282021, +91-11-23245672
e-mail: jaypee@jaypeebrothers.com

Corporate Office
4838/24, Ansari Road, Daryaganj
New Delhi 110 002, India
Phone: +91-11-43574357
Fax: +91-11-43574314
e-mail: jaypee@jaypeebrothers.com

Overseas Office
JP Medical Ltd.
83, Victoria Street, London
SW1H 0HW (UK)
Phone: +44-20 3170 8910
e-mail: info@jpmedpub.com

EU GPSR Authorised Representative
Logos Europe, 9 rue Nicolas Poussin
17000, La Rochelle, France
Phone: +33 (0) 6 67 93 73 78
e-mail: contact@logoseurope.eu

Website: www.jaypeebrothers.com
Website: www.jaypeedigital.com

© 2026, Jaypee Brothers Medical Publishers

The views and opinions expressed in this book are solely those of the original contributor(s)/author(s) and do not necessarily represent those of editor(s) or publisher of the book.

All rights reserved. No part of this publication may be reproduced, stored or transmitted in any form or by any means, electronic, mechanical, photocopying, recording or otherwise, without the prior permission in writing of the publishers.

All brand names and product names used in this book are trade names, service marks, trademarks or registered trademarks of their respective owners. The publisher is not associated with any product or vendor mentioned in this book.

Medical knowledge and practice change constantly. This book is designed to provide accurate, authoritative information about the subject matter in question. However, readers are advised to check the most current information available on procedures included and check information from the manufacturer of each product to be administered, to verify the recommended dose, formula, method and duration of administration, adverse effects and contra indications. It is the responsibility of the practitioner to take all appropriate safety precautions. Neither the publisher nor the author(s)/editor(s) assume any liability for any injury and/or damage to persons or property arising from or related to use of material in this book.

This book is sold on the understanding that the publisher is not engaged in providing professional medical services. If such advice or services are required, the services of a competent medical professional should be sought.

Every effort has been made where necessary to contact holders of copyright to obtain permission to reproduce copyright material. If any have been inadvertently overlooked, the publisher will be pleased to make the necessary arrangements at the first opportunity.

Inquiries for bulk sales may be solicited at: jaypee@jaypeebrothers.com

Treatise on Heart Disease in Indians

First Edition: **2026**

ISBN: 978-93-5696-996-4

Printed at: Samrat Offset Pvt. Ltd.

Dedication

*This book is dedicated to my father, the (late) Mathai Enas,
who instilled in me a passion for community service and learning.
He made a courageous sacrifice in sending me to medical college,
despite family opposition.*

—**Enas A Enas**

*Honoring my parents—Varkey and Mariamma.
Expressing my gratitude—to all my teachers and
especially to K Narayana Pai and Harold D Rose.*

—**Basil Varkey**

Foreword

The rise in cardiovascular diseases (CVD) is a relatively recent phenomenon, mainly over the last 60 or 70 years. This was initially documented in the richer countries, especially for myocardial infarction in Europe and North America. There was little data from other regions of the world, but it was soon recognized that strokes, especially due to hypertension, were rising in China and the Far East. Practically, no systematic data existed from South Asia although isolated case reports from the 1970s of premature coronary artery disease among South Asians who had emigrated to other countries emerged. These reports were generally (but not exclusively) among South Asians who had emigrated to wealthier countries especially those at lower socioeconomic status (e.g., workers in the Caribbean, Malaysia, Singapore or the UK) or among professionals in North America.

Dr Enas A Enas, a practicing Cardiologist of Indian origin working in the USA, took note of the several case reports of premature coronary heart disease (CHD) and observed the same phenomenon among patients in his clinical practice. This piqued his interest and he undertook a careful review of the literature and discussions with other cardiologists and epidemiologists around the world; he developed the Coronary Artery Disease among Indians (CADI) study (among over 1,000 physician volunteers) in North America and embarked on a 40-year journey to understand the causes of the rising epidemic of CHD among Indians and other South Asians in different regions of the world. Coronary heart disease is now a global threat, and high rates are seen in almost all parts of the world and among people of all ethnicities.

Dr Enas has lectured extensively around the world, especially in the US and India, and increased awareness about the growing epidemic of CHD among practicing as well as among academic doctors and researchers who established more systematic studies on the question. His interest and enthusiasm for documenting the rise in CHD and then identifying potential means of prevention are unique. It will be of value to doctors and researchers; it has increased awareness of the growing epidemic. This book is informative as it combines his personal insights over 40 years as a cardiologist and weaves them with the findings of others. In writing, organizing, and sharpening the messages, Dr Enas collaborated with a seasoned academician-Professor Emeritus, Dr Basil Varkey.

The information presented in this book on heart disease among South Asians has stimulated large prospective studies in many parts of the world (e.g., India, Canada, UK, and the USA) on South Asian populations. Consequently, in many countries mortality from CHD has started to decline among South Asians. The book is a testament to the passion and persistence of a practicing cardiologist to understand a major health problem; and find solutions for his patients and for South Asian communities at large.

Salim Yusuf
MBBS DPhil FRCP (UK and Canada)
Distinguished Professor
Department of Medicine
Emeritus Founding Executive Director
Population Health Research Institute
McMaster University and Hamilton Health Sciences, Canada
Past President, World Heart Federation (2025)

Editor's Note

In the prologue and the epilogue, Dr Enas, engagingly chronicles his journey through the field of coronary artery disease (CAD) and on his discovery of susceptibilities to and features of CAD in Indians. I am pleased to collaborate with Dr Enas, a rare breed of physician, who combined a busy practice of cardiology with sustained and impactful research that has culminated in this book. This information-packed and well-referenced book is meant to be the one-source book on coronary heart disease (coronary artery disease) for cardiologists, in particular, and to all physicians in training and students in medical colleges.

As Editor and Co-author, I have set a wider goal, beyond specialists and physicians, to reach all those who are interested, as I strongly believe that positive changes in health—specifically heart health—come from informed people. Therefore, I have taken on a seemingly impossible task, to construct a book that is useful to all while adhering to scientific rigor that is required for medical professionals. I have used teaching skills acquired over 4 decades of a rewarding teaching career to try to make this book interesting, understandable, and less forbidding. Thus, the title is heart disease (rather than coronary artery disease), and in each chapter, medical terms are explained and non-technical terms are also used in some of the tables and figures. As an example, the figure on Life's essential 8 (last chapter) in the last chapter would be a worthy addition in every home as a display to serve as a constant reminder that four of the eight factors that affect your health are under your control. An unconventional suggestion for readers without medical training is to start with the last chapter and then the chapter on diet and continue on with chapters that are of particular interest to you.

Staying on the theme of engaged and informed people, it is through individuals and their communities (panchayats, municipalities, etc.), humanitarian service organizations (Rotary Club, Lions Club, etc.), various media and social media platforms and others, that calls for changes are initiated, and efforts are led. A lot can be done to improve the cardiovascular health (heart health) of the people: To name a few—safe green spaces for daily walks and exercises, fruits and vegetables free of contamination, good nutritional programs, improved food labeling, and "Know Your Numbers" health fairs run by trained volunteer personnel to check and record blood pressure, blood glucose and cholesterol.

The vast number of references that follow each chapter of this book recognize the work of physician-scientists in clinical and laboratory research who then translate their work through scientific publications. These publications are then applied to clinical practice and to guide public health policies that benefit many. Physician-scientists expand the boundaries of medicine through research—the life blood of medical progress—but regrettably, the number of physician-scientists is declining. This brief paean is also intended to encourage those engaged in medical studies to consider this as a career path.

The work on this book has been intense, long, and sustained for over a year and I could not have done it without the understanding and steadfast support of Sheela, my life partner, for over 56 years. I am grateful. The book is done and now, readers, it is in your hands.

Basil Varkey

Prologue

All truth passes through three stages: First, it is ridiculed; Second, it is violently opposed; and Third, it is accepted as being self-evident. This quote by Arthur Schopenhauer, a 19th-century German philosopher, resonates deeply with my own 50-year journey. As one of the first to alert the United States (US) physicians and cardiologists about the heightened risk of heart disease in Indians, I encountered significant resistance and skepticism within the American cardiology community.

India and Indians face a significant burden of coronary artery disease, characterized by disproportionately high rates of heart attacks, particularly in younger individuals (under 50 years, and even under 40 years of age). Despite seemingly similar cardiovascular risk profiles across populations, Indians experience a nearly two-fold increased risk of heart attacks compared to whites, even after adjusting for traditional risk factors. The London Life Sciences Population (LOLIPOP) study, which followed 25,000 individuals (South Asians and Whites) for 20 years, further emphasizes this disparity. This landmark study revealed a persistently elevated risk of heart disease in younger South Asians, with the incidence of heart attacks among South Asian women approaching that of white European men. Notably, the risk of heart attack was highest in South Asians younger than 45 years, underscoring the urgency of this critical public health challenge.

This book delves into the heart of India's alarming heart disease epidemic—a significant public health challenge within the South Asian population. South Asians refer to people of ancestral origin from the Indian subcontinent nations, including India, Pakistan, Bangladesh, Nepal, Bhutan, and Sri Lanka, with Indians accounting for 70–75% of South Asians. Most studies among the Indian immigrants have been aggregated and commingled with other South Asians. While Pakistanis, Bangladeshis and other South Asian ethnicities exhibit even higher heart disease, this book focuses on the unique challenges and complexities of heart disease within the Indian population.

It is important to note that while vegetarianism is prevalent in India, a significant portion of the population, including vegetarians, consumes a diet high in saturated and trans fats, often found in fried foods. This can occur while simultaneously having a low intake of essential nutrients like whole grains, fruits, vegetables, nuts, seeds, and non-tropical vegetable oils.

Heart disease disproportionately accounts for two-thirds of the burden of atherosclerotic cardiovascular disease (ASCVD) in India, and ASCVD itself constitutes two-thirds of all cardiovascular diseases (CVDs) within this population. This significant burden of heart disease among Indians, compared to other CVDs like stroke, underscores the critical need to address this major health challenge. My research, spanning over five decades, has exclusively focused on understanding the specific factors contributing to the high burden of heart disease in Indians.

The catalysts for my research. As a young Resident Physician in Chicago in the early 1970s, I was deeply disturbed by the case of a fellow first-year resident physician from India who suffered a heart attack at the tender age of 29 years. He presented to the emergency department with chest pain over several days but was unfortunately and repeatedly sent home with reassurance due to his young age. This tragic event, which unfortunately still occurs today, served as a stark reminder of the vulnerability of even the healthiest individuals to this silent killer. After surviving the initial heart attack, his disease progressed relentlessly, and he tragically succumbed to heart disease before reaching 50 years of age while awaiting a heart transplant.

Another poignant case involved a 37-year-old colleague who, despite seemingly minimal initial disease, experienced a rapid and aggressive progression of coronary atherosclerosis. Within a decade, he was debilitated by severe chest pain and heart failure, ultimately requiring multiple complex surgeries (more in the Epilogue). This case underscores the potential for rapid disease progression, even in seemingly low-risk individuals.

Another 39-year-old patient was diagnosed with inoperable heart disease following his first heart attack. Tragically, he died of a stroke just over 5 years later, highlighting the close connection and shared risk factors between heart attacks and strokes.

These tragedies were further compounded by the cases of three more young Indian physicians in their forties. One experienced a devastating cascade of events, suffering a heart attack followed by an aortic dissection a year later, necessitating emergency surgery. Another, despite undergoing bypass surgery, suffered a massive heart attack within a year, resulting in permanent disability and a significant decline in his quality of life. The third suffered cardiac arrest while enroute to the hospital, narrowly surviving but sustaining significant disabilities.

Witnessing the devastating impact of heart disease on these vibrant young colleagues, most of whom were dedicated to serving others, left an indelible mark on my soul. These experiences ignited a deep sense of urgency and a burning desire to understand the underlying causes of this alarming trend and to develop effective strategies for prevention and intervention. These and other similar case studies served as the driving force behind my initiation of the landmark coronary artery disease in Indians (CADI) study.

The CADI study confirms high rates of heart disease in Indian Americans. The CADI study, a ground-breaking investigation involving nearly 2,000 Indian-American physicians and their families, conducted by the author and commissioned by the American Association of Physicians of Indian Origin (AAPI), confirmed high rates of heart disease in Indian Americans. This landmark study found that Indian American men were four times more likely to develop heart disease compared to the general US population. Furthermore, it revealed the "Indian Paradox," where traditional cardiovascular risk factors, while contributing to heart disease, do not fully explain the disproportionately high rates observed in this population, suggesting the need to explore additional, potentially genetic factors.

Elevated lipoprotein(a) [Lp(a)] found in one in four Indians. The study found that one in four Indians has elevated Lp(a) levels, a potent genetic risk factor for heart attacks. This finding, initially met with skepticism, has gained widespread recognition within the scientific and Indian communities. The evidence strongly suggests that Lp(a) is a major independent risk factor for heart attacks, particularly in young individuals (less than 50 years) and very young individuals (less than 40 years). The risk is doubled in individuals with elevated Lp(a) and further amplified to fourfold among those with other risk factors, such as diabetes or elevated LDL cholesterol.

In the INTERHEART Lp(a) study, the contribution of Lp(a) to heart attack was double in Indians than in whites (10% vs. 5%). The landmark Prospective Urban Rural Epidemiology (PURE) study has demonstrated that risk factors like high cholesterol, high blood pressure, smoking, diabetes, obesity, metabolic syndrome, physical inactivity, air pollution, and poor diet remain crucial, as these risk factors account for approximately 70% of cardiovascular disease globally.

The Global Burden of Elevated Lp(a). The 2018 special report by the National Heart, Lung, and Blood Institute (NHLBI) highlighted the global burden of elevated Lp(a), affecting approximately 1.43 billion individuals worldwide. The report revealed that 25% of Indians have high Lp(a) levels, compared to 20% of whites and 10% of Chinese. The "I" special report established the following Lp(a) classifications:

- *Normal:* <30 mg/dL
- *Moderately high:* 30–50 mg/dL
- *High:* >50 mg/dL

American guidelines embrace and incorporate seminal CADI research findings. Our research achieved a significant milestone in 2018 when the American College of Cardiology and American Heart Association (ACC/AHA) incorporated key findings from the CADI study into their Clinical Practice Guidelines. This landmark decision, recognizing both Lp(a) and South Asian ethnicity as significant risk-enhancing factors for heart disease, has profound implications. It empowers physicians to personalize treatment plans, including the use of statin therapy, based on individual risk profiles, thereby improving the prevention and management of heart disease in the Indian population.

Notably, Lp(a) levels can be measured as early as age 5–10 years, providing a crucial window of opportunity for early detection and preventive interventions, potentially averting a cardiac catastrophe decade in advance. While new medications specifically targeting Lp(a) are anticipated, the good news is that we already have the knowledge, diagnostic tools, and treatments to substantially reduce heart disease risk.

Empowering Indians with Knowledge

By combining these efforts with personalized strategies based on individual risk factor profiles, significant progress has been made in reducing heart disease rates among South Asians in Canada (personal communication with Salim Yusuf and Sonia Anand) and the US, achieving near-parity with the dominant white population. This progress is attributed to the efforts of organizations like the CADI Research Foundation, which have championed awareness and educational initiatives.

This book aims to empower individuals with the knowledge to understand heart disease and its contributing factors, enabling them to actively participate in their healthcare journey. It delves deeply into the complexities of heart disease in Indians, exploring its impact on heart attacks, strokes, and other cardiovascular events.

Across 17 chapters, this book comprehensively examines key risk factors, including tobacco use, hypertension, diabetes, cholesterol, and the critical role of Lp(a). It also explores the latest treatment strategies, including statin therapy and emerging non-statin therapies. Furthermore, the book provides extensive guidance on preventing heart attacks, managing stable angina, cardiovascular kidney metabolic syndrome, atrial fibrillation stroke, and heart failure.

Three chapters are dedicated to prevention, including one chapter focused on diet and another dedicated to "Life's Essential 8," recognizing the need for a tailored approach to heart health within this high-risk population.

While a comprehensive resource for cardiologists, this book is also written in an accessible style, making it understandable for individuals with no medical background. My sincere gratitude goes to my Co-author and Editor, Basil Varkey, whose legendary expertise and meticulous attention to detail ensured the brevity, clarity, and readability of each chapter. His invaluable contributions resulted in the book being trimmed by at least 100 pages without omitting any valuable data.

The book concludes with an epilogue, offering a personal touch as it traces the author's 50+-year journey and contributions. This blend of scientific expertise and personal reflection makes it a compelling resource for understanding and addressing heart disease in the Indian context.

Enas A Enas

Contents

1. Overview of Heart Disease in Indians 1

2. The Natural History of Heart Disease and its Diverse Manifestations 18

3. Risk Factors for Heart Disease with a Focus on Modifiable
   Factors in Indians 33

4. Tobacco Smoking 46

5. Hypertension 58

6. Diabetes Mellitus 69

7. Cholesterol and Heart Disease 84

8. Lipoprotein(a): Underrecognized Heritable Risk Factor for
   Heart Disease 99

9. Heart Disease in Women 115

10. Angina Pectoris: Shift from Invasive Treatment to
    Medical Management 128

11. Acute Coronary Syndrome: Management and Secondary Prevention 138

12. Interrelated Disorders and Diseases: Cardiovascular Kidney
    Metabolic Syndrome, Atrial Fibrillation, Stroke, and Heart Failure 151

13. Statins: Bedrock of Prevention and Treatment of Heart Disease 167

14. Nonstatins: Powerful Drugs to Fight Heart Disease 182

15. Prevention of Heart Disease: Focus on Primordial and
    Primary Prevention 195

16. Prime Importance of a Healthy Diet 205

17. Life's Essential 8 and Modifications for Indians 221

Epilogue *234*

Index *245*

CHAPTER 1

Overview of Heart Disease in Indians

■ EPIDEMIOLOGY

Epidemiology (simply stated, the study of how often diseases occur in different groups of people) forms the foundation to probe why and what to do about it. Over a long period of time, studies outside of India and in the recent past in India, to varying degrees, have shown prevalence (at any given time), incidence (new cases over a given time), increased mortality, and disability caused by heart disease [coronary artery disease (CAD)] in Indians. Of specific note and concern are the premature onset and severity of CAD. Here, we summarize the important findings of major pertinent publications.

Studies from Singapore

Singapore, a small city-state populated by a mix of ethnicities that can be considered an epidemiological laboratory, has provided many comparative case series studies as shown in **Table 1**.

Besides Singapore, a higher incidence and/or mortality from CAD in Indians compared to native-born population have been observed in many countries including the United States,[8-11] United Kingdom,[12-17] Canada,[18-20] Qatar,[21] Malaysia, Mauritius, Italy,[22] Kenya, South Africa, Fiji, New Zealand, Norway,[23] Trinidad, etc.[24] At the outset, our comments on these studies need clarification on the nomenclature as some of them are on South Asians (people who are from or have ancestry from India, Pakistan, Bangladesh, Nepal, Bhutan, Sri Lanka, and the Maldives).[25] However, 80% of South Asians are Indians.

Coronary Artery Disease in Indians (CADI) Study and Others

CADI study of Indian physicians and their family members in the US found a markedly higher prevalence of CAD than the historical control of White Americans.[8] In a large 10-year follow-up study of 341,309 patients (5,149 South Asians), conducted at Kaiser Permanente South Asian ethnicity, compared to White race, was associated with an adjusted odds ratio of 2.04 [95% confidence interval (CI): 1.83–2.28] in predicting adverse cardiovascular (CV) outcomes.[26]

Mediators of Atherosclerosis in South Asians Living in America (MASALA) study[27,28] corroborated the higher risk of heart disease in South Asians (90% were Indians). Since then, other South Asians have been enrolled in this ongoing study.

A multiethnic study in Europe showed an excess cardiovascular disease (CVD) mortality rates that were 37–91% higher among South Asians in Denmark, England, and Wales compared to the general population.[29] Immigrants from South Asia had the highest rate of heart attacks [acute myocardial infarctions (AMIs)] compared to other immigrants and the native population in Italy[22] and Norway.[30]

TABLE 1: Coronary artery disease (CAD) and acute myocardial infarction (AMI) among Indians in Singapore (1959–2019).

Author	Year	Study characteristics and findings
Danaraj[1]	1959	10,000 consecutive autopsies showed a sevenfold higher rate of coronary atherosclerosis in Indians versus Chinese
Hughes[2]	1990	The age-standardized relative risk of heart disease deaths (HDDs) among Indians versus Chinese was 3.8 for males and 3.4 for females. Notably, excess heart disease mortality decreased with age
Heng[3]	2000	The prospective Singapore Cardiovascular Cohort Study ($n = 5,920$) showed that the age-adjusted risk of developing CAD was 2.78 times for Indian males and 1.97 times for females compared to their Chinese counterparts
Mak[4]	2003	A large study ($n = 12,491$) reported that age-standardized CAD incidence was greater than threefold higher in Indians compared to Chinese
Wong[5]	2012	A study of 333 young adults with AMI < 45 years showed a threefold higher incidence of AMI in Indians than in Chinese. Indians who comprise 9% of the population accounted for 31% of AMI, while Chinese who comprise 74% of the population accounted for only 51% AMI
Gupta[6]	2018	A study ($n = 1,749$) found that second-generation Indians had double the risk of developing cardiovascular disease than the first generation
Zheng[7]	2019	Study of 16,983 consecutive ST segment elevation myocardial infarction (STEMI) patients, found that STEMI incidence was greater than twofold higher in Indians compared to Chinese (126 per 100,000 population vs. 58 per 100,000)

St. James Survey in Trinidad, West Indies

A 10-year community survey investigated the risk of CAD among people of Indian/South Asian descent. After exclusion of those with heart disease and small minority groups, 1,998 adults (786 African, 598 Indian, 147 European, and 467 adults of Mixed descent) were enrolled and followed for CAD incidence. Adults of Indian origin had higher prevalence rates of diabetes than other ethnic groups, similar to the observation in the SABRE (Southall and Brent Revisited) study.[24] The age-adjusted relative risk of any CAD event in participants free of CAD at entry was at least twice as high in Indian men and women than in other ethnic groups.[24]

Southall and Brent Revisited Study (SABRE)

The SABRE, a prospective population-based study, evaluated cardiovascular risk factors (CVRFs) in 2,049 Europeans, 1,517 South Asians, and 630 African Caribbeans (40–69 years, mean age: 52.4 ± 6.9 years from 1988 through 1991).[14] Fatal and nonfatal CAD events were captured over a median 20.5-year follow-up. Compared to Europeans, CAD incidence was greater in South Asians and less in African Caribbeans. The age- and sex-adjusted hazard ratio (HR) for South Asian versus European was 1.70 (95% CI: 1.52–1.91, $p < 0.001$). The African Caribbean versus European age- and sex-adjusted HR was 0.64 (95% CI: 0.52–0.79, $p < 0.001$). The higher risk of heart disease in South Asians and lower risk among African Caribbean remained significant when adjusted for various risk factors even though both the prevalence of diabetes in South Asians and African Caribbean was similar and more than thrice that of Europeans.[13] This study was not confined to CAD but encompassed CVD that includes strokes. Strokes were higher both in

South Asians and African Caribbeans than in Europeans. A follow-up article in 2021 showed that in South Asians the survival rate and all-cause mortality rate had markedly improved over the years.[31]

London Life Science Population Study

London Life Science Population (LOLIPOP) study followed 17,606 South Asians and 7,766 White Europeans (aged 35–75 years) from Northwest London for approximately 20 years. South Asians demonstrated a significantly higher risk of developing CAD compared to White Europeans throughout the period. **Table 2** shows the striking difference between the two populations at 5, 10, 15, and 20 years.

This marked variance is not explained by differences in risk factors as a fully adjusted multivariate model revealed that South Asians had a nearly a twofold increased HR (HR: 1.83; 95% CI: 1.63–2.06, $p < 0.0001$) of developing CAD than White Europeans after accounting for age, gender, traditional CVRFs, insulin resistance, and related metabolic disturbances **(Fig. 1)**. It should be further noted that though all four age-groups of South Asians showed an increased HR, the difference from White Europeans was most in the young with an HR of 1.88 and lessened with age (1.86 in those 45–54, 1.84 in those 55–65, and 1.67 in those >65 years old) corroborating the early 1991 report of Balarajan[16] on the increased risk of CAD in young Indians.

TABLE 2: Cumulative incidence of coronary artery disease among South Asians and Whites in the LOLIPOP study during a 20-year follow-up.[32]

	South Asians	Whites
5 years	3.81%	2.68%
10 years	7.44%	4.84%
15 years	12.73%	8.20%
20 years	17.41%	10.85%

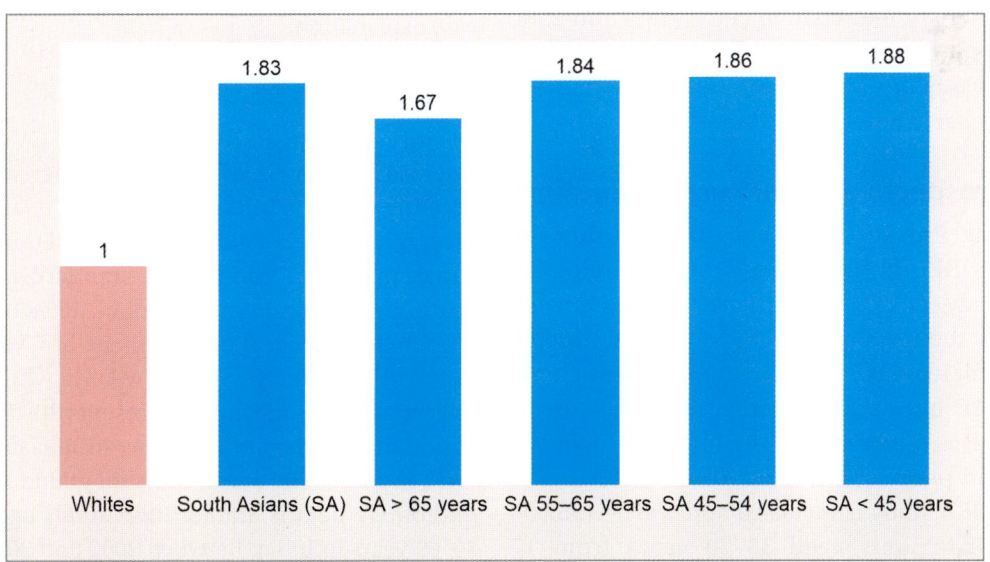

Fig. 1: Hazard ratio (risk) for coronary artery disease (CAD) incidence in South Asians versus Whites (men and women combined) in London Life Science Population (LOLIPOP) study at four distinct age-groups.
Source: Adapted from Kooner, et al.[32]

Improving Trends

Although heart disease deaths (HDDs) have been decreasing in the South Asian diaspora globally, the rate of decline was slower and the mortality rate ratio (MRR) higher than that of other populations.[33] Recent studies, though, show an improvement in these trends. A follow-up to the SABRE study in 2021 showed that in South Asians the survival rate and all-cause mortality rate had markedly improved.[31] In a large multiethnic population study in California and Hawaii reported in 2023, that CVD rate was not higher in South Asians.[34] Multiple studies report comparable or better outcomes in South Asians after major adverse cardiovascular event (MACE) and after primary percutaneous coronary intervention (PPCI) or coronary artery bypass graft (CABG).[35,36] In a large Canadian study of patients with acute coronary syndrome (ACS), 30-day and 1-year mortality were similar in South Asians and Europeans. and South Asians had improved long-term survival after CABG or percutaneous coronary intervention (PCI) (18% and 25%, respectively) than Europeans.[37] Repeat revascularization procedures, however, were higher in South Asians.

Prospective Urban Rural Evaluation

The Prospective Urban Rural Evaluation (PURE), a multinational epidemiological study of CVD,[38] is a particularly important one for the magnitude of its scope and notable conclusions. CVD encompasses not only CAD but stroke and other diseases of heart valves, heart failure, rhythm abnormalities, and peripheral arterial disease (PAD). The PURE study is inclusive and wide—155,000 participants aged 35–70 years from 17 countries, from high-income countries (HICs), middle-income countries (MICs), and low-income countries (LICs) with a long duration (median follow-up of 9.5 years).[39] Among the most notable findings of the PURE study are: (1) Cardiovascular mortality (CVM) is significantly higher in individuals of a low socioeconomic status (SES) in all countries regardless of their income status; (2) people of low SES experience a nearly threefold higher risk of CVM than those at a high SES; (3) HICs have higher levels of CVRFs but lower CVD rates, whereas LICs have lower levels of CVRF rates but higher rates of CVD; and (4) ~70% of CVD incidence and deaths were attributed to modifiable risk factors, such as hypertension, diabetes, smoking, and high non-high-density lipoprotein (HDL) cholesterol and unhealthy diets.[38]

The PURE South Asia substudy **(Fig. 2)** found CVD rates were high in both urban and rural areas (more in rural) and myocardial infarction (MI) (heart attacks) were more than double that of strokes.[39] The divergence in rates between MI and strokes (a recurring theme in other studies as well) that are diseases caused by atherosclerosis and have common risk factors (Chapter 3) escapes an easy explanation.

Million Death Study in India

Despite the mortality rate from CVDs (especially from CAD), the largest increase noted in young adults born after 1970, and divergent tracks of deaths from CAD and stroke in India,[41] the lack of standardized death registration in many Indian states has hindered an accurate assessment of CVM. The Million Death Study (MDS), which utilized verbal autopsies,[42] represents the first nationally representative effort to measure CVM in India. The researchers identified 1.3 million CV deaths among individuals aged 30–69 years in India. Between 2000 and 2015 the CV deaths among men and women aged 30–69 in India increased while CV deaths markedly decreased in the UK and in the US

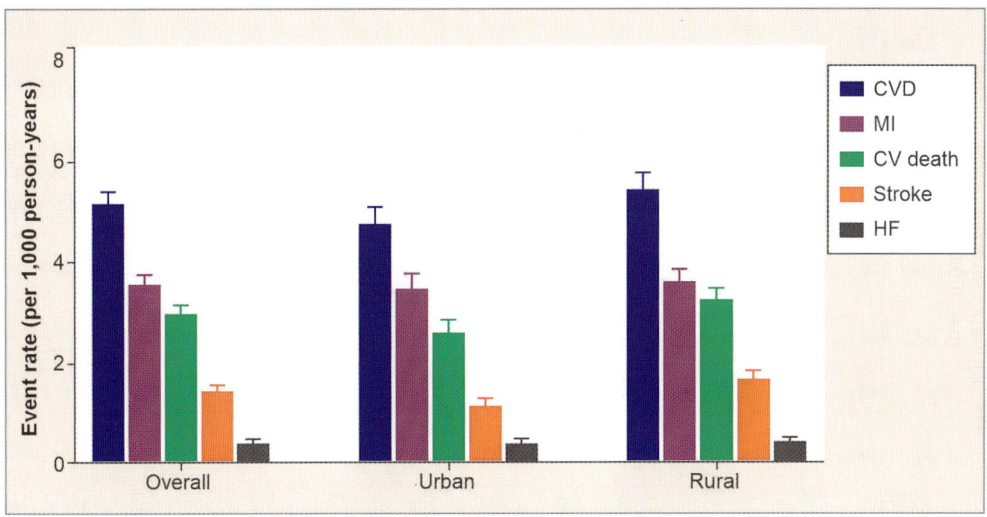

Fig. 2: The incidence of cardiovascular events in the overall South Asia cohort and the urban and rural areas in the Prospective Urban Rural Evaluation (PURE) study. (CVD: cardiovascular disease; CV death: cardiovascular death; HF: heart failure; MI: myocardial infarction)
Source: Reproduced with permission from Joseph et al.[39]

(Figs. 3A and B) while the age-standardized mortality rates of all three countries were fairly close in 2000. Thus the 2015 mortality rate in India that is more than double of UK and US reflects the marked decrease in CVM achieved in these two HICs.

Note that mortality rate from stroke (Figs. 3C and D) is much less than that of CAD and that unlike CAD rate mortality from stroke shows decrease from 2000 to 2015.

Other notable findings of the MDS in India are: (1) CAD is the leading (62%) cause of CVM, followed by stroke that accounted for 28% of deaths; (2) the observed mortality rate was lower than the global burden of disease (GBD) modeled estimate by the Institute for Health Metrics and Evaluation (IHME); (3) CAD deaths increased during the period of study in men (from 10.4 to 13.1%) and in women (from 4.8 to 6.6%) while deaths from stroke decreased slightly; (4) the rise in CVM was more in rural areas compared to urban areas; and (5) many individuals who died from CAD had not been previously diagnosed.[40]

PREMATURE CORONARY ARTERY DISEASE

There are no prospective studies focused solely on "premature" heart disease in Indians. The two major studies described earlier (PURE and MDS) were not focused on the issue of prematurity. However, there are a plethora of reports on premature coronary artery disease (PCAD) and very premature coronary artery disease (VPCAD) from within India, other South Asian countries, and from the large diaspora worldwide.[41] The source of information, the type of clinical manifestation, and the criteria used to define prematurity vary in these reports and therefore it is a challenge to cogently present them for the readers. We present the gist of larger studies in a tabular form (Table 3) and supplement them with further comments in the text.

On a historical note, credit for lighting the spark on premature heart disease in Indians goes to Littler and Lawrence[42] who in 1985,

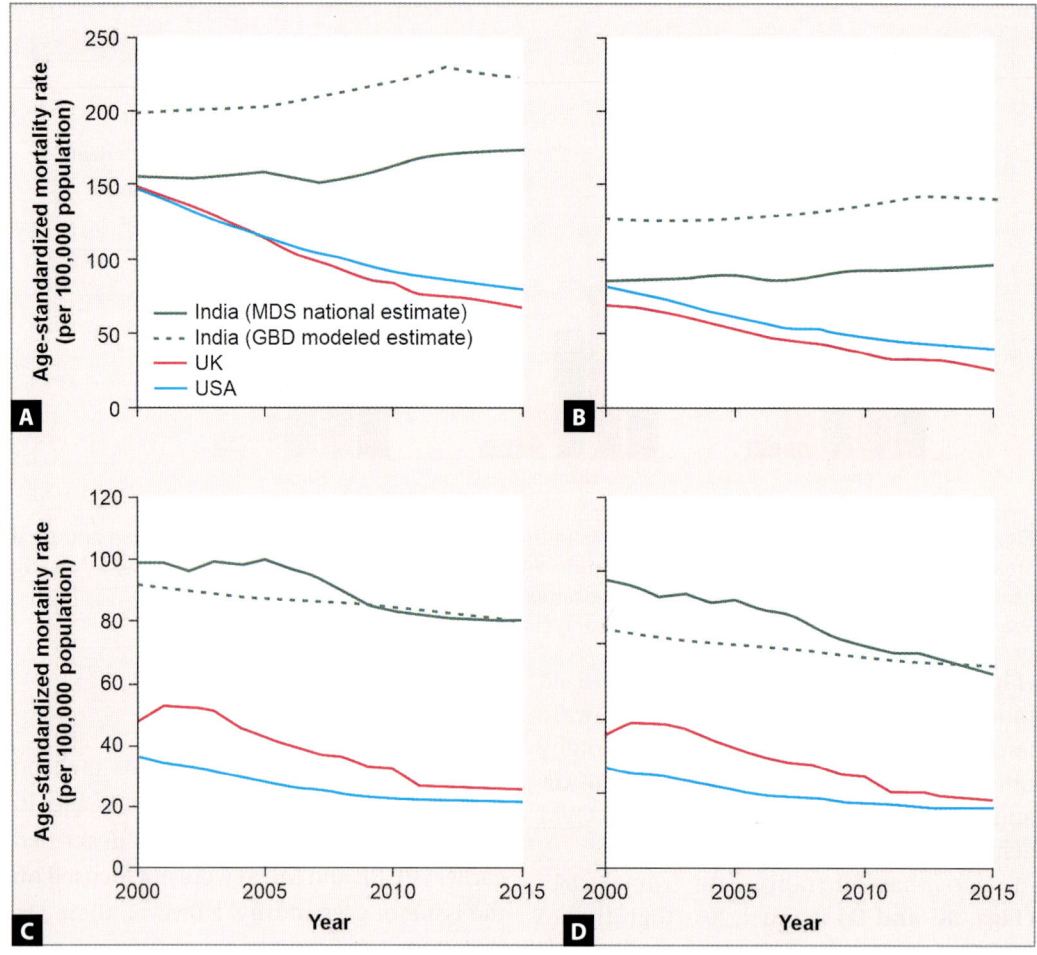

Figs. 3A to D: Secular trends in age-standardized mortality rates among men and women (aged ≥30 years), 2000–2015. Coronary artery disease in men (A) and women (B); stroke in men (C) and women (D). (GBD: global burden of disease; MDS: Million Death Study)
Source: Reproduced with permission from Ke et al.[40]

reported heart attacks in four very young (18–22 years of age) Indians and did not find any Whites in the same age-group. Balarajan[16] found that the standardized mortality rate (SMR) was higher in Indians than in Whites across a wide age range (20–69)—36% higher in men and 46% higher in women. He further noted that when younger age-groups are compared, the difference between Indians and Whites was much more pronounced (threefold higher in ages 20–29 and twofold higher in ages 30–39). Chaikhouni[21] found that 578 patients (23% of a total of 2,515) with AMI were <40 years of age and 71% of them were Indians compared to 12% Qataris (native citizens of Qatar) and 9% other Arabs.

The monumental (15,152 first AMI cases and 14,820 controls from 52 countries) INTERHEART study led by Yusuf[43] found that the median age of AMI in South Asians was 53 (compared to 63 in Western Europe and China) and that AMI under 40 years of age at 10.6% was the highest in South Asians (compared to 4.4% in Chinese, Latin

TABLE 3: Premature onset of coronary artery disease (CAD) in Indians/South Asians.

Author, Reference No.	Year	Region/country, N (number)	Source, CAD type	Definition of prematurity Age-group and comparison description
Balarajan[16]	1991	England and Wales, N = 203,341	CAD mortality registry	Definition not provided (DNP) Standardized CAD mortality rate under age 30 was over threefold higher than in Whites
Chaikhouni[21]	1993	Qatar, N = 2,515	AMI (acute myocardial infarction)	DNP 23% <40 (71% were Indians)
Yusuf[43]	2004	Global study, N = 15,152	AMI	DNP (see follow-up study under Joshi) 11% <40
Ranjith[54]	2005	South Africa, N = 2,290	ACS (acute coronary syndrome)	DNP 20% <45
Tewari[48]	2005	Lucknow, India, N = 1,971	CAG (coronary artery angiogram) registry	DNP 47% between 40 and 55; 11% <40
Joshi[55]	2007	South Asia, N = 3,936 cases and controls	AMI	DNP Mean age of first myocardial infarction (MI) 53 in South Asians versus 58.8 globally
Wong[5]	2012	Singapore, N = 333 under 45	AMI < 45	DNP AMI < 45 was threefold higher in Indians than in Chinese
Chowdhury[47]	2015	Bangladesh, N = 5,000	BRAVE (Bangladesh Risk of Acute Vascular Events)	DNP 46% <50
Deora[50]	2016	Gujarat, India, N = 8,268	CAG registry	DNP 10% <40
Agrawal[49]	2016	Varanasi, India, N = 100	AMI	DNP 27% <50
Zheng[7]	2019	Singapore, N = 16,983	STEMI (ST segment elevation MI)	DNP *Indians: 6 years younger than the Chinese*
Patil[51]	2020	Bengaluru, India, N = 628	PCAD (premature coronary artery disease) registry	*PCAD: Age <35* 100%
Sharma[52]	2022	Jaipur, India, N = 4,672	PCI (percutaneous coronary intervention) registry	*PCAD:* M (male) 40–54; F (female) 45–59 27% of M and 32% of F *VPCAD:* M < 40; F < 45 5% of M and 7% of F
Khraishah[53]	2022	Kerala, India, N = 21,374	ACS registry	DNP 22% <50

Contd...

Contd...

Author, Reference No.	Year	Region/ country, N (number)	Source, CAD type	Definition of prematurity Age-group and comparison description
Ullah[44]	2023	Pakistan, N = 15,800	CAG registry	PCAD: M40–54; F40–64 --60%
Kumar[45]	2023	Pakistan, N = 4,686	STEMI	PCAD: M < 55; F < 65 --38% VPCAD: M < 40; F < 45 --12%
Peerwani[46]	2024	Pakistan, N = 23,560	ACS	DNP 12% <45

Americans 3.7%, and overall rate of 6%). As shown on **Table 3**, studies from Pakistan,[44-46] and the prospective Bangladesh Risk of Acute Vascular Events (BRAVE) study from Bangladesh[47] reported increased incidence of heart attacks in the young. As shown in the table, studies from different regions in India such as Lucknow,[48] Varanasi,[49] Gujarat,[50] Bangalore,[51] Jaipur,[52] and Kerala[53] have corroborated the finding of PCAD in Indians.

Standardized Definition of Premature Heart Disease

The data presented in **Table 3** and discussed in the text substantiate the burden of PCAD in South Asians. However, it also brings into focus the need for standardized definitions and therefore we propose definitions [adapted from definitions and age-groups used by the World Health Organization (WHO) and the IHME that can be uniformly used. Specifically, we propose a gender-neutral definition with the following designations: (1) PCAD—between ages 50 and 69 years; (2) CAD in the young—between ages 40 and 50 years; and (3) CAD in the very young under 40 years of age.

Adoption of this definition with designations allows comparisons between countries and between states in India and is important for research on the factors involved in PCAD outside of the established CVRFs (smoking, hypertension, diabetes, high cholesterol) that would lead to improved management.

SEVERITY OF CORONARY ARTERY DISEASE

Besides the premature onset, Enas and Mehta[56] in 1995 found that CAD was very severe in Indians and termed it "malignant heart disease". As this term packed a punch, it drew much needed attention to the severity of disease in young Indians. Since then, several studies have corroborated the finding of severity of CAD in Indians, especially in the young.[43,57] In comparison, in the US and Canada less severe disease was reported in two large studies. The first, a computed tomography angiogram (CTA) evaluation of 1,420 subjects with undiagnosed chest pain from a single center found only 3% had obstructive CAD.[57] The second, by Zimmerman and associates[58] from the Coronary Artery Surgery Study (CASS) registry of 8,839 patients from the US and Canada, had 294 men <35 years and 210 women <45 years of age and found that only 504 (5.7% of the total) had obstructive heart disease.[59] Young patients generally had angiographically normal coronary arteries, nonobstructive disease or single-vessel disease. In striking contrast, Koulaouzidis and colleagues[59] reported that South

Asians compared to Caucasians had more diffuse coronary calcification, more arterial segments with obstructive ($p = 0.006$) and nonobstructive plaques ($p = 0003$), and more triple-vessel disease (TVD) ($p = 0.0004$). A comparative study of subjects of different ethnicities reported that Indians had higher SYNTAX scores, which allow a reproducible quantitative assessment of the degree and complexity of coronary atherosclerosis, than Caucasians and Chinese that persisted even after adjustment of covariates.[30,60]

A report from Jaipur, India of successive (January 2018 to June 2021) patients who underwent interventional procedures is particularly noteworthy for the severity and premature onset of CAD.[43] Findings are shown in **Table 4** and explained as follows. Of 4,672 enrolled 1,450 (30%) patients were young (premature or very premature onset) and 630 of the 1,450 (43%) had multivessel disease. In the very premature group of 212 patients multivessel disease was noted in 122 (57%). In this study, cholesterol, low-density lipoprotein cholesterol (LDL-C), and tobacco smoking were higher in the premature group compared to the non-premature group while hypertension, diabetes, and chronic kidney disease were higher in the non-premature group.[52] In another study, remnant cholesterol (very low-density lipoprotein cholesterol) that represents cholesterol in triglycerides was associated with both prematurity and severity of CAD.[61]

Others, without distinction to age-groups, have noted diabetes and metabolic syndrome (MetS) as important factors for CAD in South Asians.[62] A comparative study of asymptomatic South Asians and Whites with type 2 diabetes, matched for other traditional risk factors for

TABLE 4: Severity of premature coronary artery disease (CAD) in Indians.[52]

Indicators of severity: Vessels, stents, PCI, CABG, LVEF	Premature women 45–60 years # 299 (32%)	Very premature women <45 years # 61 (7%)	Premature men 40–55 years # 939 (25%)	Very premature men <40 years # 151 (4%)
Single-vessel disease	131 (3.8%)	25 (41%)	434 (46.2%)	65 (43%)
Double-vessel disease	110 (36.8%)	25 (41%)	330 (35.1%)	55 (36.4%)
Triple-vessel disease	55 (18.4%)	11 (18%)	13 (18.4%)	31 (20.5%)
1 stent	184 (61.5%)	42 (68.9%)	623 (66.3%)	107 (70.9%)
2 stents	84 (28.1%)	14 (23%)	238 (25.3%)	30 (19.9%)
3 or more stents	24 (8.1%)	5 (8.2%)	61.(6.5%)	9 (5.9%)
Prior percutaneous coronary intervention (PCI)	24 (8.0%)	7 (11.5%)	94 (10%)	69 (6%)
Prior coronary artery bypass grafting (CABG)	4 (1.3%)	1 (1.6%)	11 (1.2%)	0
Mean left ventricular ejection fraction (LVEF)	47.4 ± 10.2	44.2 ± 9.1	45 ± 10.1	44.8 ± 9.7
LVEF < 30%	12 (4.1%)	2 (3.3%)	37 (4%)	7 (4.7%)
LVEF 30–45%	129 (44%)	31 (50.8%)	527 (56.9%)	88 (58.7%)
LVEF > 45%	152 (41.8%)	28 (45.9%)	363 (39.2%)	55 (36.7%)

CAD, found that South Asians had more subclinical atherosclerosis as determined by Coronary Artery Calcium (CAC) score.[63] Two studies from India highlighted the correlation of MetS to diabetes and CAD. Bhatti et al.[64] found a very high prevalence (male 72%, female 86%) of type 2 diabetes in patients with MetS. Mahalle et al.[65] reported that not only those with MetS had more TVD but also that the prevalence of TVD increased in a graded fashion with the number of components of MetS (48% in those with 3 components and 77% with all 5 components).

Without diminishing the worth of the aforementioned studies, it is fair to state that the causes of both prematurity and severity of CAD in Indians are not fully known. One genetic factor, Lipoprotein (a), has emerged as a strong link to premature and severe disease[66-68] and deservedly merit further discussion (Chapter 8). A profusion of reports (many cited in this chapter) on the vast impact of CAD in South Asians led the American College of Cardiology and the American Heart Association to recognize South Asian ethnicity as a heart disease risk-enhancing factor in their 2018 ACC/AHA clinical practice guidelines.[69]

IMPACT OF CORONARY ARTERY DISEASE

To fully understand the impact of a disease on a specific population we need to consider both mortality and morbidity. For information on these we often turn to the IHME, a research organization that has a pivotal role in the GBD study.[70] IHME relies on a combination of primary and secondary data, vital statistics, disease registries, and household surveys.

As much as IHME is valued as a great resource to understand prevalence and impact of diseases globally and regionally, it must also be understood that it depends on accurate and comprehensive data from all countries. In low- and middle-income countries with deficiencies in such data, IHME uses advanced modeling techniques to estimate disease burden and cause-specific mortality rates. These limitations should be kept in mind as we present the IHME derived data **(Table 5)** on mortality and morbidity of CAD in Indians under the age of 49 with comparative figures globally and in the US.

As of 2021 the population of India was ~1.45 billion (18% of the global population), while the population of the US was ~335 million (4.23% of the global population). In 2021, a total of 609,809 CAD deaths occurred globally in the 15–49 age-group, of which India accounted for 185, 949 (30% of deaths in this age-group) and the US accounted for 13,377 (2% of deaths) **(Table 5)**. India with a population 4 times that of the US had 15 times higher rate of CAD deaths in people aged 49 and under. This vastly disproportionate number of premature deaths is not the only measure of the impact of CAD in India as disability takes a big toll too.

Disability-adjusted Life Years

Disability-adjusted life years (DALYs) provide a comprehensive measure that incorporates both years of life lost (YLL) due to premature death and years lived with disability (YLD). The latter, YLD, captures the impact of heart disease on individuals who survive but experience ongoing disability such as limitations in mobility, daily activities, and overall quality of life and is a useful metric to understand the human cost of this disease and to guide efforts to better prevention, treatment, and management strategies. As shown on **Table 4**, the pattern on DALYs is similar to that of deaths. DALYs in India were 30% of the global DALYs and 15 times higher than that of the US. The marked difference

TABLE 5: Deaths, disability-adjusted life years (DALY), years of life lost (YLL), and years lived in disability (YLD) from coronary artery disease (CAD) at ages 15–49 in the world, in India and in the US. For comparison, CAD deaths at ages 50–69 are also shown.[70]

	World		India		United States	
Mortality	Number (#) of deaths	Percentage (%)	# of deaths	% of global CAD deaths	# of deaths	% of global CAD deaths
CAD deaths All ages	8,991,637	100%	1,632,882	18.16%	495,222	5.5%
CAD deaths Ages 50–69	2,608,134	29%	661,066	25.34%	116,001	23.52%
CAD deaths Ages 15–49	609,809	6.78%	185,949	30.49%	13,377	2.19%
Morbidity	DALY #	%	DALY #	% of global DALY	DALY #	% of global DALY
DALY Ages 15–49	30,443,373	100%	9,234,826	30.33%	644,703	2.12%
	YLL #	%	YLL #	% of global YLL	YLL #	% of global YLL
YLL Ages 15–49	30,019,103	100%	9,149,875	30.48%	632,955	2.11%
	YLD #	%	YLD #	% of global YLD	YLD #	% of global YLD
YLD Ages 15–49	424,271	100%	84,951	20%	11,748	2.77%

in YLL between India and the US also merits emphasis. The number of CAD deaths in Indians under 50 years of age is under 200,000 but has a giant-size impact on YLL of >9 million compared to 633,000 in the US. This spotlights several deficiencies in awareness, diagnosis, and treatment of CAD in Indians that will be discussed in the later chapters of this book.

■ TRANSITIONS AND TRENDS

India's story, after it became an independent country in 1947, is one of remarkable progress in the health domain as life expectancy increased while deaths from communicable diseases were markedly reduced. According to the WHO data, life expectancy has shot up from 32 years to 71 years. This improvement is higher than the global average of 26 years and markedly higher than the 13-year increase in the US during the same period. India's life expectancy in 2023 of 71 years is just 8 years shy of that of the US. This remarkable epidemiological transition has rightly shifted focus from communicable diseases to noncommunicable diseases (NCDs), and in particular to heart disease. Heart disease has become the leading cause of death in India, in urban and rural areas.[39,71] The rising trend of CVD is also noted in other South Asian countries and in China. The transition of India from a low- and middle-income country to a global power with fast-paced economic growth has brought along sociocultural, nutritional, environmental, and other transitions. These are drivers that increase the risk factors for CVDs.[72]

One apparent anomaly noted is that while India has a high CAD mortality rate, India's all-cause mortality rate compares favorably with countries of the western world. This plausibly can be explained by the lower mortality rates from cancers and strokes in Indians offsetting the higher mortality rate from CAD. In the UK Biobank population-based study of ~500,000 people, South Asians had a 20% lower cancer incidence and 41% lower cancer mortality compared to Whites.[73] Other studies from the US, India, and UK have also reported lower rates of cancer incidence and mortality among Indians and other South Asians.[74,75] As was noted earlier, both in PURE South Asia substudy and MDS, strokes were much less than CADs in Indians and deaths from MI far exceeded those from stroke.

The challenge posed by the magnitude and impact of heart disease in India is formidable but not insurmountable as exemplified by the success of the US in combating heart disease. In 1990, the US had the highest age-standardized death rate (ASDR) for heart disease driven by uncontrolled risk factors and high rates of premature deaths. The nearly 50% decline in ASDR for heart disease in the US in the following three decades was not an accidental happening but was a deliberate one that focused on (1) identification and control of three major risk factors (tobacco use, hypertension, and high cholesterol), and (2) better care of patients with ACS, and (3) secondary prevention.[76]

India needs to act on all levels of pre-vention (Chapters 15, 16, and 17) and recognition and management of risk factors and fast and optimal care of acute events (discussed in various chapters of this book). The first step is to know more about atherosclerosis, the cause of CAD, and other CVDs. In the next chapter, we explain atherosclerosis—the process of plaque formation, vulnerable plaques, its insidious nature, the gamut of clinical manifestations—and stress the importance of early detection of heart disease that is often silent.

■ KEY TAKEAWAYS

- Many studies have reported increased risk of heart disease (CAD) and heart attacks (AMIs) in Indians/South Asians compared to other ethnic populations.
- Though there are no large prospective studies focused on prematurity, premature onset of heart disease in Indians (outside and within India) are reported in numerous studies **(Table 3)**. As the definitions used to define "prematurity" are varied, a gender-neutral standardized definition is proposed.
- Besides prematurity, the severity of CAD in South Asians/Indians is more than in other populations according to some studies.
- In a large study in India **(Table 4)** of successive patients who underwent PCI 30% were premature or very premature. Of the very premature (women <age 45, men age <40), more than one half of them (57%) had double- or triple-vessel disease.
- Based on the number of sources of reports on the incidence, prematurity, and severity of CAD in South Asians, the American College of Cardiology and the American Heart Association recognized South Asian ancestry as a risk-enhancing factor for CAD.
- The causes for premature and severe CAD in Indians are not fully understood. Genetic factors play a role but what they are and to what extent they cause CAD are areas that are currently being explored and these are discussed in subsequent chapters.
- India is disproportionately impacted by heart disease. 18% of CAD deaths in the world are in India (compared to 5.5% in the US). The disproportion is markedly more when CAD deaths under 50 years of age are compared: 30% in India versus 2% in the US.

- Besides mortality, to fully understand how India is impacted by CAD, morbidity should also be considered. Measure of DALYs incorporates both YLL due to premature death and YLD. DALYs in India are 30% of the global DALYs and 15× (times) of the US as per IHME data (limitations noted in the text).
- Since India became an independent country in 1947, life expectancy has shot up to a level close to that of the US and deaths from communicable diseases have been markedly controlled. Heart disease has become the leading cause of death in India and it markedly increases the YLD in survivors.

REFERENCES

1. Danaraj TJ, Acker M, Danaraj W, Wong HO, Tan BY. Ethnic group differences in coronary heart disease in Singapore: an analysis of necropsy records. Am Heart J. 1959;58:516-26.
2. Hughes K, Lun KC, Yeo PP. Cardiovascular diseases in Chinese, Malays, and Indians in Singapore. I. Differences in mortality. J Epidemiol Community Health. 1990;44(1):24-8.
3. Heng DM, Lee J, Chew SK, Tan BY, Hughes K, Chia KS. Incidence of ischaemic heart disease and stroke in Chinese, Malays and Indians in Singapore: Singapore Cardiovascular Cohort Study. Ann Acad Med Singap. 2000;29(2):231-6.
4. Mak KH, Chia KS, Kark JD, Chua T, Tan C, Foong BH, et al. Ethnic differences in acute myocardial infarction in Singapore. Eur Heart J. 2003;24(2):151-60.
5. Wong CP, Loh SY, Loh KK, Ong PJ, Foo D, Ho HH. Acute myocardial infarction: Clinical features and outcomes in young adults in Singapore. World J Cardiol. 2012;4(6):206-10.
6. Gupta P, Gan ATL, Man REK, Fenwick EK, Tham YC, Sabanayagam C, et al. Risk of Incident Cardiovascular Disease and Cardiovascular Risk Factors in First and Second-Generation Indians: The Singapore Indian Eye Study. Sci Rep. 2018;8(1):14805.
7. Zheng H, Pek PP, Ho AF, Wah W, Foo LL, Li JQ, et al. Ethnic Differences and Trends in ST-Segment Elevation Myocardial Infarction Incidence and Mortality in a Multi-Ethnic Population. Ann Acad Med Singap. 2019;48(3):75-85.
8. Enas EA, Garg A, Davidson MA, Nair VM, Huet BA, Yusuf S. Coronary heart disease and its risk factors in first-generation immigrant Asian Indians to the United States of America. Indian Heart J. 1996;48(4):343-53.
9. Palaniappan L, Garg A, Enas E, Lewis H, Bari S, Gulati M, et al. South Asian Cardiovascular Disease & Cancer Risk: Genetics & Pathophysiology. J Community Health. 2018; 43(6):1100-14.
10. Vijayaraghavan K, Brown A. South Asian ancestry as a risk enhancer for ASCVD: Merits and challenges. J Clin Lipidol. 2019;13(4):522-4.
11. Volgman AS, Palaniappan LS, Aggarwal NT, Gupta M, Khandelwal A, Krishnan AV, et al.; American Heart Association Council on Epidemiology and Prevention; Cardiovascular Disease and Stroke in Women and Special Populations Committee of the Council on Clinical Cardiology; Council on Cardiovascular and Stroke Nursing; Council on Quality of Care and Outcomes Research; and Stroke Council. Atherosclerotic Cardiovascular Disease in South Asians in the United States: Epidemiology, Risk Factors, and Treatments: A Scientific Statement From the American Heart Association. Circulation. 2018;138(1):e1-e34.
12. Forouhi NG, Sattar N, Tillin T, McKeigue PM, Chaturvedi N. Do known risk factors explain the higher coronary heart disease mortality in South Asian compared with European men? Prospective follow-up of the Southall and Brent studies, UK. Diabetologia. 2006;49(11):2580-8.
13. Tillin T, Hughes AD, Mayet J, Whincup P, Sattar N, Forouhi NG, et al. The relationship between metabolic risk factors and incident cardiovascular disease in Europeans, South Asians, and African Caribbeans: SABRE (Southall and Brent Revisited)—a prospective population-based study. J Am Coll Cardiol. 2013;61(17):1777-86.
14. Tillin T, Sattar N, Godsland IF, Hughes AD, Chaturvedi N, Forouhi NG. Ethnicity-specific

obesity cut-points in the development of Type 2 diabetes - a prospective study including three ethnic groups in the United Kingdom. Diabet Med. 2015;32(2):226-34.
15. McKeigue PM. Coronary heart disease in Indians, Pakistanis and Bangladeshis: aetiology and possibilities of prevention. Br Heart J. 1992;67:341-2.
16. Balarajan R. Ethnic differences in mortality from ischaemic heart disease and cerebrovascular disease in England and Wales. BMJ. 1991;302(6776):560-4.
17. Wang J, Tillin T, Hughes AD, Chaturvedi N. Associations between family history and coronary artery calcium and coronary heart disease in British Europeans and South Asians. Int J Cardiol. 2020;300:39-42.
18. Anand SS, Yusuf S. Risk factors for cardiovascular disease in Canadians of South Asian and European origin: a pilot study of the Study of Heart Assessment and Risk in Ethnic Groups (SHARE). Clin Invest Med. 1997;20(4):204-10.
19. Sheth T, Nair C, Nargundkar M, Anand S, Yusuf S. Cardiovascular and cancer mortality among Canadians of European, south Asian and Chinese origin from 1979 to 1993: An analysis of 1.2 million deaths. C Med J. 1999;161(2):132-8.
20. Bainey KR, Gupta M, Ali I, Bangalore S, Chiu M, Kaila K, et al. The Burden of Atherosclerotic Cardiovascular Disease in South Asians Residing in Canada: A Reflection From the South Asian Heart Alliance. CJC Open. 2019;1(6):271-81.
21. Chaikhouni A, Chouhan L, Pomposiello C, Banna A, Mahrous F, Thomas G, et al. Myocardial infarction in Qatar: the first 2515 patients. Clin Cardiol. 1993;16(3):227-30.
22. Fedeli U, Cestari L, Ferroni E, Avossa F, Saugo M, Modesti PA. Ethnic inequalities in acute myocardial infarction hospitalization rates among young and middle-aged adults in Northern Italy: high risk for South Asians. Intern Emerg Med. 2018;13(2):177-82.
23. Rabanal KS, Selmer RM, Igland J, Tell GS, Meyer HE. Ethnic inequalities in acute myocardial infarction and stroke rates in Norway 1994-2009: a nationwide cohort study (CVDNOR). BMC Public Health. 2015;15:1073.
24. Miller GJ, Beckles GL, Maude GH, Carson DC, Alexis SD, Price SG, et al. Ethnicity and other characteristics predictive of coronary heart disease in a developing community: principal results of the St James Survey, Trinidad. Int J Epidemiol. 1989;18(4):808-17.
25. Stefil M, Bell J, Calvert P, Lip GY. Heightened risks of cardiovascular disease in South Asian populations: causes and consequences. Expert Rev Cardiovasc Ther. 2023;21(4):281-91.
26. Pursnani S, Merchant M. South Asian ethnicity as a risk factor for coronary heart disease. Atherosclerosis. 2020;315:126-30.
27. Shah H, Garacci E, Behuria S, Cainzos-Achirica M, Kandula NR, Kanaya AM, et al. Cardiovascular risk-enhancing factors and coronary artery calcium in South Asian American adults: The MASALA study. Am J Prev Cardiol. 2023;13:100453
28. Shah NS, Talegawkar SA, Jin Y, Hussain BM, Kandula NR, Kanaya AM. Cardiovascular Health by Life's Essential 8 and Associations With Coronary Artery Calcium in South Asian American Adults in the MASALA Study. Am J Cardiol. 2023;199:71-7.
29. Rafnsson SB, Bhopal RS, Agyemang C, Fagot-Campagna A, Harding S, Hammar N, et al. Sizable variations in circulatory disease mortality by region and country of birth in six European countries. Eur J Public Health. 2013;23(4):594-605.
30. Gijsberts CM, Seneviratna A, Hoefer IE, Agostoni P, Rittersma SZ, Pasterkamp G, et al. Inter-Ethnic Differences in Quantified Coronary Artery Disease Severity and All-Cause Mortality among Dutch and Singaporean Percutaneous Coronary Intervention Patients. PLoS One. 2015;10(7): e0131977.
31. Vyas MV, Chaturvedi N, Hughes AD, Marmot M, Tillin T. Cardiovascular disease recurrence and long-term mortality in a tri-ethnic British cohort. Heart. 2021;107(12):996-1002.
32. Kooner A, Kooner JS, Kooner IK, Misra S, et al. Cumulative incidence of coronary heart disease (CHD) among UK South

Asians-- results of the prospective follow-up of the London life sciences population (LOLIPOP) cohort of 25,372 participants at 20 years. 2024. Heart (British Cardiac Society) 110 (Suppl 3):A213-A215 DOI:10.1136/heartjnl-2024-BCS.198

33. Rabanal KS, Lindman AS, Selmer RM, Aamodt G. Ethnic differences in risk factors and total risk of cardiovascular disease based on the Norwegian CONOR study. Eur J Prev Cardiol. 2013;20(6):1013-21.

34. Waitzfelder B, Palaniappan L, Varga A, Frankland TB, Li J, Daida YG, et al. Prevalence of cardiovascular disease among Asian, Pacific Islander and multi-race populations in Hawai'i and California. BMC Public Health. 2023;23(1):885.

35. Deb S, Tu JV, Austin PC, Ko DT, Rocha R, Mazer CD, et al. Impact of South Asian Ethnicity on Long-Term Outcomes After Coronary Artery Bypass Grafting Surgery: A Large Population-Based Propensity Matched Study. J Am Heart Assoc. 2016;5(7)e003941.

36. Krishnamurthy A, Keeble C, Burton-Wood N, Somers K, Anderson M, Harland C, et al. Clinical outcomes following primary percutaneous coronary intervention for ST-elevation myocardial infarction according to sex and race. Eur Heart J Acute Cardiovasc Care. 2019;8(3):264-72.

37. Kaila KS, Norris CM, Graham MM, Ali I, Bainey KR. Long-term survival with revascularization in South Asians admitted with an acute coronary syndrome (from the Alberta Provincial Project for Outcomes Assessment in Coronary Heart Disease Registry). Am J Cardiol. 2014;114(3):395-400.

38. Yusuf S, Joseph P, Rangarajan S, Islam S, Mente A, Hystad P, et al. Modifiable risk factors, cardiovascular disease, and mortality in 155 722 individuals from 21 high-income, middle-income, and low-income countries (PURE): a prospective cohort study. Lancet. 2020;395(10226):795-808.

39. Joseph P, Kutty VR, Mohan V, Kumar R, Mony P, Vijayakumar K, et al. Cardiovascular disease, mortality, and their associations with modifiable risk factors in a multi-national South Asia cohort: a PURE substudy. Eur Heart J. 2022;43(30):2831-40.

40. Ke C, Gupta R, Xavier D, Prabhakaran D, Mathur P, Kalkonde YV, et al.; Million Death Study Collaborators. Divergent trends in ischaemic heart disease and stroke mortality in India from 2000 to 2015: a nationally representative mortality study. Lancet Glob Health. 2018;6(8):e914-e923.

41. Ahmed ST, Rehman H, Akeroyd JM, Alam M, Shah T, Kalra A, et al. Premature Coronary Heart Disease in South Asians: Burden and Determinants. Curr Atheroscler Rep. 2018; 20(1):6.

42. Littler WA, Lawrence RE. Acute myocardial infarction in Asians and Whites in Birmingham. Br Med J (Clin Res Ed). 1985; 290:1472.

43. Yusuf S, Hawken S, Ounpuu S, Dans T, Avezum A, Lanas F, et al.; INTERHEART Study Investigators. Effect of potentially modifiable risk factors associated with myocardial infarction in 52 countries (the INTERHEART study): case-control study. Lancet. 2004;364(9438):937-52.

44. Ullah W, Malik R, Bashir F, Khan M, Khan S, Alam M, et al. Comparison of Premature, Extremely Premature, and Older Adults With Coronary Artery Disease in Pakistan. JACC Asia. 2023;3(1):164-5.

45. Kumar R, Ammar A, Qayyum D, Mujtaba M, Siddiqui MN, Khan MQ, et al. Increasing Incidence of ST-Elevation Acute Coronary Syndrome in Young South Asian Population, a Challenge for the World? An Assessment of Clinical and Angiographic Patterns and Hospital Course of Premature Acute Myocardial Infarction. Am J Cardiol. 2023; 205:190-7.

46. Peerwani G, Hanif B, Rahim KA, Kashif M, Virani SS, Sheikh S. Presentation, management, and early outcomes of young acute coronary syndrome patients- analysis of 23,560 South Asian patients from 2012 to 2021. BMC Cardiovasc Disord. 2024;24(1): 378.

47. Chowdhury R, Alam DS, Fakir II, Adnan SD, Naheed A, Tasmin I, et al. The Bangladesh

Risk of Acute Vascular Events (BRAVE) Study: objectives and design. Eur J Epidemiol. 2015;30(7):577-87.
48. Tewari S, Kumar S, Kapoor A, Singh U, Agarwal A, Bharti BB, et al. Premature coronary artery disease in North India: an angiography study of 1971 patients. Indian Heart J. 2005;57(4):311-8.
49. Agrawal V, Lohiya BV, Sihag BK, Prajapati R. Clinical Profile with Angiographic Correlation in Naive Acute Coronary Syndrome. J Clin Diagn Res. 2016;10(9):OC10-OC14.
50. Deora S, Kumar T, Ramalingam R, Manjunath CN. Demographic and angiographic profile in premature cases of acute coronary syndrome: analysis of 820 young patients from South India. Cardiovasc Diagn Ther. 2016;6(3):193-8.
51. Patil RS, Shetty LH, Krishnan S, Trivedi AS, Raghu TR, Manjunath CN. Profile of coronary artery disease in Indian rural youth (< 35 yrs). Indian Heart J. 2020;72(5):394-7.
52. Sharma SK, Makkar JS, Bana A, Sharma K, Kasliwal A, Sidana SK, et al. Premature coronary artery disease, risk factors, clinical presentation, angiography and interventions: Hospital based registry. Indian Heart J. 2022; 74(5):391-7.
53. Khraishah H, Karout L, Jeong SY, Alahmad B, AlAshqar A, Belanger MJ, et al. Clinical characteristics and cardiovascular outcomes among young patients with acute myocardial infarction in Kerala, India: A secondary analysis of ACS QUIK trial. Atheroscler Plus. 2022;50:25-31.
54. Ranjith N, Pegoraro RJ, Naidoo DP. Demographic data and outcome of acute coronary syndrome in the South African Asian Indian population. Cardiovasc J S Afr. 2005;16(1):48-54.
55. Joshi P, Islam S, Pais P, Reddy S, Dorairaj P, Kazmi K, et al. Risk factors for early myocardial infarction in South Asians compared with individuals in other countries. JAMA. 2007;297(3):286-94.
56. Enas EA, Mehta J. Malignant coronary artery disease in young Asian Indians: thoughts on pathogenesis, prevention, and therapy. Clin Cardiol. 1995;18:131-5.
57. Agha AM, Bryant JP, Marquez M, Butt K, Feranec N, Sensakovic WF, et al. The Frequency of Premature Coronary Artery Disease Identified on Coronary CT Angiography Among Patients Presenting With Chest Pain at a Single Institution. JACC Cardiovasc Imaging. 2019;12(2):372-4.
58. Zimmerman FH, Cameron A, Fisher LD, Ng G. Myocardial infarction in young adults: angiographic characterization, risk factors and prognosis (Coronary Artery Surgery Study Registry). J Am Coll Cardiol. 1995;26(3):654-61.
59. Koulaouzidis G, Nicoll R, Charisopoulou D, McArthur T, Jenkins PJ, Henein MY. Aggressive and diffuse coronary calcification in South Asian angina patients compared to Caucasians with similar risk factors. Int J Cardiol. 2013;167(6):2472-6.
60. Serruys PW, Onuma Y, Garg S, Sarno G, van den Brand M, Kappetein AP, et al. Assessment of the SYNTAX score in the Syntax study. EuroIntervention. 2009;5(1):50-6.
61. Goliasch G, Wiesbauer F, Blessberger H, Demyanets S, Wojta J, Huber K, et al. Premature myocardial infarction is strongly associated with increased levels of remnant cholesterol. J Clin Lipidol. 2015;9(6):801-6. e1.
62. Enas EA, Mohan V, Deepa M, Farooq S, Pazhoor S, Chennikkara H. The metabolic syndrome and dyslipidemia among Asian Indians: a population with high rates of diabetes and premature coronary artery disease. J Cardiometab Syndr. 2007;2(4): 267-75.
63. Gobardhan SN, Dimitriu-Leen AC, van Rosendael AR, van Zwet EW, Roos CJ, Oemrawsingh PV, et al. Prevalence by Computed Tomographic Angiography of Coronary Plaques in South Asian and White Patients With Type 2 Diabetes Mellitus at Low and High Risk Using Four Cardiovascular Risk Scores (UKPDS, FRS, ASCVD, and JBS3). Am J Cardiol. 2017;119(5):705-11.
64. Bhatti GK, Bhadada SK, Vijayvergiya R, Mastana SS, Bhatti JS. Metabolic syndrome and risk of major coronary events among the urban diabetic patients: North Indian

Diabetes and Cardiovascular Disease Study-NIDCVD-2. J Diabetes Complications. 2016;30(1):72-8.
65. Mahalle N, Garg MK, Naik SS, Kulkarni MV. Association of metabolic syndrome with severity of coronary artery disease. Indian J Endocrinol Metab. 2014;18(5):708-14.
66. Enas EA, Chacko V, Senthilkumar A, Puthumana N, Mohan V. Elevated lipoprotein(a)—a genetic risk factor for premature vascular disease in people with and without standard risk factors: a review. Dis Mon. 2006;52(1):1-50.
67. Enas EA, Varkey B, Dharmarajan TS, Pare G, Bahl VK. Lipoprotein(a): An independent, genetic, and causal factor for cardiovascular disease and acute myocardial infarction. Indian Heart J. 2019;71(2):99-112.
68. Enas EA, Varkey B, Dharmarajan TS, Pare G, Bahl VK. Lipoprotein(a): An underrecognized genetic risk factor for malignant coronary artery disease in young Indians. Indian Heart J. 2019;71(3):184-98.
69. Grundy SM, Stone NJ, Bailey AL, Beam C, Birtcher KK, Blumenthal RS, et al. 2018 AHA/ACC/AACVPR/AAPA/ABC/ACPM/ADA/AGS/APhA/ASPC/NLA/PCNA Guideline on the Management of Blood Cholesterol: Executive Summary: A Report of the American College of Cardiology/American Heart Association Task Force on Clinical Practice Guidelines. J Am Coll Cardiol. 2019;73(24):3168-209.
70. Institute for Health Metrics and Evaluation (IHME). GBD Compare Data Visualization. Seattle, WA: IHME, University of Washington, 2024. Available from http://vizhub.healthdata.org/gbd-compare [Last accessed May, 2025].
71. Roth GA, Mensah GA, Johnson CO, Addolorato G, Ammirati E, Baddour LM, et al.; GBD-NHLBI-JACC Global Burden of Cardiovascular Diseases Writing Group. Global Burden of Cardiovascular Diseases and Risk Factors, 1990-2019: Update From the GBD 2019 Study. J Am Coll Cardiol. 2020;76(25):2982-3021.
72. Kalra A, Jose AP, Prabhakaran P, Kumar A, Agrawal A, Roy A, et al. The burgeoning cardiovascular disease epidemic in Indians – perspectives on contextual factors and potential solutions. Lancet Reg Health Southeast Asia. 2023;12:100156.
73. Muilwijk M, Ho F, Waddell H, Sillars A, Welsh P, Iliodromiti S, et al. Contribution of type 2 diabetes to all-cause mortality, cardiovascular disease incidence and cancer incidence in white Europeans and South Asians: findings from the UK Biobank population-based cohort study. BMJ Open Diabetes Res Care. 2019;7(1):e000765.
74. Hebbar S, Fuggle WJ, Nevill AM, Veitch AM. Colorectal cancer incidence and trend in UK South Asians: a 20-year study. Colorectal Dis. 2012;14(6):e319-22.
75. Tran HN, Udaltsova N, Li Y, Klatsky AL. Low Cancer Risk of South Asians: A Brief Report. Perm J. 2018;22:17-095.
76. Nabel EG, Braunwald E. A tale of coronary artery disease and myocardial infarction. N Engl J Med. 2012;366(1):54-63.

CHAPTER 2
The Natural History of Heart Disease and its Diverse Manifestations

■ INTRODUCTION

Atherosclerotic cardiovascular disease (ASCVD), which comprises coronary artery disease (CAD), cerebrovascular disease, peripheral arterial disease (PAD), and aortic aneurysm, is the primary cause of morbidity and mortality globally.[1] While atherosclerosis is the dominant cause of cardiovascular disease (CVD), a minority of other nonatherosclerotic diseases (e.g., congenital, valvular, myocardial, atrial fibrillation) also fall under the designation of CVD. Among ASCVDs the most common one is CAD, also known as coronary heart disease and commonly known as heart disease.

Within our body the silent, stealthy, and relentless siege of atherosclerosis is going on in our coronary arteries that carry blood to our heart. Left unchecked, atherosclerotic plaque progression culminates in a terrifying climax: Sudden cardiac death (SCD) or the life-altering devastation of a heart attack. Understanding this silent threat is important for all and particularly for Indians as they are prone to early and severe heart disease. This chapter unveils the natural history of CAD and explains its diverse clinical presentations.

■ ATHEROSCLEROSIS

Atherosclerosis, a gradual buildup of fatty deposits (plaques) on artery walls, is the root cause of two leading causes of death: Acute myocardial infarction (AMI, or heart attack) and strokes. In the US as well as in many countries heart attacks are the leading cause of death. Atherosclerosis has been with us from ancient times, as traces of the disease were found in the arteries of Egyptian pharaohs preserved through mummification. However, only in recent decades have we fully grasped its alarming impact, claiming over a third of all deaths in Western nations[2] and causing an increasing number of deaths in other populous countries. The danger of atherosclerosis lies not just in isolated blockages but in its systemic nature. Contrary to the commonly held view, plaque is not confined to a single segment of an artery; but can affect the entire vascular system impacting vital organs (especially the heart and the brain). Hence there is the need for a comprehensive approach to understanding, preventing, and treating this pervasive disease.[2]

What exactly is plaque? Plaque, which looks and feels a bit like pizza cheese, is a sticky paste made up of atherogenic lipoproteins (ALPs), fat, blood platelets, calcium, waste products from cells, blood-clotting fibrin, and other blood substances deposited within an artery's lining. Atherosclerosis involves a complex interaction of processes in which ALPs gradually oxidize—essentially, rust—to form fatty streaks, and ultimately a plaque with a cover over it. Plaque hardens and thickens the artery wall and—what is even more dangerous is the bursting of a clot that causes a heart attack.[3]

Central Role of Lipids in Atherosclerosis

Atherosclerosis is caused mainly by three ALPs—low-density lipoprotein cholesterol (LDL-C), remnant cholesterol (remnant-C) formerly known as very low-density lipoprotein (VLDL), and lipoprotein(a) [Lp(a)]—and each of them contains a molecule of apolipoprotein B (ApoB).[4] The contribution of remnant-C to atherosclerosis is less than the other two and the contribution of a fourth one—intermediate-density lipoprotein (IDL) to atherosclerosis is small.[5] It is important to appreciate that atherosclerosis can occur when ALPs [especially LDL-C and Lp(a)] are elevated even in the absence of other cardiovascular risk factors (CVRFs). Recent data show the primacy of LDL-C as atherosclerosis can develop in nonsmoking adults with LDL-C levels >60 mg/dL with normal levels of blood pressure.[6] Notably, the non-lipid risk factors may contribute but do not cause atherosclerosis and by extension, heart disease. Atherosclerosis increases incrementally with the number of these atherogenic particles in the bloodstream and the number and severity of other CVRFs. **Figure 1** depicts the key players in the initiation and progression of atherosclerosis.

Atherosclerosis is an insidious process; if it were not so and coronary arteries narrowed

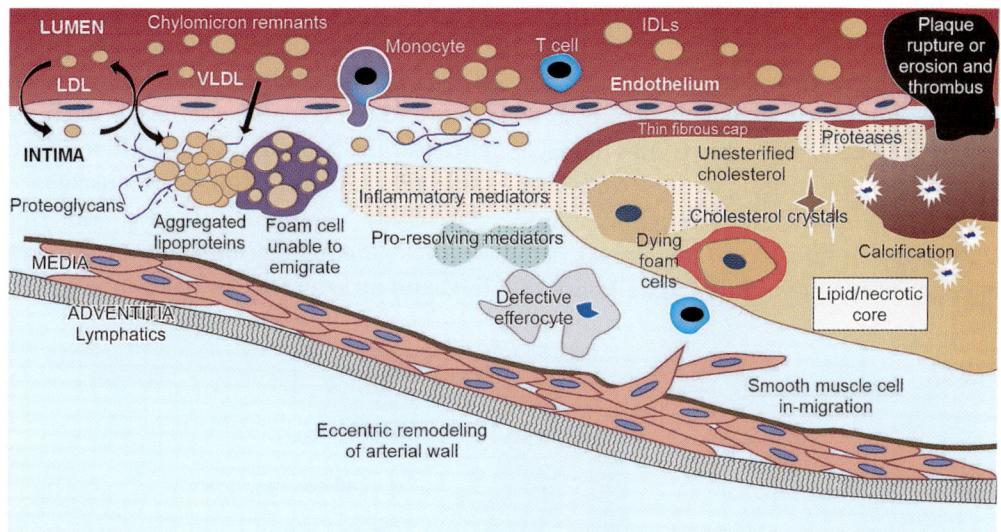

Fig. 1: High plasma concentrations of ApoB lipoproteins [LDL, IDL, VLDL, chylomicron remnants, Lp(a)] increase entry into intima and retention. ApoB lipoproteins bind to proteoglycans and begin aggregating, a process that accelerates once plaque begins. Retention is influenced by particle composition and diet, among other factors. Retention leads to a maladaptive cellular response leading to increased inflammation, fibrosis, and necrosis. The lipid/necrotic core forms when normal phagocytic processes and efferocytosis are overwhelmed by continued retention and accumulation of "toxic" ApoB lipoproteins. Plaque rupture or erosion can lead to formation of overlying thrombus, which can precipitate an acute clinical event.
[Apo: apolipoprotein; IDL: intermediate-density lipoprotein; LDL: low-density lipoprotein; Lp(a): lipoprotein(a); VLDL: very low-density lipoprotein]
Source: Reproduced with permission from Robinson et al.[4]

as soon as the buildup of plaques started then many people, even in their twenties and thirties, would get chest pain and seek medical attention. The danger of atherosclerosis is that in the first several decades of life plaques grow slowly, do not narrow the arteries, and cause pain as the arteries expand in diameter to compensate for this narrowing until they are stretched to their limit and can expand no more. There is worse: The large, hardened, highly visible plaques that narrow one's arteries and generate chest pain are not the most dangerous plaques.

THE SILENT BATTLE WITHIN: HOW ENDOTHELIAL DAMAGE FUELS HEART DISEASE

Imagine your arteries as smooth water pipes lined with a thin but crucial layer called the endothelium. This "active" layer regulates blood flow, keeps LDL out, and prevents clots. However, high blood pressure, diabetes, smoking, and other CVRFs damage this endothelium, turning it into a "diseased lining". This endothelial dysfunction allows LDL to seep in and form fatty streaks, the first signs of plaque buildup, a hallmark of atherosclerosis. Atherosclerosis is not just plaque buildup; it is an inflammatory battle. Early fatty streaks trigger inflammation that weakens the artery lining, further worsening the situation. This weakened defense allows LDL to accumulate, forming unstable plaque prone to rupture. When such plaque ruptures, it triggers blood clot formation, often silently, blocking blood flow to the heart and causing a heart attack. This highlights the importance of preventing endothelial dysfunction and inflammation, not just treating blockages.

ANATOMY OF THE CORONARY ARTERIES (FIG. 2)

The two main coronary arteries are the left main coronary artery (LMCA) and the right coronary artery (RCA). The LMCA supplies blood to the left side (atrium and ventricle). It divides into the left anterior descending (LAD) branch that supplies blood to the front and the circumflex artery branch that encircles the heart and supplies blood to the outer side and back of the heart muscle.

The RCA supplies blood to the right ventricle, the right atrium, and the sinoatrial (SA) and atrioventricular (AV) nodes, which

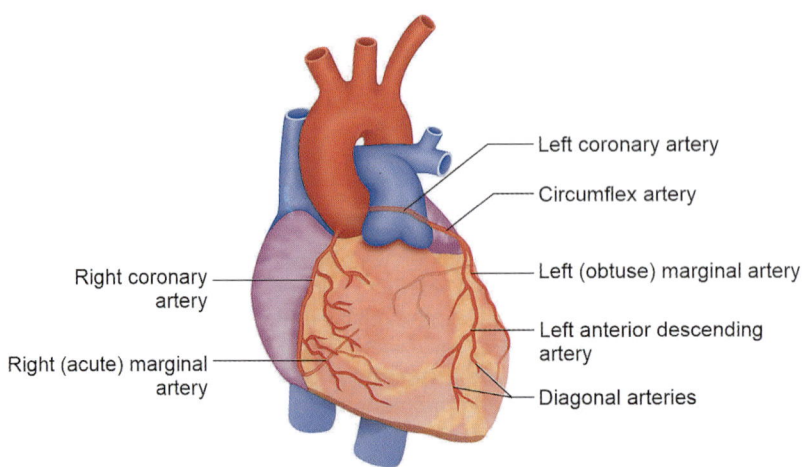

Fig. 2: Anatomy of the main coronary arteries.

regulate the heart rhythm. RCA divides into smaller branches, including the right posterior descending artery and the acute marginal artery. Together with the LAD artery, the RCA helps supply blood to the middle or septum of the heart. Smaller branches of the coronary arteries include obtuse marginal (OM), septal perforator (SP), and diagonals.

PROGRESSION OF CORONARY ATHEROSCLEROSIS

A Swedish study tracked nearly 16,300 coronary artery segments over 15 years, revealing that narrowing (stenosis) overall is a slow process.[7] However, the key takeaway is this: Risk factors like high blood pressure and diabetes significantly accelerate progression, from nonobstructive (<50% stenosis) to obstructive lesion (>50% stenosis). Research studies have shown an eightfold increase in progression **(Fig. 1)** for those with the four major CVRFs.[7]

Additionally, disease progression was seen more in men and in those with previously established obstructive disease. Specific arteries and segments that are more prone to faster narrowing were also identified **(Fig. 3)**: The left coronary artery is more prone than the RCA; proximal segments are more prone than the distal segments especially in the LAD (almost a third of progression of obstructive CAD). The natural history of coronary atherosclerosis underscores the importance of managing CVRFs to slow disease progression and potentially avoid future interventions like coronary artery bypass graft (CABG) surgery or percutaneous coronary intervention (PCI) commonly known as an angioplasty.

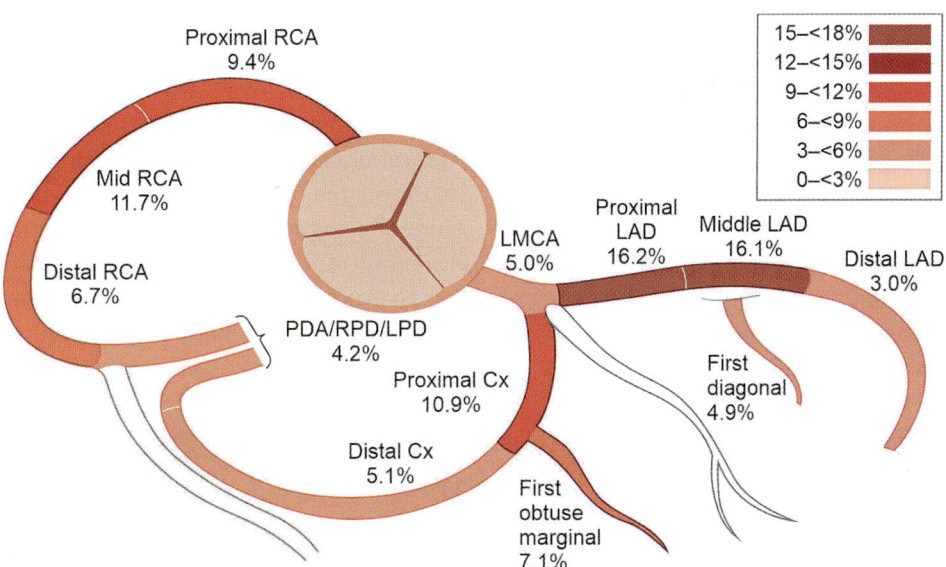

Fig. 3: Distribution of coronary atherosclerosis in different branches and segments of coronary arteries color-coded for the degree of stenosis. (Cx: left circumflex artery; LAD: left anterior descending artery; LMCA: left main coronary artery; LPD: left posterior descending artery; PDA: posterior descending artery; RCA: right coronary artery; RPD: right posterior descending artery)
Source: Reproduced with permission from Mohammad MA et al.[7]

A SILENT THREAT: UNDETECTED ATHEROSCLEROSIS IN YOUNG PEOPLE

In light of the natural history of coronary atherosclerosis it should not come as a surprise that autopsies of young people, even under 30 years of age, who died in wars—Korea, Vietnam, and Iraq—have revealed significant plaque deposits.[8] It is important to understand that this disease is an invisible threat to life, undetected by physical examination and routine tests and therefore the emphasis should be on prevention (i.e., knowing risk factors, identifying them early, and effective interventions).

PLAQUES

Two types of plaques, stable and vulnerable, and their characteristics and clinical import are listed in **Table 1**.[9] Hard, stable plaques have little risk of rupturing. They can progressively narrow the channel of a coronary artery, but this is more likely to cause chest pain well before it causes a heart attack. The large, hard, visually noticeable plaques that show up impressively on an angiogram are not your greatest worry because they give advanced warning of their danger by causing chest pain when they narrow an artery. On the other hand, vulnerable plaques, silent, soft, and hidden, are dangerous. Like a volcanic mountain rumbling far beneath the surface, soft buried plaque can be very active. It can suddenly erupt, spewing its contents directly into the lumen of the artery and trigger the formation of a potentially dangerous blood clot that causes a heart attack.

Plaque rupture exposes the highly thrombogenic necrotic core of a vulnerable plaque to the blood, activating the platelets and other blood-clotting factors. This activation triggers the formation of a platelet-rich thrombus that adheres to the damaged vessel wall. The activated platelets release various procoagulant factors, including thrombin. Thrombin is a powerful enzyme that converts fibrinogen to fibrin, forming the mesh of the fibrin-rich thrombus. This fibrin-rich thrombus is further stabilized by the incorporation of platelets and other blood-clotting factors. The best strategy to try to convert a vulnerable plaque to stable plaque is by statin therapy that reduces the lipid core and thickens the fibrous cap of the plaque (Chapter 13).

Counterintuitively, a vulnerable plaque may not rupture at the minimum lumen area (MLA). In fact, over two-thirds of plaque ruptures involve sites away from MLA. The thrombus can then propagate upstream and/or downstream, occluding the coronary artery and reducing blood flow to the heart muscle. Imaging modalities such as intravascular ultrasound (IVUS) can help to identify vulnerable plaques before they rupture and cause acute coronary syndrome (ACS).[10]

TABLE 1: Differences between stable plaque and vulnerable plaque.[9]

Stable plaque	Vulnerable plaque
• Less likely to rupture	• More likely to rupture
• Protected by thick fibrous cap	• Have a thin fibrous cap
• Hard and calcified; large sclerotic component with a small lipid core	• High macrophage density and inflammation
• Grow over time and narrow the artery	• Large soft and thrombogenic lipid core
• Can produce angina during exertion	• Can cause heart attacks or strokes
• Angiographically moderate to severe stenosis	• Angiographically mild stenosis

There are other host factors that increase the risk of a plaque rupture and of a heart attack. These include factors of the blood, of the heart, and multiple risk factors and social determinants of health (SDOH) of the patient. Prothrombotic factors (factors that promote blood clot) are smoking, high levels of Lp(a), fibrinogen, triglycerides (details in later chapters), and certain medications. An example is Vioxx (rofecoxib), a pain relief medication, that was withdrawn from the market because of increased risk of heart attack or stroke. Previous cardiac arrest or heart attack increases the risk of ventricular arrhythmia that may lead to a cardiac arrest. Surviving a cardiac catastrophe is clearly welcome news, but the point is that it is far better not to have had such an event at all in the first place, because that very history places one at a greater future risk. Like a bone that has been broken before, a post-coronary event heart may never quite fully regain its earlier robustness.[10]

Plaque Progression, Rupture, and Coronary Artery Remodeling

The fundamental theme that ASCVD is an insidious process over many years was introduced earlier. Within the coronary arteries what starts as foam cells and fatty streak, with the passage of time forms lipid-rich plaque with a lipid core and a fibrous cap. This progression and plaque rupture are schematically depicted on **Figure 4**. The tears in the hardened plaque lining of arteries may go unnoticed. While the body at times heals these tears, this "healing" often leads to rapid plaque growth and a higher risk of future ruptures. Coronary artery remodeling is the process by which the coronary arteries expand to maintain the coronary lumen for blood flow **(Fig. 5)**. However, outward remodeling can also make the artery wall weaker and more vulnerable to rupture.[11] Lipid-lowering therapy (LLT) is effective in preventing heart attack and reducing the size

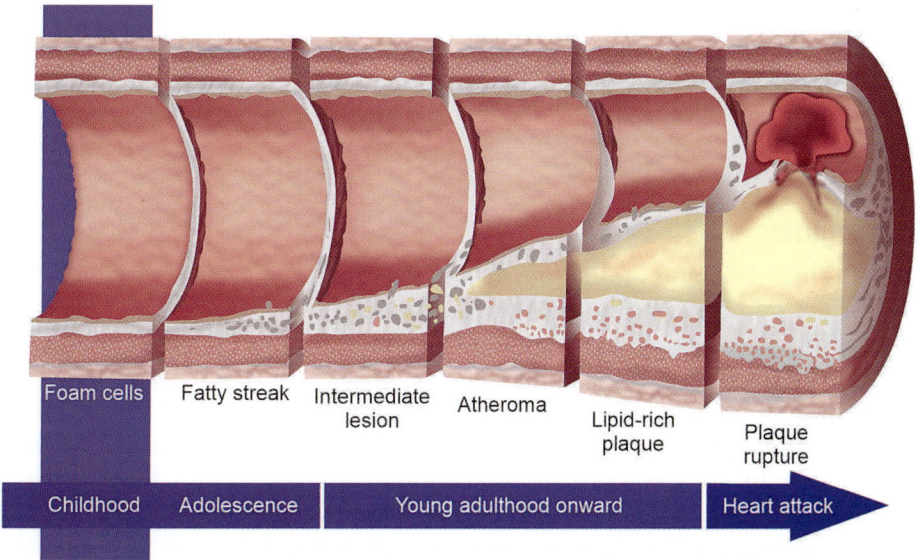

Fig. 4: The progression of coronary atherosclerosis through many years and the changes within the coronary artery. Of particular note is plaque growth with outward remodeling and plaque rupture.

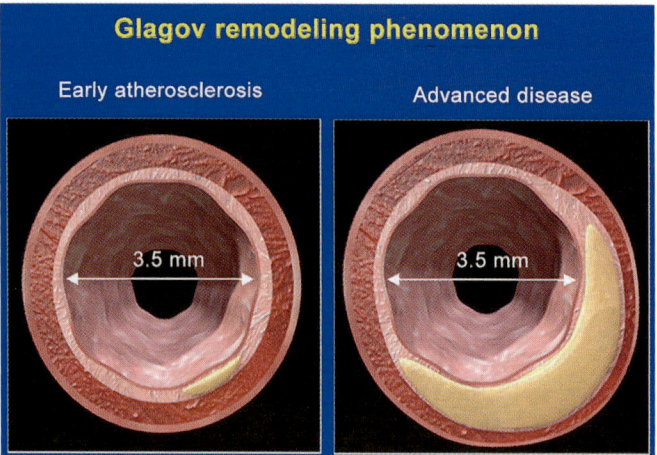

Fig. 5: Despite the large amount of plaque in advanced disease the lumen size is identical to that of early atherosclerosis and blood flow preserved to the same extent.
Source: Reproduced with permission from Professor Steven E. Nissen, Cleveland Clinic, Ohio.[12]

and vulnerability of plaques (Chapters 13 and 14), including even small plaques not visible on an angiogram.

SYMPTOMS AND MANIFESTATIONS OF CORONARY ARTERY DISEASE

The clinical manifestations of heart disease are listed in **Table 2**. Among these, angina is the most characteristic one and acute coronary syndrome (ACS) is the most important one. As implied in the term "silent" myocardial ischemia due to CAD is asymptomatic.

Stable Angina

Stable angina is chest discomfort (characteristics depicted in **Figure 6**) due to ischemia that occurs when the coronary arteries are narrowed by >70% by large, stable plaque limiting blood flow to the heart especially during exertion or stress.

Note the features that increase the probability of angina. If the probability is low consider noncardiac chest pain (gastroesophageal, pleuropulmonary, chest wall, etc.). Angina typically feels like tightness, pressure, or squeezing in the center of your chest, sometimes radiating to the shoulders, arms, neck, jaw, or back. It can also manifest as heaviness or tightness centrally. Activities like exercise, stress, cold weather, or a big meal can trigger these symptoms. While sharp, fleeting pain especially located

TABLE 2: Clinical manifestations of heart disease.

Stable angina	*Refer to text and* **Figure 6**
Acute coronary syndrome (ACS)	Unstable angina *Acute myocardial infarction (AMI):* • STEMI (ST-elevation MI) • NSTEMI (non-ST-elevation MI) Sudden cardiac arrest (SCA) and sudden cardiac death (SCD)
Silent myocardial ischemia	Coronary Artery Calcium (CAC) score **(Box 1)** useful in detection
Heart failure (HF)	HF has multiple causes (Chapter 12) and one among them CAD. It is usually a late manifestation of CAD

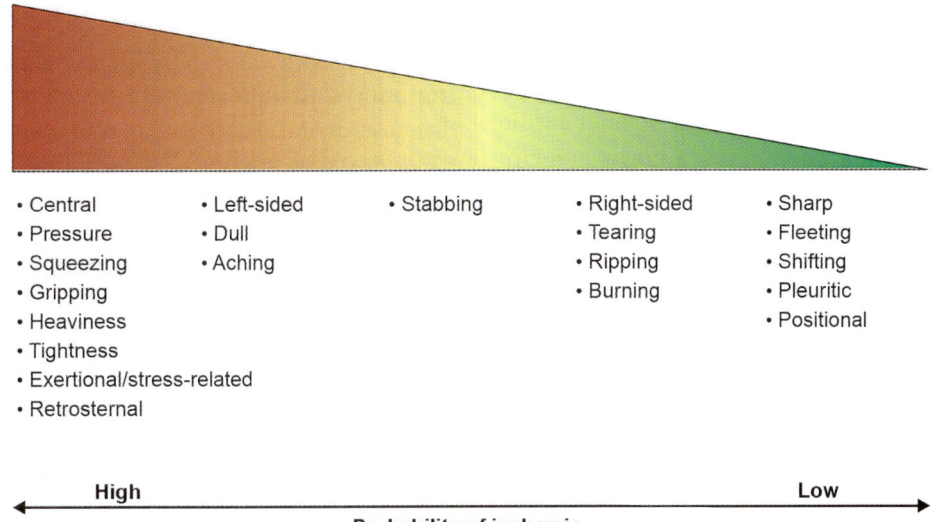

Fig. 6: Probability of ischemia based on common descriptions of chest discomfort.
Source: Reproduced with permission from Gulati et al.[13]

> **BOX 1:** Coronary Artery Calcium (CAC) score (heart scan).[21-26]
>
> - CAC scoring is noninvasive and safe and is a relatively inexpensive test ($30 to $100), compared to stress tests and especially with imaging
> - A zero CAC score is excellent news for those with or without symptoms as it markedly reduces the probability of a heart attack in the following 10 years. However, it is not a free pass as CVRFs continue to influence the development and progression of heart disease
> - The likelihood of having a CAC score above zero increases significantly with age, jumping from 30% in individuals aged 45–55 to 70% for those between 55 and 85
> - A CAC score between 1 and 99 is not to be ignored especially in young women under 50. This seemingly low score can still double one's risk of heart attack compared to someone with a zero score. It is a wake-up call to prioritize heart-healthy habits like exercise, diet, and stress management
> - A score above 100 suggests moderate plaque buildup, even without symptoms. This is a wake-up call for aggressive lifestyle changes and potentially statin therapy
> - For young adults with a family history (Hx) of heart disease, a CAC score above 100 is a significant indicator of future risk of a heart attack even without other CVRFs
> - CAC scores above 300 indicate a steeper increase in risk of heart attack, stroke, or bypass surgery. For scores exceeding 1,000, the terrain becomes a sheer cliff. The risk of cardiovascular events skyrockets (fivefold), demanding immediate and aggressive intervention to prevent a potential plunge
> - As many as one in eight young adults (20–30 years old) with multiple CVRFs (like high blood pressure, cholesterol, smoking, obesity, or diabetes) may have a CAC score above 1. This seemingly small amount of plaque buildup grows in the continuing presence of risk factors and increases the risk of heart attack and stroke. Early detection through CAC scoring allows for preventive measures, treatment and intervention
> - Multiple CVRFs at a young age is most concerning; by 40–50 years of age, approximately 1 of every 4 men with hypertension, dyslipidemia, diabetes, smoking, or a family Hx of CAD would have CAC > 0. Premature CAC (before age 50) precedes premature MI by 20–30 years[27]
>
> (CAD: coronary artery disease; CVRFs: cardiovascular risk factors; MI: myocardial infarction)

on the right side is unlikely to be angina. Rest or medication usually relieves angina within minutes. An important point to emphasize is that neither a normal cardiovascular examination nor a normal electrocardiogram (ECG) rules out angina pectoris or heart disease. Stable angina does worsen over time. Angina should not be ignored as it is a harbinger of ACS.

Acute Coronary Syndrome

Acute coronary syndrome is a broad designation that encompasses unstable angina, AMI and sudden cardiac arrest (SCA).

Unstable Angina

Unstable angina has the characteristics of angina (Chapter 10) but is severe and lasts longer, many minutes (typically >10) and is not completely relieved by nitroglycerin (the usual angina medication) and may happen at rest or mild exertion. The intensity of symptoms do not always reflect the severity of blockage. Unstable angina is a life-threatening emergency and needs immediate medical intervention to avoid a heart attack (AMI). Some practical points of vital importance when one has chest pain are:
- Do not ignore it and do not delay in calling Emergency Medical System (EMS) for help. Call 911 (in the US) or the emergency response system number in your region as every second counts when it comes to treating a heart attack.
- The EMS staff who respond to 911 are well trained to recognize heart attacks and are equipped to provide emergency care and they alert the hospital for fast-track care.
- Do not attempt to drive to the hospital and risk a cardiac arrest enroute (happens in 1 in 300).

Acute Myocardial Infarction

In patients with chest pain, blood tests (e.g., troponin) and abnormal ECG establish the diagnosis of AMI. Those with new ST elevation, ST depression, or new left bundle branch block (LBBB) should be treated according to STEMI (ST-elevation myocardial infarction) and NSTEMI (non-STEMI) guidelines for ACS. **Table 3** defines and describes STEMI and NSTEMI and other types of MI.

ST-elevation myocardial infarction type MI is a critical situation and early diagnosis is of paramount importance. It is caused by a complete blockage of a coronary artery, typically due to a blood clot that forms at the site of a ruptured plaque. A complete blockage of a coronary artery starves the heart muscle, leading to potential complications like arrhythmias, heart failure, and even shock. Treatment focus is on rapidly opening the blocked artery with angioplasty or clot-busting medication to minimize damage.

Non-STEMI is due to plaque rupture and thrombus formation that result in incomplete blockage of the involved artery and has varying degrees of troponin elevation and ECG changes but not ST elevation. Thrombolytic therapy is contraindicated in NSTEMI. This type of MI is considered a mild heart attack.

Sudden Cardiac Arrest

Sudden cardiac arrest is when the heart abruptly stops beating and is a medical emergency requiring immediate cardiac pulmonary resuscitation (CPR) and defibrillation. SCD is death resulting from SCA within 60 minutes of symptoms (or no symptoms at all). Shockingly, for up to a third of heart disease patients, SCA may be their first, last, and only manifestation. However, SCA can strike even those without known heart disease. Intriguingly, about

TABLE 3: Types of myocardial infarctions (MI).[14]

Type 1 MI	This is the most common type of heart attack (75–80%), resulting from a blood clot stemming from a ruptured coronary artery plaque that blocks blood flow to the heart muscle. It can be STEMI or NSTEMI
Type 2 MI	Type 2 MI NSTEMI, unlike the blockage in Type 1 MI, stems from an imbalance between demand and supply: The heart muscle either needs more oxygen than it is getting (high demand) or the supply is limited (low supply). This mismatch can be caused by various issues like abnormal heart rhythms, anemia, low blood pressure, or even artery problems (constriction, clots, narrowing)
Type 3 MI	Silent heart attack leading to sudden death; no time for blood tests
Type 4 MI	Type of heart attack that is associated with percutaneous coronary intervention (PCI)
Type 5 MI	Also known as periprocedural myocardial infarction (PPMI) after cardiac or noncardiac surgery; Type 5 MI is a serious complication of surgery that can lead to death. Type 5 MI often occurs usually within 72 hours of surgery, but it can occur at any time during the recovery period. The symptoms are the same as the symptoms of a classic heart attack
Silent MI	As implied in the name, this type is often an accidental observation on an ECG and the high-risk groups are the elderly, those with diabetes, and or chronic kidney disease. People with silent MI, which may be as high as 20% of heart attacks, are at high risk for major cardiovascular adverse events (MACEs) such as heart attack, ischemic stroke, and sudden death

(ECG: electrocardiogram; NSTEMI: non-ST-elevation myocardial infarction; STEMI: ST-elevation myocardial infarction)

TABLE 4: Decrease in the age- and sex- adjusted rate of acute myocardial infarctions (AMIs) and profound decrease in ST-elevation MI (STEMI) in the United States.[17]

	2000	2002	2004	2006	2008
AMI	285	275	260	230	203
STEMI	120	105	80	70	48
Non-STEMI	165	170	180	160	155

one half of SCDs classified as arrhythmic (caused by abnormal heart rhythm) show no clear abnormality during autopsy. This phenomenon is known as "hearts too good to die" and is so far unexplained.

HEART ATTACK: HOW FAR WE HAVE COME

Before 1912, a heart attack (AMI) was a death sentence, only diagnosed after death. James Herrick revolutionized this by describing heart attack symptoms of patients enabling diagnosis without autopsy and in proposing blood clots in coronary arteries as the cause.[9] Though Herrick's work was initially met with skepticism, it paved the way for earlier diagnosis, treatment, and ultimately saved countless lives.

Thanks to risk factor control, early diagnosis and medical advancements such as coronary perfusion, the case-fatality rates from AMI have plummeted from over 50% to <5% in the US.[8,15,16] In the US, 805,000 AMIs occur annually, with men at higher risk until age 75 and women taking the lead after 85. **Table 4** shows the overall decrease of AMIs and the profound decrease in the more serious STEMI type in the US between 2000 and 2008.[17]

Better management of major risk factors like high blood pressure, cholesterol, and smoking has contributed to a 60% decrease in STEMI in the US in 8 years. Additionally, the widespread use of high-sensitivity troponin allows for earlier diagnosis of smaller heart muscle injuries, previously often diagnosed as unstable angina. This earlier detection can lead to more timely treatment and potentially prevent future heart attacks.

A Tale of Two Countries

While the US has seen a significant decrease in AMIs due to better control of risk factors like smoking, high blood pressure, and cholesterol, India has not witnessed the same decline. Control of CVRFs, with the exception of smoking, have been poor in India.[18] The control of CVRFs like hypertension and cholesterol is <15% in India, compared to >50% in the US. People in the US have a lower lifetime exposure to these risk factors compared to their Indian counterparts.[18] The positive trend of decreasing AMI rates in the US is an objective lesson in the importance of prioritizing effective control of CVRFs.[8]

DIAGNOSTIC TESTS FOR HEART DISEASE

Heart disease's greatest threat lies in its ability to go undetected for years. Plaque builds in the arteries often without warning signs and may first manifest as a heart attack. Nearly one half of high-risk persons may have reduced blood flow to their heart muscles (silent myocardial ischemia). Notably, checkups such as routine blood tests and ECGs and even stress tests may miss impending danger as outward expansion of the plaque can advance while the lumen for blood flow is preserved ("Glagov phenomenon"), depicted in **Figure 5**.[12]

Therefore, tests that can detect coronary plaques before the occurrence of symptoms are of greater use **(Fig. 7)** as medications and interventions can be used to avert a heart attack.[19]

Stress Tests With or Without Nuclear Imaging

Stress tests evaluate how the heart functions under exertion. There are two main types: Exercise stress tests and nuclear stress tests. During an exercise stress test, a patient walks on a treadmill with increasing intensity while the physician monitors the heart's electrical activity (ECG), heart rate, blood pressure, and breathing. A positive test is one with abnormal changes in ECG, indicative of ischemia. A nuclear stress test uses a small amount of radioactive tracer to create detailed images of blood flow to the heart muscle, both at rest and during exertion that shows areas with reduced blood flow due to narrowed arteries (coronary stenosis)—a sign of silent ischemia.

Stress Echocardiography

Stress echocardiography, a noninvasive alternative to nuclear stress tests, uses ultrasound to visualize heart function at rest and during exertion. Unlike nuclear imaging, it involves no radiation and is often less expensive. During the test, an ultrasound technician captures images of the heart before and after exercise on a treadmill or bike. These images are then compared to identify any changes in size, shape, or pumping efficiency that potentially indicate ischemia. While it offers cost- and radiation-free benefits, stress echocardiography has limitations as up to 60% of results may be inconclusive or less accurate due to factors like preexisting heart abnormalities or obesity.

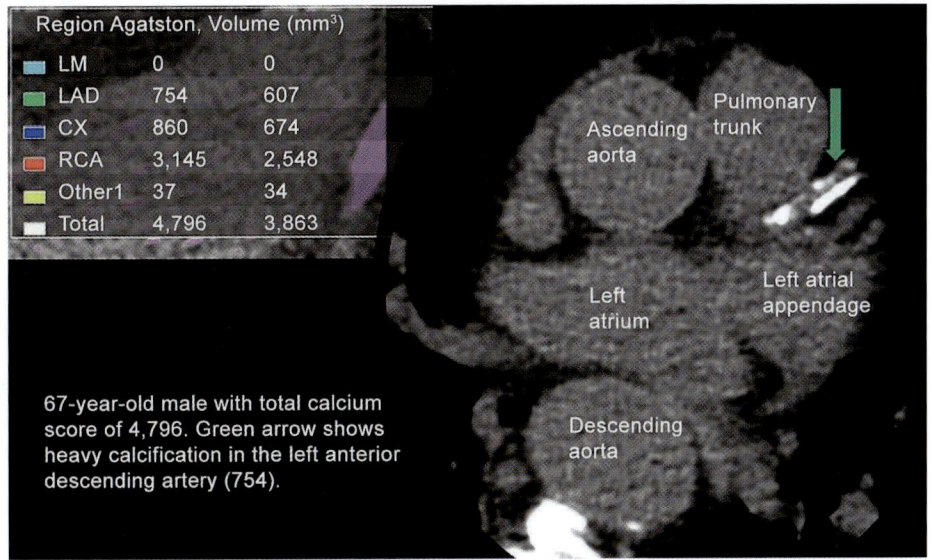

Fig. 7: Heavy calcium deposition in the left anterior descending (LAD) artery. (CX: circumflex artery ; LM: left main artery; RCA: right coronary artery)
Courtesy: Dr Mariam Thomas, Clinical Professor of Radiologic Sciences, David Geffen School of Medicine at UCLA, CA.

Coronary Angiography

Coronary angiography is a minimally invasive procedure by injecting dye through an intra-arterial catheter inserted into coronary arteries with the guidance of radiologic imaging. The coronary arteries and the flow of dye through them are visualized. Though the plaque itself is not seen, its impact on the arterial lumen and to the flow through the vessel are seen. Fifty percent or more of a coronary artery narrowing is considered obstructive CAD. Left main coronary stenosis of 50% or more or anatomically significant stenosis of 70% or more of 3 vessels are considered high-risk CAD. Severe blockages are easily detected but mild plaques and diffuse buildup of plaques in small coronary arteries may be missed.

Coronary Artery Calcium Scoring

Unlike other tests, Coronary Artery Calcium (CAC) scoring directly measures plaque buildup in the coronary arteries.[20] **Figure 7** depicts the appearance of calcium in the anterior descending branch of the LCA and the **Box 1** that follows lists the features of CAC scoring.

Computed Tomographic Coronary Angiography and Fractional Flow Reserve CT

Computed tomographic coronary angiography (CTCA) and fractional flow reserve CT (FFRCT) are cutting-edge radiographic tests that provide a detailed view of the coronary arteries without the need for an intravascular catheter. The scan is completed quickly, typically within minutes and provides high-resolution 3D images to assess the size and shape of the arteries and any blockages, especially high-risk plaques or any other abnormalities within the arteries. While CTCA might eventually replace traditional coronary angiography, the goal is to find refinements in CTCA for early detection of atherosclerosis that allows early start of preventive measures that not only reduce the need for invasive procedures but importantly prevent heart attacks. Reports from developed countries already note that these tests have halved the need for invasive coronary angiography (ICA) and reduced the need for PCI in those who underwent ICA.[28-31]

A consequential randomized controlled Prevent Coronary Artery Disease (PRECAD) trial has been developed to assess the potential benefit of aggressive control of CVRFs—blood pressure, blood sugar, and LDL-C (<70 mg/dL), which would prevent the onset of atherosclerosis and/or progression in young healthy adults. The primary endpoint would be change in the total plaque volume, as a surrogate for CVD, measured by noninvasive measures.[32]

In this chapter we have expounded on the basic disease—atherosclerosis—and the stealthy nature of coronary atherosclerosis with plaques, its clinical presentations, and the diagnostic tests for CAD. In Chapter 11, the management of ACS is detailed. The marked reduction achieved in heart attacks in the US is an object lesson on the importance of focusing on controlling CVRFs. In the next chapter we will enumerate and explain these risk factors and focus on the important modifiable CVRFs in Indians.

■ KEY TAKEAWAYS

- Atherosclerosis, an insidious process that leads to plaque formation in the coronary arteries, is the root cause of heart disease. High LDL-C promotes vulnerable plaque, even in seemingly open arteries. Statins can stabilize this plaque, reducing rupture risk, even if arteries remain narrowed.
- Stable plaques narrow arteries over time, reducing blood flow and potentially causing chest pain (angina). However, unlike vulnerable plaque, they pose a less immediate threat.
- Nonobstructive plaque buildup may progress slowly, but multiple risk factors (like high blood pressure, cholesterol, diabetes, smoking) can accelerate the process and increase the risk of future blockages and major adverse cardiovascular events. This emphasizes the need to manage all CVRFs, not just the plaque.
- While angina is the common symptom of heart disease, the most important manifestations are grouped together as ACS.
- Acute chest pain should not be ignored. Chest pain, specifically unstable angina, is a prodrome of a heart attack and is a medical emergency. Time is of essence and the patient needs to be transported to a hospital immediately.
- *Heart attack types:* STEMI, caused by a complete blockage, triggers rapid and severe heart muscle damage, showing up clearly on an ECG. NSTEMI, from a partial blockage, results in less extensive, potentially slower damage and may not show on a standard ECG. This distinction is critical for swift diagnosis and tailored treatment.
- No chest pain does not mean no heart disease (CAD). Delaying diagnosis can be risky; early detection is crucial for optimal management. Silent but scary: Up to 20% of heart attacks (AMIs) strike silently, without immediate pain, damaging the heart and raising future health risks.
- The threat of an SCA is not confined to just those with known heart disease. While smoking and a history of heart problems increase the risk, two-thirds of SCA victims have no prior diagnosis of heart disease. Early detection through screenings and lifestyle modifications can be the difference between life and death.
- Normal stress tests can be misleading as up to half may have hidden atherosclerotic plaque buildup as detected and measured by coronary artery calcification (CAC score). Therefore the need for better (sensitive and specific) tests that can identify disease early, stratify risks, and guide optimal treatment.
- CAC score above 100 is a trigger for statin therapy, even with normal LDL, and scores exceeding 300 indicate very high risk to guide and intensify treatment.

REFERENCES

1. Tsao CW, Aday AW, Almarzooq ZI, Anderson CAM, Arora P, Avery CL, et al.; American Heart Association Council on Epidemiology and Prevention Statistics Committee and Stroke Statistics Subcommittee. Heart Disease and Stroke Statistics-2023 Update: A Report From the American Heart Association. Circulation. 2023;147(8):e93-e621.
2. Gibbons GH, Seidman CE, Topol EJ. Conquering Atherosclerotic Cardiovascular Disease - 50 Years of Progress. N Engl J Med. 2021;384(9):785-8.
3. Libby P. Vascular biology of atherosclerosis: overview and state of the art. Am J Cardiol. 2003;91(3A):3A-6A.
4. Robinson JG, Williams KJ, Gidding S, Borén J, Tabas I, Fisher EA, et al. Eradicating the Burden of Atherosclerotic Cardiovascular Disease by Lowering Apolipoprotein B Lipoproteins Earlier in Life. J Am Heart Assoc. 2018;7(20):e009778.
5. Richardson TG, Sanderson E, Palmer TM, Ala-Korpela M, Ference BA, Davey Smith G, et al. Evaluating the relationship between circulating lipoprotein lipids and apolipoproteins with risk of coronary heart disease: A multivariable Mendelian randomisation analysis. PLoS Med. 2020; 17(3):e1003062.
6. Fernandez-Friera L, Fuster V, López-Melgar B, Oliva B, García-Ruiz JM, Mendiguren J, et al. Normal LDL-Cholesterol Levels Are Associated With Subclinical Atherosclerosis in the Absence of Risk Factors. J Am Coll Cardiol. 2017;70(24):2979-91.
7. Mohammad MA, Stone GW, Koul S, Olivecrona GK, Bergman S, Persson J, et al. On the Natural History of Coronary Artery Disease: A Longitudinal Nationwide Serial Angiography Study. J Am Heart Assoc. 2022; 11(21):e026396.
8. Dalen JE, Alpert JS, Goldberg RJ, Weinstein RS. The epidemic of the 20(th) century: coronary heart disease. Am J Med. 2014;127(9):807-12.
9. Libby P, Buring JE, Badimon L, Hansson GK, Deanfield J, Bittencourt MS, et al. Atherosclerosis. Nat Rev Dis Primers. 2019; 5(1):56.
10. Stone PH, Libby P, Boden WE. Fundamental Pathobiology of Coronary Atherosclerosis and Clinical Implications for Chronic Ischemic Heart Disease Management-The Plaque Hypothesis: A Narrative Review. JAMA Cardiol. 2023;8(2):192-201.
11. Libby P. Current concepts of the pathogenesis of the acute coronary syndromes. Circulation. 2001;104(3):365-72.
12. Nissen SE. Personal unpublished collection. (with permission from the author).
13. Gulati M, Levy PD, Mukherjee D, Amsterdam E, Bhatt DL, Birtcher KK, et al. 2021 AHA/ACC/ASE/CHEST/SAEM/SCCT/SCMR Guideline for the Evaluation and Diagnosis of Chest Pain: Executive Summary: A Report of the American College of Cardiology/American Heart Association Joint Committee on Clinical Practice Guidelines. Circulation. 2021;144(22):e368-e454.
14. Thygesen K, Alpert JS, Jaffe AS, Chaitman BR, Bax JJ, Morrow DA, et al.; Executive Group on behalf of the Joint European Society of Cardiology (ESC)/American College of Cardiology (ACC)/American Heart Association (AHA)/World Heart Federation (WHF) Task Force for the Universal Definition of Myocardial Infarction. Fourth Universal Definition of Myocardial Infarction (2018). J Am Coll Cardiol. 2018;72(18):2231-64.
15. Martin SS, Aday AW, Almarzooq ZI, Anderson CAM, Arora P, Avery CL, et al.; American Heart Association Council on Epidemiology and Prevention Statistics Committee and Stroke Statistics Subcommittee. 2024 Heart Disease and Stroke Statistics: A Report of US and Global Data From the American Heart Association. Circulation. 2024;149(8):e347-e913.
16. Maddox TM, Stanislawski MA, Grunwald GK, Bradley SM, Ho PM, Tsai TT, et al. Nonobstructive coronary artery disease and risk of myocardial infarction. JAMA. 2014;312(17):1754-63.
17. Yeh RW, Sidney S, Chandra M, Sorel M, Selby JV, Go AS. Population trends in the incidence

and outcomes of acute myocardial infarction. N Engl J Med. 2010;362(23):2155-65.
18. Gupta R, Khedar RS, Gaur K, Xavier D. Low quality cardiovascular care is an important coronary risk factor in India. Indian Heart J. 2018;70 Suppl 3:S419-S430.
19. Libby P, Aikawa M. Mechanisms of plaque stabilization with statins. Am J Cardiol. 2003; 91(4A):4B-8B.
20. Greenland P, Lloyd-Jones DM. Coronary Artery Calcium Test for Heart Disease Risk Assessment. JAMA Cardiol. 2022;7(10): 1083.
21. Adelhoefer S, Uddin SMI, Osei AD, Obisesan OH, Blaha MJ, Dzaye O. Coronary Artery Calcium Scoring: New Insights into Clinical Interpretation-Lessons from the CAC Consortium. Radiol Cardiothorac Imaging. 2020;2(6):e200281.
22. Grandhi GR, Mirbolouk M, Dardari ZA, Al-Mallah MH, Rumberger JA, Shaw LJ, et al. Interplay of Coronary Artery Calcium and Risk Factors for Predicting CVD/CHD Mortality: The CAC Consortium. JACC Cardiovasc Imaging. 2020;13(5):1175-86.
23. Kanaya AM, Kandula NR, Ewing SK, Herrington D, Liu K, Blaha MJ, et al. Comparing coronary artery calcium among U.S. South Asians with four racial/ethnic groups: the MASALA and MESA studies. Atherosclerosis. 2014;234(1):102-7.
24. Osei AD, Uddin SMI, Dzaye O, Achirica MC, Dardari ZA, Obisesan OH, et al. Predictors of coronary artery calcium among 20-30-year-olds: The Coronary Artery Calcium Consortium. Atherosclerosis. 2020;301:65-8.
25. Cainzos-Achirica M, Bittencourt MS, Osei AD, Haque W, Bhatt DL, Blumenthal RS, et al. Coronary Artery Calcium to Improve the Efficiency of Randomized Controlled Trials in Primary Cardiovascular Prevention. JACC Cardiovasc Imaging. 2021;14(5):1005-16.
26. Budoff MJ, Kinninger A, Gransar H, Achenbach S, Al-Mallah M, Bax JJ, et al.; CONFIRM Investigators. When Does a Calcium Score Equate to Secondary Prevention?: Insights From the Multinational CONFIRM Registry. JACC Cardiovasc Imaging. 2023;16(9):1181-9.
27. Dzaye O, Razavi AC, Dardari ZA, Shaw LJ, Berman DS, Budoff MJ, et al. Modeling the Recommended Age for Initiating Coronary Artery Calcium Testing Among At-Risk Young Adults. J Am Coll Cardiol. 2021;78(16): 1573-83.
28. Knuuti J, Ballo H, Juarez-Orozco LE, Saraste A, Kolh P, Rutjes AWS, et al. The performance of non-invasive tests to rule-in and rule-out significant coronary artery stenosis in patients with stable angina: a meta-analysis focused on post-test disease probability. Eur Heart J. 2018;39(35):3322-30.
29. van den Hoogen IJ, van Rosendael AR, Lin FY, Bax JJ, Shaw LJ, Min JK. Coronary Computed Tomography Angiography as a Gatekeeper to Coronary Revascularization: Emphasizing Atherosclerosis Findings Beyond Stenosis. Curr Cardiovasc Imaging Rep. 2019;12(6):24.
30. Knuuti J, Wijns W, Saraste A, Capodanno D, Barbato E, Funck-Brentano C, et al.; ESC Scientific Document Group. 2019 ESC Guidelines for the diagnosis and management of chronic coronary syndromes. Eur Heart J. 2020;41(3):407-77.
31. Adamson PD, Newby DE. The SCOT-HEART Trial. What we observed and what we learned. J Cardiovasc Comput Tomogr. 2019; 13(3):54-8.
32. Devesa A, Ibanez B, Malick WA, Tinuoye EO, Bustamante J, Peyra C, et al. Primary Prevention of Subclinical Atherosclerosis in Young Adults: JACC Review Topic of the Week. J Am Coll Cardiol. 2023;82(22):2152-62.

CHAPTER 3

Risk Factors for Heart Disease with a Focus on Modifiable Factors in Indians

◼ INTRODUCTION

The rightful start of any discussion on cardiovascular risk factors (CVRFs) is the Framingham Heart Study (FHS) that started in 1948 with the mission "to study the expression of coronary artery disease (CAD) in a "normal" or unselected population and to determine the factors predisposing to the development of the disease through clinical and laboratory exam and long-term follow-up."[1-4] Now, 75 years and 3 generations of enrollees later, we honor this classic study that gave us evidence-based results on CVRFs with a wide range prevention, treatment, lifestyle, public policy, etc.—of applications that were instrumental in reducing the mortality and morbidity of heart disease in the US and other countries. The initial phase of FHS identified hypertension and high cholesterol as risk factors and as the study progressed tobacco smoking and diabetes were added to this list.

◼ MAJOR RISK FACTORS AND INDIAN PARADOX

All major studies since then have substantiated the risk posed by hypertension, high cholesterol, tobacco smoking, and diabetes, hence, these four factors are accepted as major (at times referred to as "traditional" or "established") CVRFs. Based on FHS and subsequent studies, atherosclerotic cardiovascular disease (ASCVD) risk calculators have been developed and refined. However, standard risk ASCVD calculators developed in the western countries based largely on their native population underestimate the risk and are insufficient to understand the aggressive nature of CAD (early onset, severe disease, and premature deaths) in Indians. Moreover, the heightened risk and aggressive nature of CAD in Indians are observed despite lower traditional risk factors (the "Indian paradox"). **Figures 1A to C** from the UK Biobank Prospective Cohort Study is illustrative of this paradox.[5] Of particular note, as shown in the figure, South Asians have increased risk for ASCVD compared to Europeans despite having comparable risk by both Pooled Cohort and QRISK equations.

Why this paradox? To answer this one must understand that the genesis and progression of CAD, besides the major CVRFs, are also influenced by diverse elements such as genes, environment, lifestyle, and metabolism. Raj Bhopal[6] analyzed several theories (genes, fat storage, life and dietary style, developmental, and intergenerational effects) and could not single out one among them as the sole culprit. It follows that multiple factors are at play in combination(s) and may be interwoven. Identifying all the modifiable risk factors, in all categories, is essential to implement effective prevention and intervention strategies.[7,8]

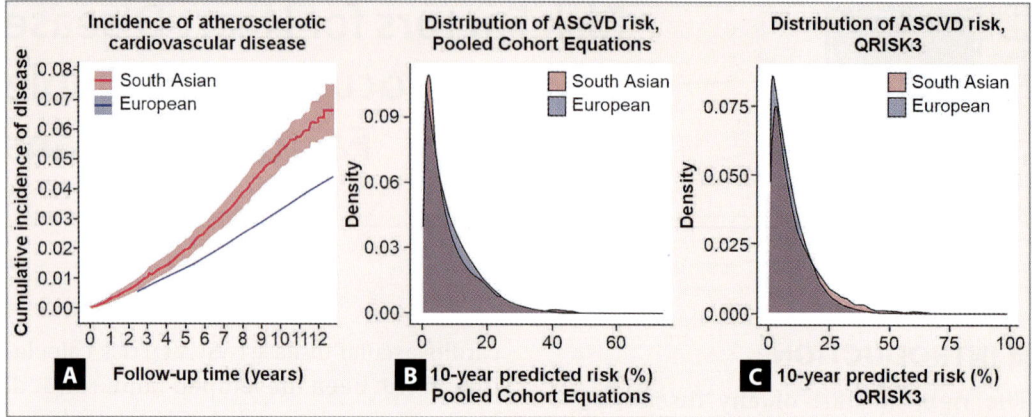

Figs. 1A to C: Observed and predicted incidence of atherosclerotic cardiovascular disease (ASCVD) in individuals of South Asian versus European ancestry: (A) Unadjusted cumulative incidence of initial ASCVD events over the length of follow-up stratified by South Asian or European ancestry; (B) Distribution of unadjusted 10-year predicted risk of ASCVD by the American Heart Association/American College of Cardiology Pooled Cohort Equations, stratified by individuals of South Asian and European ancestry; and (C) Distribution of unadjusted 10-year predicted risk of ASCVD by the QRISK 3 equations, stratified by individuals of South Asian and European ancestry.
Source: Reproduced with permission from Patel AP.[5]

BEYOND THE MAJOR RISK FACTORS LOOKING INTO RISK FACTORS ACROSS DIFFERENT COUNTRIES

Two very large studies, notable for their global scope and the wide range of factors examined, have provided very useful and actionable information. The INTERHEART study in 52 countries reported that nine risk factors (the four major risk factors and five others) explained >90% of acute myocardial infarctions (AMI) **(Table 1)**.[9,10] The other five factors were abdominal obesity, psychosocial factors, reduced fruit and vegetable consumption, alcohol use, and physical inactivity. More recently, the Prospective Urban Rural Epidemiology (PURE) study reported that a dozen risk factors explained >65–70% of incident cardiovascular (CVD) events in low, middle, and high-income countries **(Table 1 and Fig. 2)**.[11] The four major risk factors feature here too. Note that in two of them—Nonhigh density lipoprotein cholesterol (NHDL-C) and diabetes—the population attributable fractions (PAF) are higher in South Asians compared to the global population and these two are covered in detail in subsequent chapters. Here we spotlight the risk factors, beyond the major (established) ones, that were identified in this study.

LIFESTYLE FACTORS

Unhealthy Diets

Laden with bad fats, refined carbohydrates, added sugar, and excessive salt are high on the list of modifiable risk factors even more than tobacco use and inactivity combined. Notably, high carbohydrate diets in India appear to have a stronger tie to high triglycerides and

TABLE 1: Important coronary artery disease (CAD) risk factors from cross-sectional INTERHEART and prospective PURE studies.

Risk factors	INTERHEART	PURE
Lifestyle factors	• Unhealthy diet • Tobacco smoking • Physical inactivity • Alcohol	• Unhealthy diet and sodium intake • Tobacco smoking • Physical inactivity • Household air pollution
Metabolic factors	• Hypertension • Diabetes • Abnormal lipids (ApoB/ApoA1) • Abdominal obesity • Lipoprotein(a)	• Hypertension • Diabetes • High NHDL-C (Nonhigh density lipoprotein cholesterol) • Abdominal obesity • Grip strength
Social factors	• Psychosocial stress • Depression	• Psychosocial stress • Depression • Low education

Source: Adapted from Sharma,[7] Yusuf.[9,10]

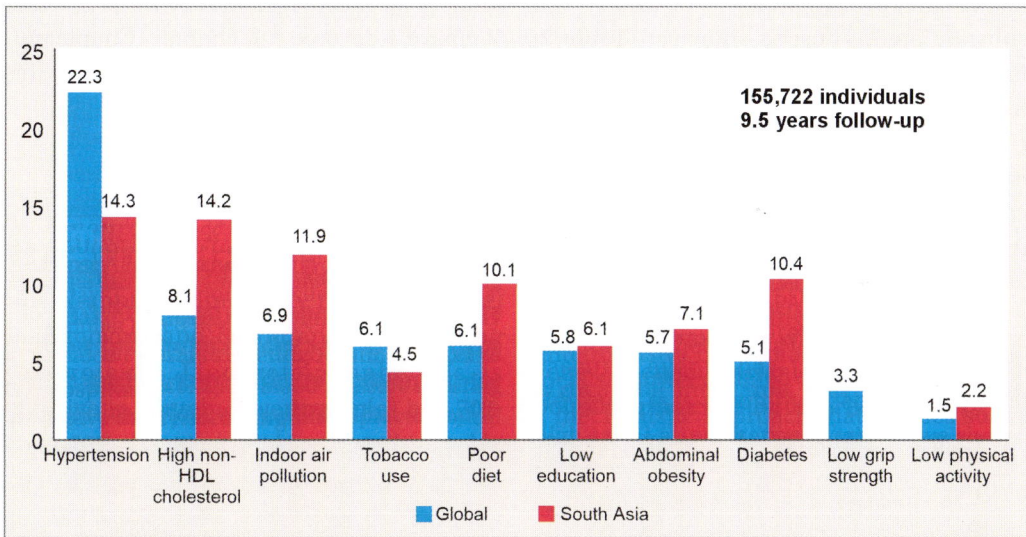

Fig. 2: Population attributable fractions (percent) for various cardiovascular risk factors in the Prospective Urban Rural Epidemiology (PURE) study.
Source: Reproduced with permission Sharma S, Gaur K, Gupta R. Indian Heart J. 2024.[10]

diabetes than genetics, with fried foods and trans fats further amplifying this risk. Traditional, whole plant-based vegetarianism is a heart-healthy cornerstone of Indian cuisine. However, unhealthy adaptations loaded with refined carbohydrates, tropical oils (coconut oil and palm oil) that are rich in saturated fats (SFA), and high-heat cooking methods make it unhealthy. Important points to note are:[12]

- High-heat cooking and reused oils generate harmful trans fats and advanced glycation end products (AGE).
- *Saturated fat-rich oils:* Palm oil, coconut oil, and ghee elevate cholesterol levels.
- The worst effect occurs when trans fats (TFA) replace SFA.
- Low protein intake weakens the immune system and increases heart disease risk.
- Excessive sugar and refined carbohydrates contribute to weight gain, diabetes, and heart disease. Refined carbohydrates may be as detrimental as SFAs for Indian hearts.[6,10]

The substantial benefit in using monounsaturated fats (MUFA) or polyunsaturated fats (PUFA) over that of TFA or SFA is well substantiated. Thus, as shown in **Table 2**, isocaloric substitution of 5% calories from SFA with PUFA lowers cardiovascular risk by 28% and with MUFA by 15%. An isocaloric substitution of 5% of calories from carbohydrates to PUFA lowers CV risk by 22%. Also to note that the simple step of replacing refined carbohydrates with whole grains reduces CV risk by 10%.

Many of the food items attractively displayed in grocery stores are ultra-processed foods that are mass produced in factories with added sugar, salt, and fat and are competitively priced to healthier alternatives. Clear labeling of constituents, warning labels, and increase in taxes are being effectively used in several countries to reduce the sales of unhealthy food. In 2016, Chile mandated food manufacturers to use the octagonal shaped STOP sign on warning labels of packaged foods that are high in calories, sodium, saturated fat, and added sugar and eight other countries followed suit. These measures along with ongoing public education and affordable healthy food choices are needed to reduce heart disease. We have a devoted full chapter (Chapter 16) on the prime importance of diet later in this book.

Tobacco Use

Impressive strides have been made in India, reducing smoking rates from 25 to 9%

TABLE 2: Reduction in cardiovascular risk with isocaloric substitution of 5% of the calories from saturated fats (A) or carbohydrates from refined carbohydrates/added sugars (B) with MUFA, PUFA, and unrefined (whole grain) carbohydrates.

A. From saturated fat to		
MUFA	5%	−15%
PUFA	5%	−28%
Carbohydrates from whole grains	5%	−8%
B. From refined carbohydrates/added sugars by equivalent to		
Saturated fat 5%	5%	−1%
MUFA	5%	−5%
PUFA	5%	−22%
Carbohydrates from whole grains	5%	−10%

(MUFA: monounsaturated fats; PUFA: polyunsaturated fats)
Source: Adapted from Li Y, et al.[12]

(smoking rates in Indian immigrants in the US are 5% in men and 1% in women), but continued action is needed to eliminate this scourge. Bidis and smokeless tobacco, especially chewing tobacco, remain a deadly threat in South Asia, with India leading the world in chewing tobacco-related deaths. Electronic cigarettes and secondhand smoke add to this pervasive public health issue.[11,12] Quitting nicotine use, in any form, is the single most important step to reduce risks of heart disease, cancer, and lung diseases (Chapter 4).

Physical Inactivity

Physical inactivity is linked to a rise in heart disease, diabetes, and even cancer. The overall physical inactivity in Indians is 21% and as high as 71% urban women.[13,14] The World Health Organization (WHO) recommends 150 minutes of moderate-intensity exercise weekly. Cultural norms and lack of appropriate facilities can be barriers, but simple solutions like daily 10,000 steps (especially for non-obese individuals) and wearable fitness trackers can significantly boost activity levels and life expectancy. The target of 10,000 steps daily may be hard for some, especially for senior citizens; if so, aim for 4,000 and keep in mind that every step counts![14] In 2019, an estimated 832,000 premature deaths and 15.7 million disability-adjusted life years (DALYs) were attributed to physical inactivity.[14,15] Though the cardiovascular benefits of physical activity are confirmed, excessive amounts of exercise (high volume and frequency) are not recommended and have not shown to impact the progression of coronary artery calcium (CAC) scores.[16]

Alcohol Use

Alcohol use is harmful in excess (defined by western standards as seven (in women) and 14 (in men) drinks a week). In the United States, one "standard" drink (or one alcoholic drink equivalent) contains roughly 14 g of pure alcohol, which is found in: 12 ounces of regular beer, which is usually about 5% alcohol; 5 ounces of wine, which is typically about 12% alcohol; 1.5 ounces of distilled spirits, which is about 40% alcohol. A standard American drink pour of distilled spirit is 45 mL, compared to a standard European drink (peg) of 30 mL. In India, a standard drink, mistakenly called "a peg" is 60 mL and may lead to unintentional overuse of alcohol. Besides alcohol usage is a socially accepted norm in western countries while it is not in South Asian countries where binge drinking is more common. These are possible explanations for the INTERHEART study finding alcohol use as a risk factor in South Asians but not in western populations. Another important health risk was brought to the attention of the public recently by the US Surgeon General on the causal link between alcohol consumption and seven different types of cancers.

Household Air Pollution

The PURE study revealed that over 40% of participants relied on solid fuels for cooking, exposing them to household air pollution, which increased the risk of heart disease and death by 14% compared to cleaner fuels like gas or electricity. Given that this issue impacts a staggering 2.5 billion people globally, with women disproportionately affected due to their greater exposure while cooking. The problem is particularly severe in India, where air pollution levels far exceed the World Health Organization (WHO) limits and contribute to nearly 40% of all air pollution-related deaths, many of them premature.[11,17-19]

METABOLIC FACTORS

Hypertension and *diabetes* are discussed in detail in Chapter 5 and Chapter 6.

High cholesterol is one of the earliest major CVRFs identified and as fractionation became available, abnormal lipids and high Non-HDL cholesterol (NHDL-C) were specifically identified as the key agents in CAD **(Table 1)**. Befitting its importance, this topic is detailed in Chapter 7. Lipoprotein (a) is explained in Chapter 8.

Abdominal Obesity

Indians face an underappreciated risk from abdominal fat storage, even for those with a normal BMI. BMI, though widely used, is an imperfect metric that does not account for racial, ethnic, and cultural differences and does not differentiate people with abdominal (visceral and subcutaneous) fat. Indians have lower thresholds for abdominal obesity, overweight, and obesity compared to the WHO criteria **(Table 3)**.[20-22]

This means Indians can be more susceptible to health problems despite having BMIs considered healthy elsewhere. A major study in New Delhi highlights this, showing abdominal obesity rates in Indian men and women as high as 70% using Indian criteria, compared to 20% (men) and 35% (women) with standard BMI >30 thresholds.[23] Importantly, for Indians, maintaining a healthy weight (ideally BMI 19–23) and reducing abdominal fat are crucial for good health, achievable with simple lifestyle changes in diet, exercise, and waist measurement.[24]

The "thin fat" Indian body type is a paradox. Despite a normal BMI, these individuals have high abdominal fat and metabolic risks such as diabetes and high blood fats. This paradox is particularly striking in urban Indians, who are 5-9 times more likely to exhibit dysglycemia (abnormal blood sugar) and dyslipidemia (abnormal lipids) within the "healthy" BMI range compared to other ethnicities.[25]

The magnitude of risk posed by abdominal obesity, a component of metabolic syndrome, is driven home by the results of a recent study **(Table 4)** by Anjana and colleagues.[26] In this study, abdominal obesity was defined as a waist circumference >90 cm for men and >80 cm for women (based on the WHO Asia Pacific guidelines).

Abdominal obesity was more common than diabetes, dysglycemia, or hypertension. Generalized obesity was defined as a BMI >25 kg/m^2. Dysglycemia was defined as the presence of prediabetes or diabetes. Hypercholesterolemia was defined as total cholesterol (TC) >200 mg/dL and low density lipoprotein-cholesterol (LDL-C) >130 mg/dL was defined as high. Hypertension was found in more than one-third (nearly two-thirds by the American College of Cardiology/American Heart Association (ACC/AHA) criteria), and obesity in nearly a third of the population.

TABLE 3: Difference in criteria for obesity and abdominal obesity in Indians and Americans.[20]

Weight	Indians	Americans
Overweight	Body mass index >23	Body mass index >25
Obese	Body mass index >25	Body mass index >30
Male waist circumference	>90 cm or >35 inches	>102 cm or >40 inches
Female waist circumference	>80 cm or >31 inches	>88 cm or >34.6 inches

TABLE 4: Burden of noncommunicable diseases in India.[26]

Abdominal obesity	351.0 million
Generalized obesity	254.2 million
Hypertension	315.5 million
Dysglycemia	236.4 million
Prediabetes	136.0 million
Diabetes	101.3 million
High cholesterol	213.3 million
High low density lipoprotein (LDL) cholesterol	185.7 million

■ SOCIAL FACTORS

Psychosocial stress, particularly from work and relationships, increases CVD risk. Two-fold increases in heart disease risk are linked to specific stressors such as job strain and work reward imbalance. In essence, one's social environment and how one reacts to its challenges can significantly impact heart health.[27,28] Psychosocial stress also triggers physical and mental responses such as headaches, fatigue, anxiety, and depression, and these adverse manifestations may be more common in women.

Depression is associated with risk for heart disease even after accounting for lifestyle factors and medical disorders.[29] A meta-analysis of eight prospective cohort and case-controlled studies has shown a 60% higher adjusted risk of CVD in patients with depression.[30] Depression and CVD can be considered as two-way streets as CVD is increased in depression and depression is increased in CVD. Depression is present in one of five patients with CVD,[9] and is associated with 2.5-3.5-fold increased risk of myocardial infarction (MI) even after adjusting for lifestyle factors and other medical disorders.[8,9] Depression is associated with decreased adherence to lifestyle changes and medications, worsening risk factors, increased mortality, excess disability, greater health care expenditures, and reduced quality of life.[29] For these reasons, standardized screening pathways for depression in patients with CVD offer the potential for early identification and optimal management of depression to improve health outcomes.[31]

Low education is a risk factor in South Asia, especially in women as nearly two-thirds of women have less than high school education. It is associated with a two-fold risk of CVD incidence and a three-fold risk of CVD death. Both paternal and maternal low education are associated with higher mortality, regardless of other markers of socioeconomic status.[11,32]

■ RISK-ENHANCING FACTORS

In addition to the well-established major CVRFs discussed earlier the 2018 Cholesterol Clinical Practice Guidelines of ACC and AHA recognized several risk-enhancing factors (RENFs) as noted in **Box 1**, that are useful in refining and improving risk assessment and importantly on initiation of statin therapy.[33] This is particularly relevant to Indians and other South Asians as Pooled Cohort Equations (PCE) based calculators underestimate their ASCVD risk.

South Asian ethnicity (ancestry from India, Pakistan, Bangladesh, Sri Lanka, Nepal, Bhutan, and Maldives) gained formal acceptance as a risk-enhancing factor based on the accumulated evidence presented in previous chapters. The significance of this cannot be understated as it positively impacts early screening tests and diagnosis, preventive measures, lifestyle modifications, and timely treatment and interventions.[32]

Family history of premature heart disease is a risk-enhancer and is of pointed importance to Indians. Early screening

> **BOX 1:** ASCVD risk-enhancing factors as per 2018 ACC/AHA Multisociety Cholesterol Clinical Practice Guidelines.
>
> - South Asian ancestry
> - Family history of premature ASCVD (males <55 years and females <65 years)
> - Chronic kidney disease (Stages 2–4)
> - Chronic inflammation (rheumatoid arthritis, systemic lupus erythematosus, psoriasis, HIV/AIDS, etc.)
> - Premature (<40 years) menopause
> - Pregnancy-related (gestational diabetes, preeclampsia, recurrent pregnancy loss, and stillbirth)
> - Metabolic syndrome (Met S)
> - Lipids and triglycerides (LDL-C ≥160 mg/dL, non-HDL-C ≥190 mg/dL, fasting triglycerides ≥175 mg/dL)
> - Biomarkers [Lipoprotein A (Lp(a)) ≥50 mg/dL or ≥125 nmol/L, apolipoprotein B (Apo B) ≥130 mg/dL, C-reactive protein ≥2 mg/dL]
> - Ankle brachial index <0.9
>
> (AIDS: Acquired immunodeficiency syndrome; ASCVD: atherosclerotic cardiovascular disease; LDL-C: low density lipoprotein cholesterol; HDL-C: high density lipoprotein cholesterol; HIV: Human immunodeficiency virus)
> *Source:* Grundy S, et al.[33]

[lipid panel, Lp(a) test] as young as age 5–10 and a coronary calcium scan after the age of 30 can help assess risk and guide primary preventive measures. A history of a heart attack (myocardial infarction) in a parent before the age of 60 years increases the risk of CAD by 1.5–2-fold.[34] Therefore, a family history of heart disease calls for careful assessment and treatment of treatable risk factors such as hypertension, dyslipidemia, and diabetes.

Medical conditions that enhance the risk of ASCVD with specific descriptors and qualifiers are as noted on the table and are mostly self-explanatory. However, metabolic syndrome (Met S) because of its frequency and mostly asymptomatic nature merits further explanation.

Metabolic Syndrome

The core abnormality is an imbalance between intake (anabolism) and catabolism of nutrients (overnutrition)[35] and its correction is focused on caloric restriction and increased physical activity. According to the INTERHEART study,[36] its incidence is high among Indians, as much as one in three men and one in two women and markedly increases their risk for type 2 diabetes mellitus (T2D) and increases the risk for heart disease. Recent guidelines use a three out of five criteria [fasting glucose (>100 mg/dL), triglycerides >150 mg/dL], HDL (<40 mg/dL men, <50 mg/dL women), blood pressure (BP) (>130/85 mm Hg), abdominal obesity (waist circumference of >90 cm in men, >80 cm in women)] for diagnosis.[21,37] Waist circumference measure is an acceptable proxy for visceral fat estimation in South Asians in lieu of computed tomography (CT) scans.[38,39]

Biomarkers

Four of them are listed on the table as RENFs. Lipoprotein(a), in our studied opinion, is more than a biomarker and is elaborated on in Chapter 8. Apo B, which encompasses all atherogenic lipids when elevated, has emerged as a reliable predictor of risk for heart disease (Chapter 7). High-sensitivity C-reactive protein (Hs-CRP) is a good marker for chronic inflammatory conditions but is not cardiospecific. Ankle-brachial index (ABI) is calculated for each lower limb by dividing the ankle systolic BP by the highest systolic BP in both arms. This test to detect peripheral artery disease has been in use for a long time and is now recognized as an ASCVD risk-enhancing factor (ABI <9).[33]

EFFORTS TO IMPROVE THE ACCURACY OF RISK PREDICTION

A natural extension to the successful efforts to identify additional (to the four established CVRFs) factors and the RENFs is to try various combinations of these to improve the accuracy of predicting ASCVD, its progression, and a major adverse cardiac event (MACE). Of the many studies undertaken in this regard, two major ones yielded particularly noteworthy results.

Akintoye and co-researchers[40] pooled data from three epidemiological cohorts [involving 22,942 participants from Atherosclerosis Risk In Communities (ARIC), Cardiovascular Health Study (CHS), and Multiethnic Study of Atherosclerosis (MESA)].[40] Over a period of 19 years a total of 1,960 individuals (8.5%) experienced MACE. Of the 10 factors evaluated, six helped predict MACE **(Table 5)**, independent of the PCE. Each factor individually lacked enough predictive strength but combining any three of them predicted a 10-year MACE risk >7.5%—the threshold for statin treatment in the US. Consequently, individuals identified by this method could reap the proven benefits in risk reduction with statin therapy (Chapter 13).

Coronary Artery Calcium Score

In analysis of data from pooled individual-level data of 22,942 participants (56% women, mean age 59 years), Akintoye[40] evaluated the predictive ability of the risk enhancers and CAC score for ASCVD. As shown in **Table 6**,

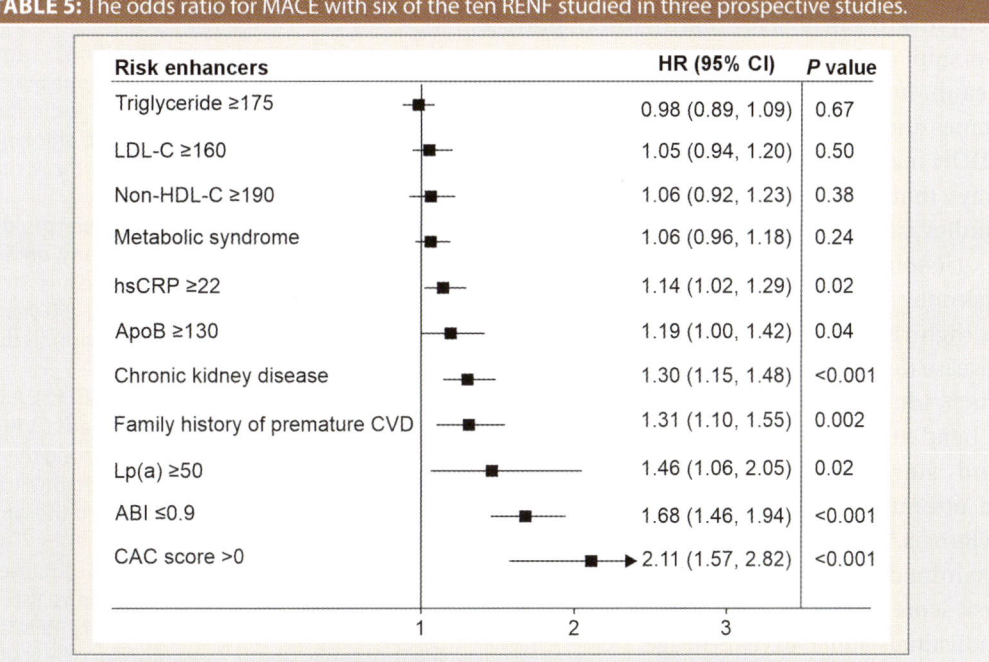

TABLE 5: The odds ratio for MACE with six of the ten RENF studied in three prospective studies.

Risk enhancers	HR (95% CI)	P value
Triglyceride ≥175	0.98 (0.89, 1.09)	0.67
LDL-C ≥160	1.05 (0.94, 1.20)	0.50
Non-HDL-C ≥190	1.06 (0.92, 1.23)	0.38
Metabolic syndrome	1.06 (0.96, 1.18)	0.24
hsCRP ≥22	1.14 (1.02, 1.29)	0.02
ApoB ≥130	1.19 (1.00, 1.42)	0.04
Chronic kidney disease	1.30 (1.15, 1.48)	<0.001
Family history of premature CVD	1.31 (1.10, 1.55)	0.002
Lp(a) ≥50	1.46 (1.06, 2.05)	0.02
ABI ≤0.9	1.68 (1.46, 1.94)	<0.001
CAC score >0	2.11 (1.57, 2.82)	<0.001

(ABI: Ankle-brachial index; ApoB: Apolipoprotein B; CAC: coronary artery calcium; Lp(a): Lipoprotein A; hsCRP: High-sensitivity C-reactive protein; LDL-C: low density lipoprotein cholesterol; HDL-C: high density lipoprotein cholesterol; MACE: major adverse cardiac event; RENF: risk-enhancing factors)
Source: Reproduced with permission from Akintoye et al.[40]

TABLE 6: Synergistic effect of ASCVD risk-enhancing factors and CAC score.[40]

Number of risk-enhancing factors	CAC score = 0	CAC score = ≥1
<3 risk-enhancing factors	3.5%	9.8%
≥3 risk-enhancing factors	9.7%	14.2%

(ASCVD: atherosclerotic cardiovascular disease; CAC: coronary artery calcium)

participants with three or more RENFs and a CAC score of ≥1 had a four-fold greater risk of adverse cardiac events compared to those with <3 RENFs and a CAC score of 0. Besides, prior studies have shown that CAC progression markedly increases the risk of MACE.[41-43]

■ OTHER RISK CONTRIBUTORS

Social determinants of health (SDOH) are gaining more attention in general and on cardiovascular health in particular. SDOH are the conditions in the environment where people are born, live, learn, work, play, worship, and age that affect a wide range of health, functioning, and quality of life outcomes and risks.[44,45] Individual and area-level SDOH may capture social factors in different ways that represent distinct influences on cardiovascular diseases and their outcomes.

Genome-wide polygenic score for CAD risk may be useful to identify individuals at high risk for extremely premature heart disease decades before a cardiac catastrophe. Such identification can give individuals a head start in adopting lifestyle changes and starting pharmacological therapy to attenuate the development of atherosclerosis.[46] However, to date, no study has examined the clinical utility of polygenic risk score in risk stratification of ASCVD in individuals under 40 years of age.

Understanding the risk factors of heart disease in Indians is the first and necessary step in prevention and treatment. Our discussion of risk factors in this chapter firstly, affirms the major risk factors (detailed in chapters to follow), moves on to the two major studies with substantial South Asian participants that identified additional risk factors, then to the RENFs recognized by multiple organizations, and finally to the fruitful efforts to improve predictive accuracy by combining many factors. We emphasize that most of the risk factors for heart disease in Indians are modifiable and therefore they should be targeted for immediate, concerted, and sustained action.

■ KEY TAKEAWAYS

- Hypertension, tobacco smoking, high cholesterol, and diabetes are the four major (established) risk factors for CAD. India has made progress in reducing tobacco smoking but not in the control of the other three risk factors.
- Commonly used ASCVD risk calculators do not fully explain the incidence, early onset, severity, and premature deaths in Indians. 30% of global premature heart disease (<50 years of age) are in Indians out of proportion to the global rate of 8%.
- Results generated by the landmark INTERHEART and PURE studies have identified CVRFs additional to the four major ones. Among them are modifiable factors: Unhealthy diet, physical inactivity, abdominal obesity, tobacco use, and alcohol use.
- Cholesterol Clinical Practical Guidelines developed by multiple organizations listed several ASCVD risk-enhancing factors (RENFs). Most notably, South Asian ancestry by itself was formally recognized as RENF. Among the RENFs of particular note are—family history of premature ASCVD, lipoprotein(a), and metabolic syndrome.

- India bears a large burden of noncommunicable disorders—obesity, hypertension, diabetes, and high cholesterol. Obesity, in particular abdominal obesity, is a key feature of metabolic syndrome. Metabolic syndrome affects one in three Indian men and one in two Indian women. Metabolic syndrome markedly increases the risk of developing diabetes and increases the risk of heart disease and heart attacks.
- Use of various combinations of aforementioned risk factors and others to improve the accuracy of predicting MACE has produced actionable results: (1) Three factors combined could predict people with a 10-year MACE risk of 7.5% (meeting the US threshold for statin treatment), (2) CAC score >1 combined with three or more RENFs predicted a four-fold risk of heart events compared to those with a CAC score of 0 and <3 RENFs.

REFERENCES

1. Kannel WB, Dawber TR, Kagan A, Revotskie N, Stokes J, 3rd. Factors of risk in the development of coronary heart disease—six year follow-up experience. The Framingham Study. Ann Intern Med. 1961;55:33-50.
2. Kannel WB. Contributions of the Framingham Study to the conquest of coronary artery disease. Am J Cardiol. 1988;62(16):1109-12.
3. Kannel WB. Fifty years of Framingham Study contributions to understanding hypertension. J Hum Hypertens. 2000;14(2):83-90.
4. Kannel WB, Neaton JD, Wentworth D, Thomas HE, Stamler J, Hulley SB, et al. Overall and coronary heart disease mortality rates in relation to major risk factors in 325,348 men screened for the MRFIT. Multiple Risk Factor Intervention Trial. Am Heart J. 1986;112(4):825-36.
5. Patel AP, Wang M, Kartoun U, Ng K, Khera AV. Quantifying and understanding the higher risk of atherosclerotic cardiovascular disease among South Asian individuals: Results From the UK Biobank Prospective Cohort Study. Circulation. 2021;144(6):410-22.
6. Bhopal R. Epidemic of Cardiovascular Disease and diabetes: Explaining the phenomenon in South Asians worldwide. Oxford: Oxford University Press; 2019.
7. Global Cardiovascular Risk C, Magnussen C, Ojeda FM, Leong DP, Alegre-Diaz J, Amouyel P, Aviles-Santa L, et al. Global effect of modifiable risk factors on cardiovascular disease and mortality. N Engl J Med. 2023;389(14):1273-85.
8. Yusuf S, Joseph P, Rangarajan S, Islam S, Mente A, Hystad P, et al. Modifiable risk factors, cardiovascular disease, and mortality in 155 722 individuals from 21 high-income, middle-income, and low-income countries (PURE): a prospective cohort study. Lancet. 2020;395(10226):795-808.
9. Yusuf S, Hawken S, Ounpuu S, Dans T, Avezum A, Lanas F, et al. Effect of potentially modifiable risk factors associated with myocardial infarction in 52 countries (the INTERHEART study): case-control study. Lancet. 2004;364(9438):937-52.
10. Sharma S, Gaur K, Gupta R. Trends in epidemiology of dyslipidemias in India. Indian Heart J. 2024;76(Suppl 1):S20-8.
11. Joseph P, Kutty VR, Mohan V, Kumar R, Mony P, Vijayakumar K, et al. Cardiovascular disease, mortality, and their associations with modifiable risk factors in a multinational South Asia cohort: a PURE substudy. Eur Heart J. 2022;43(30):2831-40.
12. Li Y, Hruby A, Bernstein AM, Ley SH, Wang DD, Chiuve SE, et al. Saturated fats compared with unsaturated fats and sources of carbohydrates in relation to risk of coronary heart disease: a prospective cohort study. J Am Coll Cardiol. 2015;66(14):1538-48.
13. Lee IM, Shiroma EJ, Lobelo F, Puska P, Blair SN, Katzmarzyk PT; Lancet Physical Activity Series Working Group. Effect of physical inactivity on major noncommunicable diseases worldwide: an analysis of burden of disease and life expectancy. Lancet. 2012;380(9838):219-29.
14. Roth GA, Mensah GA, Johnson CO, Addolorato G, Ammirati E, Baddour LM, et al. Global burden of cardiovascular diseases and risk factors, 1990-2019: Update From the GBD 2019 Study. J Am Coll Cardiol. 2020;76(25):2982-3021.
15. Blair SN, Kampert JB, Kohl HW 3rd, Barlow CE, Macera CA, Paffenbarger RS Jr, et al.

Influences of cardiorespiratory fitness and other precursors on cardiovascular disease and all-cause mortality in men and women. JAMA. 1996;276(3):205-10.
16. Shuval K, Leonard D, DeFina LF, Barlow CE, Berry JD, Turlington WM, et al. Physical activity and progression of coronary artery calcification in men and women. JAMA Cardiol. 2024;9(7):659-66.
17. Hystad P, Duong M, Brauer M, Larkin A, Arku R, Kurmi OP, et al. Health effects of household solid fuel use: findings from 11 countries within the prospective urban and rural epidemiology study. Environ Health Perspect. 2019;127(5):57003.
18. Fatmi Z, Coggon D. Coronary heart disease and household air pollution from use of solid fuel: a systematic review. Br Med Bull. 2016;118(1):91-109.
19. India State-Level Disease Burden Initiative Air Pollution C. The impact of air pollution on deaths, disease burden, and life expectancy across the states of India: the Global Burden of Disease Study 2017. Lancet Planet Health. 2019;3(1):e26-e39.
20. Misra A, Chowbey P, Makkar BM, Vikram NK, Wasir JS, Chadha D, et al. Consensus statement for diagnosis of obesity, abdominal obesity and the metabolic syndrome for Asian Indians and recommendations for physical activity, medical and surgical management. J Assoc Physicians India. 2009; 57:163-70.
21. Alberti KG, Eckel RH, Grundy SM, Zimmet PZ, Cleeman JI, Donato KA, et al. Harmonizing the metabolic syndrome: a joint interim statement of the International Diabetes Federation Task Force on Epidemiology and Prevention; National Heart, Lung, and Blood Institute; American Heart Association; World Heart Federation; International Atherosclerosis Society; and international association for the Study of Obesity. Circulation. 2009;120(16):1640-5.
22. World Health Organization, Western Pacific Regional office, WPRO IRIS. The Asia-Pacific perspective: Redefining obesity and its treatment 2000. [online] Available from http://iris.wpro.who.int/handle/10665.1/5379 [Last accessed May, 2025].
23. Huffman MD, Prabhakaran D, Osmond C, Fall CH, Tandon N, Lakshmy R, et al. Incidence of cardiovascular risk factors in an Indian urban cohort results from the New Delhi birth cohort. J Am Coll Cardiol. 2011;57(17):1765-74.
24. Enas EA, Singh V, Munjal YP, Bhandari S, Yadave RD, Manchanda SC. Reducing the burden of coronary artery disease in India: challenges and opportunities. Indian Heart J. 2008;60(2):161-75.
25. Patel SA, Shivashankar R, Ali MK, Anjana RM, Deepa M, Kapoor D, et al. Is the "South Asian Phenotype" Unique to South Asians?: comparing cardiometabolic risk factors in the CARRS and NHANES studies. Glob Heart. 2016;11(1):89-96 e3.
26. Anjana RM, Unnikrishnan R, Deepa M, Pradeepa R, Tandon N, Das AK, et al. Metabolic non-communicable disease health report of India: the ICMR-INDIAB national cross-sectional study (ICMR-INDIAB-17). Lancet Diabetes Endocrinol. 2023;11(7):474-89.
27. Santosa A, Rosengren A, Ramasundarahettige C, Rangarajan S, Gulec S, Chifamba J, et al. Psychosocial risk factors and cardiovascular disease and death in a population-based cohort from 21 Low-, Middle-, and High-Income countries. JAMA Netw Open. 2021; 4(12):e2138920.
28. Lavigne-Robichaud M, Trudel X, Talbot D, Milot A, Gilbert-Ouimet M, Vézina M, et al. Psychosocial stressors at work and coronary heart disease risk in men and women: 18-year Prospective Cohort Study of Combined Exposures. Circ Cardiovasc Qual Outcomes. 2023;16(10):e009700.
29. Carmin CN, Ownby RL, Fontanella C, Steelesmith D, Binkley PF. Impact of mental health treatment on outcomes in patients with heart failure and ischemic heart disease. J Am Heart Assoc. 2024;13(7):e031117.
30. Van der Kooy K, van Hout H, Marwijk H, Marten H, Stehouwer C, Beekman A. Depression and the risk for cardiovascular diseases: systematic review and meta analysis. Int J Geriatr Psychiatry. 2007;22(7):613-26.
31. Rafiei S, Raoofi S, Baghaei A, Masoumi M, Doustmehraban M, Nejatifar Z, et al.

Depression prevalence in cardiovascular disease: global systematic review and meta-analysis. BMJ Support Palliat Care. 2023;13(3):281-9.
32. Rosengren A, Subramanian SV, Islam S, Chow CK, Avezum A, Kazmi K, et al. Education and risk for acute myocardial infarction in 52 high, middle and low-income countries: INTERHEART case-control study. Heart. 2009;95(24):2014-22.
33. Grundy SM, Stone NJ, Bailey AL, Beam C, Birtcher KK, Blumenthal RS, et al. 2018 AHA/ACC/AACVPR/AAPA/ABC/ACPM/ADA/AGS/APhA/ASPC/NLA/PCNA guideline on the management of blood cholesterol: executive summary: A Report of the American College of Cardiology/American Heart Association Task Force on Clinical Practice Guidelines. J Am Coll Cardiol. 2019;73(24):3168-209.
34. Dugani SB, Hydoub YM, Ayala AP, Reka R, Nayfeh T, Ding JF, et al. Risk factors for premature myocardial infarction: a systematic review and meta-analysis of 77 studies. Mayo Clin Proc Innov Qual Outcomes. 2021;5(4):783-94.
35. Mente A, Yusuf S, Islam S, McQueen MJ, Tanomsup S, Onen CL, et al. Metabolic syndrome and risk of acute myocardial infarction a case-control study of 26,903 subjects from 52 countries. J Am Coll Cardiol. 2010;55(21):2390-8.
36. Grundy SM. Metabolic syndrome pandemic. Arterioscler Thromb Vasc Biol. 2008;28(4):629-36.
37. Enas EA, Mohan V, Deepa M, Farooq S, Pazhoor S, Chennikkara H. The metabolic syndrome and dyslipidemia among Asian Indians: a population with high rates of diabetes and premature coronary artery disease. J Cardiometab Syndr. 2007;2(4):267-75.
38. Mongraw-Chaffin M, Gujral UP, Kanaya AM, Kandula NR, Carr JJ, Anderson CAM. Relation of ectopic fat with atherosclerotic cardiovascular disease risk score in South Asians Living in the United States [from the Mediators of Atherosclerosis in South Asians Living in America (MASALA) Study]. Am J Cardiol. 2018;121(3):315-21.
39. Gulati S, Misra A. Abdominal obesity and type 2 diabetes in Asian Indians: dietary strategies including edible oils, cooking practices and sugar intake. Eur J Clin Nutr. 2017;71(7):850-7.
40. Akintoye E, Afonso L, Bengaluru Jayanna M, Bao W, Briasoulis A, Robinson J. Prognostic Utility of Risk Enhancers and Coronary Artery Calcium Score Recommended in the 2018 ACC/AHA Multisociety Cholesterol Treatment Guidelines Over the Pooled Cohort Equation: Insights From 3 Large Prospective Cohorts. J Am Heart Assoc. 2021;10(12):e019589.
41. Shah H, Garacci E, Behuria S, Cainzos-Achirica M, Kandula NR, Kanaya AM, et al. Cardiovascular risk-enhancing factors and coronary artery calcium in South Asian American adults: The MASALA study. Am J Prev Cardiol. 2023;13:100453.
42. Budoff MJ, Tayek J. Coronary artery calcium progression: Increasing CAC is associated with increased events. JACC Cardiovasc Imaging. 2018;11(3):517-8.
43. Cardarelli R, Hall A, Rankin W. Coronary artery calcium progression is associated with cardiovascular events among asymptomatic individuals: From the North Texas Primary Care Practice-based Research Network (NorTex-PBRN). J Am Board Fam Med. 2017;30(5):592-600.
44. Wang Z, Pu B. Joint effects of depression and social determinants of health on mortality risk among U.S. adults: a cohort study. BMC Psychiatry. 2024;24(1):752.
45. Shah NS, Huang X, Petito LC, Bancks MP, Ning H, Cameron NA, et al. Social and psychosocial determinants of racial and ethnic differences in cardiovascular health in the United States population. Circulation. 2023;147(3):190-200.
46. Gray MP, Berman Y, Botta G, Grieve SM, Ho A, Hu J, et al. Incorporating a polygenic risk score-triaged coronary calcium score into cardiovascular disease examinations to identify subclinical coronary artery disease (ESCALATE): protocol for a prospective, nonrandomized implementation trial. Am Heart J. 2023;264:163-73.

CHAPTER 4

Tobacco Smoking

■ INTRODUCTION

Tobacco smoking takes its ignominious place alongside wars, pestilence, famine, and natural disasters as the greatest threats to human lives. Its systemic adverse effects are insidious and the toll of disease, morbidity, and death disproportionately affect men and people who are socioeconomically disadvantaged. Over 80% of the world's 1.3 billion tobacco users live in low- and middle-income countries (LMICs). Tobacco use is the leading cause of preventable death in the world killing over 8 million people each year.[1] More than 7 million of those deaths are the result of direct tobacco use while around 1.2 million are the result of nonsmokers being exposed to secondhand smoke (SHS).[2] On a brighter note, there is impressive progress, over the years, in the multifront efforts to curb tobacco use as depicted in **Figures 1A and B**.

The decline in cigarette smoking in the US to 11% of adults in 2024,[3] is even more impressive than the global trend. This drop in smoking rates to a historic low coincides with the 60th anniversary of the landmark US Surgeon General's report on Smoking and Health.[4] To give the readers a snapshot of the prevalent tobacco culture of the mid to late 60s, when we (authors) were resident physicians, the cars had cigarette lighters, smoking was a norm in physician offices, hospitals, and ash trays were built in or provided in medical student classrooms and conference rooms and nearly 40% of nurses smoked. Given the tenor of the times, it took courage for the Surgeon General (Dr Luther Terry) to warn the nation that smoking causes lung cancer and is the most important cause of chronic bronchitis and may be a causative factor in emphysema, cardiovascular disease, and various types of cancer (based on the review of over 7,000 scientific articles by his advisory committee). The importance of this report cannot be overstated as it sparked the passage of the Cigarette Labeling and Advertising Act of 1965 (warning labels on cigarette packages), antismoking initiatives, and was instrumental in changing the culture of tobacco smoking in the US. A brief review of seminal studies dating back to 1950 and a few since then follows.

■ SEMINAL STUDIES ON HEALTH RISKS OF TOBACCO SMOKING

Early Reports in 1950

A report in the British Medical Journal "Smoking and carcinoma of the lung; preliminary report," by Doll and Hill is widely credited as the first to sound the alarm on risks of smoking.[5] In this report, the authors cite Wynder and Graham from the US, on suggesting smoking as a possible cause of lung cancer.[6] Doll followed up the preliminary report with the British Doctors Study that convincingly established the health risks of smoking.

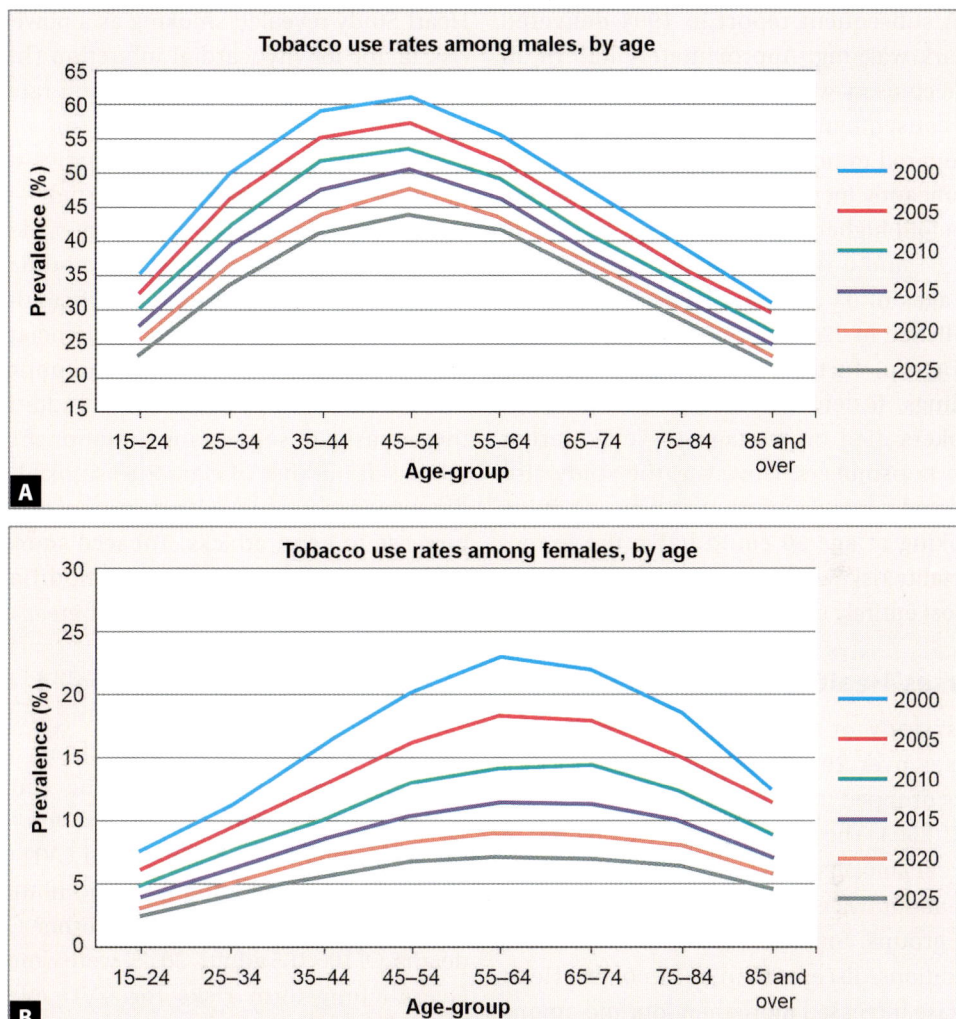

Figs. 1A and B: Global trends in age pattern of tobacco use in: (A) Males (upper panel); (B) Females (lower panel) 2000–2025.[2]

British Doctors Study

This landmark cohort study of 50,000 doctors for over 50 years provided the first robust statistical evidence linking smoking to an increased risk of lung cancer. The study revealed that men who smoked 25 cigarettes per day had a 25-fold increased risk of developing lung cancer compared to nonsmokers. The annual lung cancer rate among smokers was 3.15 per 1,000, while it was a mere 0.07 for nonsmokers. The study also demonstrated a significant reduction in lung cancer risk among doctors who quit smoking. Beyond lung cancer, the study uncovered a strong association between smoking and increased risks of coronary artery disease (CAD) and chronic bronchitis. Smokers, on average, experienced a shortened lifespan of approximately 10 years compared to nonsmokers.[7-12]

A subsequent report in 1994 delivered a stark warning: Approximately half of all tobacco users would ultimately succumb to the consequences of their smoking habit. Compared to nonsmokers, smokers faced a significantly increased mortality rate, with a threefold higher risk between the ages of 45 and 64 and a twofold higher risk between the ages of 65 and 84.[7-12] The final report, published in 2004 after 50 years of rigorous follow-up, further solidified the study's findings. It demonstrated that continuous smokers died on average 10 years earlier than nonsmokers. However, the study also reported hopeful and positive news. Quitting smoking at age 50 could halve the excess mortality risk, while quitting at age 30 could almost entirely eliminate it.[7-12]

Nurses' Health Study

This study of 237,648 female registered nurses over 20 years found that smoking rates dropped from 33.2% in 1976 to 8.4% in 2002/2003. The mortality rate was higher in current smokers than in former smokers and was about twice that of never-smokers in all age groups. Smokers had more comorbid conditions/diseases than nonsmokers. Heart disease increased more than fourfold among female nurse smokers over never-smokers. This large prospective study reinforced one of the important conclusions of the British Doctors Study that quitting smoking makes a difference as nurses who quit smoking had a lower mortality rate than those who continued to smoke.[13]

Studies on Smoking and Cardiovascular Disease

The British Doctors Study, as was mentioned earlier, also found that smoking increased the risk of coronary thrombosis. Framingham Heart Study revealed smoking as a powerful risk factor for myocardial infarction (heart attack), and that smoking cessation rapidly and markedly reduces risk for myocardial infarction.[14] Two large studies—the INTERHEART study and the PURE study—that were discussed in the previous chapter, identified tobacco smoking as a key modifiable risk factor that contributed significantly to myocardial infarctions and this association was consistent across different populations of different countries.[15,16] In addition, there was a dose-response relationship—increased number of cigarettes smoked per day was associated with a proportionate increase in heart attacks. Tobacco smoking also adversely affects other modifiable risk factors—hypertension, diabetes, and cholesterol (atherogenic lipids).

Khan and associates[17] pooled and analyzed data on current smoking status, covariates, and CVD outcomes from nine population-based cohorts in the United States. They examined the association between smoking status and total CVD and CVD subtypes, including fatal and nonfatal CAD, stroke, heart failure, and other CVD deaths. Of 106,165 adults, 50.4% were women. Overall long-term risks for CVD events were 46.0% [95% confidence interval (CI), 44.7–47.3] and 34.7% (95% CI, 33.3–36.0) in middle-aged men and women, respectively. In middle-aged men who reported smoking compared with those who did not smoke, competing hazard ratios (HRs) were higher for the first presentation being a fatal CVD event [HR, 1.79 (95% CI, 1.68–1.92)], with a similar pattern among women [HR, 1.82 (95% CI, 1.68–1.98)] **(Figs. 2A and B)**.

Smoking was associated with earlier CVD onset by 5.1 and 3.8 years in men and women. Similar patterns were observed in younger and older adults. Those who reported smoking

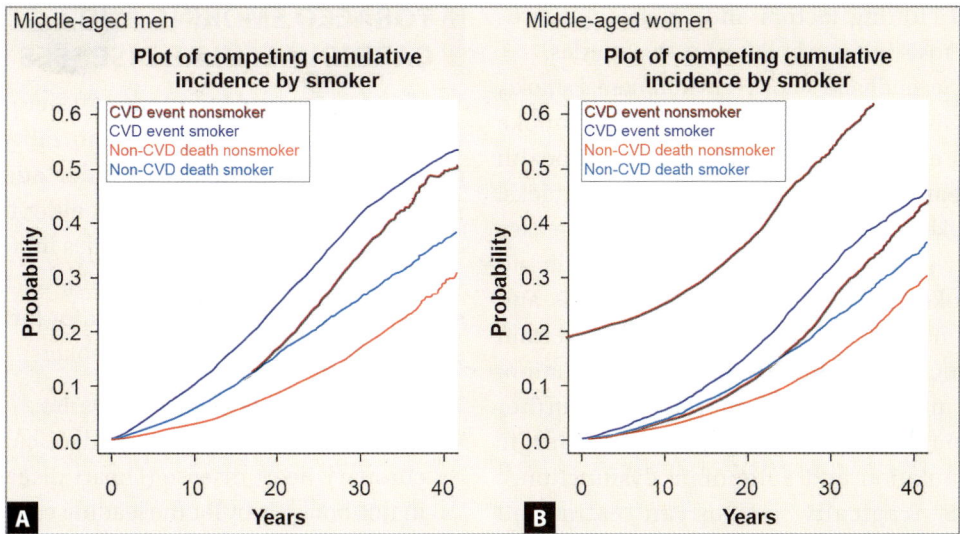

Figs. 2A and B: Cumulative incidence of cardiovascular disease (CVD) morbidity and mortality among middle-aged adults (40–59 years of age). Risk of cardiovascular disease in (A) Men and (B) Women based on smoking status and adjusted for competing risks of noncardiovascular death.[17]

had, on average, earlier onset of CVD and shorter overall survival across the life course. A new and important finding was that current smoking was associated with a fatal event as the first manifestation of clinical CVD. Thus, smoking cessation efforts at individual and wider population levels should inform the increased risk of cardiovascular disease across the lifetime and particularly stress the higher risk of cardiovascular death as the first presentation among those who smoke.[17]

Agbaje[18] in a large study of healthy children (n = 1,931) followed for 14 years showed a large increase in smoking rates from 2% at age 13 to 24% by age 17. This early smoking was linked to a 33–52% increased risk of premature heart damage. By age 24, 8% had developed left ventricular hypertrophy (LVH) and 17% had left ventricular diastolic dysfunction.[18] This study highlighted the serious and potentially irreversible consequences of early smoking on young people's cardiovascular health.

VIRTUALLY EVERY ORGAN IN SMOKERS ARE AFFECTED NONSMOKERS SUFFER CONSEQUENCES OF SECONDHAND SMOKE

All forms of tobacco use are unhealthy and there is no safe level of exposure. Cigarette smoking is the most common form of combustible tobacco use. Other forms include pipe, waterpipe tobacco, cigars, cigarillos, tobacco, roll-your-own, and bidis. Combustible tobacco products produce mainstream smoke inhaled and exhaled by the smoker and sidestream smoke from the burning end of the cigarette. Among >7,000 chemicals in cigarette smoke, many components are known to mediate the pathophysiology of CVD.[19] Chemicals such as carbon monoxide, polycyclic aromatic hydrocarbons (PAHs), nicotine, and heavy metals, and their oxides have toxic effects on vascular endothelium, blood lipids, and clotting factors and promote atherosclerosis (plaque buildup) in the arteries.

Secondhand smoke (environmental smoke, passive smoking) from sidestream smoke and exhaled smoke poses a serious health threat, increasing the risk of heart attacks, stroke, and other cardiovascular diseases by 25–30% in nonsmokers.[20] Secondhand smoke (SHS) induces oxidative stress and promotes vascular inflammation. Apart from vasoconstriction and thrombus formation, the myocardial oxygen balance is further impaired by SHS-induced adrenergic stimulation and autonomic dysfunction.[21] SHS tragically causes an estimated 1.3 million CVD deaths globally. Given the dangers of SHS, healthcare providers must routinely inquire about patients' exposure and advise them on avoidance strategies. While smoke-free policies have reduced SHS exposure in public spaces, homes remain a primary source, particularly for children, underscoring the need for ongoing education and awareness.[22-24]

Widespread Harmful Effects

Tobacco smoking adversely affects nearly every organ and every system in the body. Respiratory, cardiac, vascular, gastrointestinal, genitourinary lungs, heart, blood vessels, and others. Besides lung cancer, smoking is a risk factor for oral cancer, esophageal cancer, pancreatic cancer, bladder cancer, and cervical cancer. It is the most important risk factor for chronic obstructive pulmonary disease (COPD) that includes chronic bronchitis, emphysema, and asthma. Smoking increases the risk for pregnancy complications (miscarriage, stillbirth) and risks for fetuses and infants (birth defects, low birth weight, and sudden infant death syndrome).[1]

TOBACCO SMOKING AND CARDIOVASCULAR DISEASES

Smoking is an independent predictor of all-cause and cardiovascular mortality in general and in particular in older adults. Pooled data on >500,000 persons older than age 60 years) from 25 cohort studies indicate more than a doubling of risk for current smokers and a 37% increased risk for former smokers compared with never-smokers.[25]

Tobacco smoking associated CVDs are:

- Coronary artery disease also called coronary heart disease ("heart disease," in this book), is by far the leading cause of mortality and morbidity among all CVDs. The clinical manifestations of CAD (e.g., angina pectoris, myocardial infarction) are described in Chapter 2.
- Cerebrovascular disease (Chapter 12)
- Heart failure (Chapter 12). Meta-analysis of seven studies, based on 42,759 participants and 4,826 heart failure cases, revealed that current smokers had a greater risk of heart failure incidence compared with nonsmokers (never or former smokers) (HR = 1.609, 95% CI, 1.470–1.761). Additionally, former smokers had a greater risk of heart failure incidence compared with never smokers (HR = 1.209, 95% CI, 1.084–1.348).[26]
- Kidney disease (Chapter 12)
- Atrial fibrillation (Chapter 12) and other arrhythmias
- Aortic disease—including aneurysms that may enlarge over time and possibly rupture.
- Peripheral arterial disease—intermittent claudication (pain on walking) limits mobility and could possibly lead to gangrene. Tobacco smoking, the major risk factor for thromboangiitis obliterans

(Buerger's disease), is a rare inflammatory condition primarily affecting the small and medium-sized arteries and veins in the extremities, is tobacco smoking. Younger men are predisposed to this disease and Indians may also be predisposed.
- Impotence—may result from internal pudendal and penile atherosclerosis.

PATHOGENETIC MECHANISMS

How does tobacco smoke cause and promote atherosclerosis? The multifront processes involved are complex and interconnected.[27] Among the numerous components of tobacco smoke are nicotine, carbon monoxide (CO), several oxidant gases, and other toxic chemicals. Nicotine causes sympathetic stimulation, increased myocardial oxygen demand coronary vasoconstriction, and decreased oxygen supply that lead to myocardial ischemia while CO decreases oxygen supply to the myocardium. Oxidant gases and other toxic chemicals activate platelets and prothrombotic factors and endogenous activation of free radicals with increased oxidative stress and reduced nitric oxide (a vasodilator). The confluence of inflammation from increased cytokines, endothelial dysfunction, prothrombotic state, and insulin resistance leads to plaque formation and progression of coronary atherosclerosis.[27]

TOBACCO USE IN INDIA: HEARTENING TRENDS BUT CHALLENGES REMAIN

India has achieved remarkable progress in reducing tobacco use, as the number of smokers have decreased markedly from 250 to 120 million as per surveys over 20 years **(Fig. 3)**. This progress is substantially from India's commitment to the World Health Organization (WHO) Framework Convention on Tobacco Control (FCTC) treaty that came into force in 2005. Smoke-free laws and increased tobacco taxation are proving to be powerful tools in preventing future cardiovascular deaths in India.[28] However,

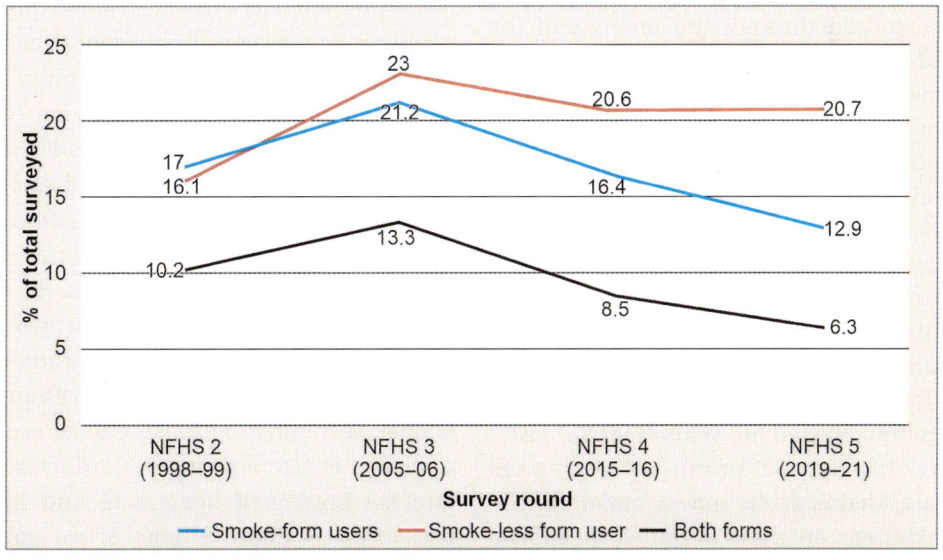

Fig. 3: Trend of tobacco use among males across different rounds of National Family Health Surveys (NFHS 2, NFHS 5).[29]

the use of smokeless tobacco (ST) continues to be a major challenge as while smoking in Indian men declined, ST use has not **(Fig. 3)**.

Bidi use is a serious health issue in India and other countries in South Asia as about one-half of the tobacco smokers in India are bidi smokers. These hand-rolled products of tobacco are wrapped in tendu leaf (*Diospyros melanoxylon*) and are less expensive. In economically disadvantaged parts of the country, it is more commonly used and is rooted in cultural patterns. It is a common misconception that as bidis are smaller and less expensive than cigarettes, they are also less harmful. Bidis are as harmful as cigarettes and can cause death from lung and heart disease.[30] Bidi smoking is linked to severe respiratory impairment, increased mortality risk, and adverse cardiorespiratory outcomes.[30-34]

Smokeless tobacco use is a global health threat, with over 300 million users who are predominantly Asians (South and Southeast). ST products—various forms of chewing tobacco, snuff, snus, and others—are absorbed through the mucosa of the mouth or nose. They contain a large array of chemicals, including nicotine, nitrosamines, nitrosamine acids, PAHs, aldehydes, and metals. Cancers linked to the use of ST use include that of head and neck (mouth, tongue, cheek, and gums), esophagus, and pancreas.[2]

Geographically, over 85% of the ST-related disease burden is concentrated in South and Southeast Asia, with India accounting for a substantial 70%, followed by Pakistan (7%) and Bangladesh (5%) in terms of deaths and disability-adjusted life years (DALYs) lost.[35] Many different ST products—pan, paan masala, khaini, sarda, mawa, gutka, mishri, gudakhu, etc., are chewed, snuffed, or applied to the teeth and gums. The more commonly used ones by Indians contain tobacco-lime mixture, tobacco, lime, areca nut mixture, and tobacco with betel quid. Bharathi and colleagues used data from the Longitudinal Aging Study in India (LASI) wave 1, a nationally representative cross-sectional study collected in 2017–2018, to analyze the use and demographic characteristics of current and previous users of smokeless tobacco.[36] The type of occupation, type of employer, place of work, kind of business, and workload were found to be significantly associated with ST use. Similarly, education and occupation were found to be important predictors of ST use in another study from India.[37] These studies provide valuable information for governmental control policies and treatment plans to target the population at high risk.

Electronic cigarette (e-cigarette) use has increased in teenagers and young adults. This electronic delivery system heats a liquid (types include with nicotine and without nicotine and various additives, flavors, and chemicals) to form aerosols. It was promoted as a harmless aid in quitting smoking of conventional cigarettes and those promotions were questioned and subjected to scrutiny.[38] It has also fallen short as a smoking cessation aid and in some persons may even have increased smoking (dual smoking) or served as a gateway to cigarette use. E-cigarette associated lung injury (EVALI) has been reported in the US.[39] E-cigarette emissions contain varying amounts of nicotine, that is highly addictive and long-term effects of all additives are not known. Secondhand exposure to aerosols to nonusers is also a concern. Cardiovascular effects—increased heart rate and blood pressure—as acute effects of e-cigarette smoking have been reported. So far, there have been no large-scale studies that link e-cigarette use to heart attacks. E-cigarettes are aggressively promoted to appeal to children and teenagers, with sleek designs and thousands of flavors. They are sold in open markets in many countries that have no minimum age requirement or no regulations at all.

Economic Impact

A press release from the Ministry of Commerce and Industry of India, posted on January 1, 2025, cites the large contribution of tobacco exports and production. During 2023–2024, the value of Indian tobacco exports reached a record high INR 12,005.89 crore, an export growth of 87% over the previous 5 years. Tobacco farmers' income doubled over the last 5 years. India is the second largest producer of tobacco in the world after China is the second largest exporter after Brazil. In India, tobacco is cultivated on 0.45 million hectares, accounting for 0.27% of the net cultivated area, and yields approximately 750 million kilograms of tobacco leaf.

This large contribution to the national economy should be viewed in light of the costs of human lives and disability. In 2017, an estimated 267 million Indians above 15 years of age used tobacco products (smoking or smokeless). This widespread use exacts a devastating toll, resulting in approximately 3,500 tobacco-related deaths daily. The economic burden of tobacco-related healthcare and lost productivity is immense, estimated at INR 1,773 billion (US $ 22.17 billion).[40]

■ CONTROL MEASURES

A 2024 study, in collaboration with the WHO, offered a compelling case for prioritizing tobacco control measures in India. By implementing a 10% reduction in tobacco consumption through a targeted increase in tobacco taxes (11% for bidis, 29% for cigarettes, and 30% for ST), the study projected that 3.08 million tobacco-related deaths could be averted from 2021 to 2026, and that 1.36 million new jobs could be created over those 5 years resulting in a net 0.22% increase in the GDP.[40]

Effective tobacco control requires a comprehensive strategy. Smokers need accessible cessation programs with strong support from healthcare providers with availability of multiple channels, personalized counseling, and medication support (nicotine replacement therapy).

The cardiovascular benefits of quitting smoking should be a central message to every smoker. Within 2 years after quitting smoking, the risk of heart attack drops sharply. The risk is reduced by half 5–10 years after quitting, and 15 years after quitting the risk of CAD drops to near the level of a nonsmoker.[41]

On a global scale, the WHO introduced the MPOWER package in 2008, as a set of six evidence-based policy interventions, to help countries [182 countries have ratified the Framework Convention on Tobacco Control (FCTC) treaty as of December 2024] meet their obligations to reduce tobacco use.[42]

The acronym MPOWER stands for:
- *M*onitor tobacco use and prevention policies
- *P*rotect people from exposure to tobacco smoke
- *O*ffer help to quit tobacco use
- *W*arn about the dangers of tobacco
- *E*nforce bans on tobacco advertising, promotion, and sponsorship
- *R*aise taxes on tobacco products

The 2024 Global Burden of Disease (GBD) study projected that, if current smoking trends continue, an estimated 2,040 million years of life would be lost to smoking between 2022 and 2050 (83% of them in men).[1] In contrast, if tobacco use is eliminated by 2050, the outlook would be dramatically different with far fewer years of life lost and an increase in life expectancy reaching 77.6 years for men and 81.0 years for women by 2050.[1,43-48] However, to eliminate tobacco use is not an easy task because of the strong opponents to the WHO recommended policies. Most formidable of the opponents is the tobacco industry that has a history of using front groups, influencing politicians, and other tactics. They have enormous financial resources and their goal of maximizing profits through sales and business expansion is directly in conflict with public health goals. To counter the power and influence of tobacco companies, more resources, educational initiatives, strong support from healthcare providers, informed public, professional and advocacy organizations, and innovative strategies are needed.[49]

■ KEY TAKEAWAYS

- Tobacco smoking is the leading cause of preventable death in the world killing over 8 million people each year. More than 7 million deaths are the result of direct tobacco use while around 1.2 million are the result of nonsmokers being exposed to secondhand smoke.
- Morbidity and mortality are disproportionately more on men and on people who are socioeconomically disadvantaged.
- Smoking rates have fallen globally and in the US the rate of 11% tied the all-time low in 2024, coinciding with the historic warning, 60 years earlier, by the Surgeon General on the adverse health effects of smoking.
- The pioneering British Doctors Study and other seminal studies (Nurses' Health Study, Framingham Heart Study, INTERHEART, PURE study, etc.) unequivocally linked smoking with heart disease, heart attacks, and deaths. Cessation of smoking markedly reduced adverse outcomes.
- Nearly every organ and every system in the body, respiratory, cardiac, vascular, gastrointestinal, genitourinary lungs, heart, blood vessels, and others are adversely affected by tobacco smoking.
- Smoking increases the risk for coronary artery disease, cerebrovascular disease, peripheral arterial disease, aortic disease, heart failure, etc.
- India's progress in curbing tobacco smoking has been commendable, as the number of smokers have more than halved over 20 years. This progress is substantially from India's commitment to the WHO FCTC treaty that came into force in 2005.
- In contrast to tobacco smoking, ST use has not decreased. Control measures require interventions targeted to high-risk populations.
- Effective tobacco control programs for smokers require committed healthcare providers, councilors, good communication channels, and medication support (nicotine replacement therapy).
- The MPOWER package introduced by the WHO is a set of six evidence-based policy interventions to help countries meet their obligations to reduce tobacco use. Notably, 182 countries have ratified the FCTC treaty as of December 2024.
- The goal to eliminate tobacco use by the year 2050 is laudable as it will markedly reduce years of lives lost, especially in men, and increase life expectancy in both genders. However, this is not easy as governments and people will have to balance the loss of revenue from tobacco farming and exports and successfully combat the money, power, and influence of tobacco companies and other vested interests.

■ REFERENCES

1. G.B.D Tobacco Forecasting Collaborators. Forecasting the effects of smoking prevalence scenarios on years of life lost and life expectancy from 2022 to 2050: a systematic analysis for the Global Burden of Disease Study 2021. Lancet Public Health. 2024;9(10):e729-44.
2. World Health Organization. (2025). Global report on trends in tobacco use; key facts: 2000-2025, 3rd edition. [online] Available

from https://www.who.int/publications/i/item/who-global-report-on-trends-in-prevalence-of-tobacco-use-2000-2025-third-edition [Last accessed May, 2025].
3. Jones JM. (2024). Consumption habits: Cigarette smoking rates in the U.S ties 80-year low; results from the Gallop Poll. [online] Available from https://news.gallup.com/poll/648521/cigarette-smoking-rate-ties-year-low.aspx [Last accessed May, 2025].
4. Report USG. Smoking and Health: Report of the Advisory Committee of the Surgeon General of the Public Health Service. Washington, DC: Public Health Service Publication No. 1103; 1964.
5. Doll R, Hill AB. Smoking and carcinoma of the lung; preliminary report. Br Med J. 1950;2(4682):739-48.
6. Wynder EL, Graham EA. Tobacco smoking as a possible etiologic factor in bronchogenic carcinoma; a study of 684 proved cases. J Am Med Assoc. 1950;143(4):329-36.
7. Doll R, Hill AB. The mortality of doctors in relation to their smoking habits; a preliminary report. Br Med J. 1954;1(4877):1451-5.
8. Doll R, Hill AB. Mortality in relation to smoking: Ten years' observations of British doctors. Br Med J. 1964;1(5396):1460-7 CONCL.
9. Doll R, Peto R. Mortality in relation to smoking: 20 years' observations on male British doctors. Br Med J. 1976;2(6051):1525-36.
10. Doll R, Peto R, Hall E, Wheatley K, Gray R. Mortality in relation to consumption of alcohol: 13 years' observations on male British doctors. BMJ. 1994;309(6959):911-8.
11. Doll R, Peto R, Boreham J, Sutherland I. Mortality in relation to smoking: 50 years' observations on male British doctors. BMJ. 2004;328(7455):1519.
12. Di Cicco ME, Ragazzo V, Jacinto T. Mortality in relation to smoking: the British Doctors Study. Breathe (Sheff). 2016;12(3):275-6.
13. Sarna L, Bialous SA, Jun HJ, Wewers ME, Cooley ME, Feskanich D. Smoking trends in the Nurses' Health Study (1976-2003). Nurs Res. 2008;57(6):374-82.
14. Grundy SM, Balady G, Criqui M, Fletcher G, Greenland P, Hiratzka LF, et al. Primary prevention of coronary heart disease: guidance from Framingham: A statement for healthcare professionals from the AHA Task Force on Risk Reduction. American Heart Association. Circulation. 1998;97(18):1876-87.
15. Yusuf S, Hawken S, Ounpuu S, Dans T, Avezum A, Lanas F, et al. Effect of potentially modifiable risk factors associated with myocardial infarction in 52 countries (the INTERHEART study): case-control study. Lancet. 2004;364(9438):937-52.
16. Yusuf S, Joseph P, Rangarajan S, Islam S, Mente A, Hystad P, et al. Modifiable risk factors, cardiovascular disease, and mortality in 155 722 individuals from 21 high-income, middle-income, and low-income countries (PURE): a prospective cohort study. Lancet. 2020;395(10226):795-808.
17. Khan SS, Ning H, Sinha A, Wilkins J, Allen NB, Vu THT, et al. Cigarette smoking and competing risks for fatal and nonfatal cardiovascular disease subtypes across the life course. J Am Heart Assoc. 2021;10(23): e021751.
18. Agbaje AO. Incidental and progressive tobacco smoking in childhood and subsequent risk of premature cardiac damage. J Am Coll Cardiol. 2025;85(5):546-9.
19. Borgerding M, Klus H. Analysis of complex mixtures--cigarette smoke. Exp Toxicol Pathol. 2005;57(Suppl 1):43-73.
20. Fischer F, Kraemer A. Meta-analysis of the association between second-hand smoke exposure and ischaemic heart diseases, COPD and stroke. BMC Public Health. 2015; 15:1202.
21. Raupach T, Schafer K, Konstantinides S, Andreas S. Secondhand smoke as an acute threat for the cardiovascular system: a change in paradigm. Eur Heart J. 2006;27(4):386-92.
22. US Surgeon General' report. (2024). Eliminating Tobacco-Related Disease and Death. [online] Available from https://www.hhs.gov/sites/default/files/2024-sgr-tobacco-related-health-disparities-exec-summary.pdf [Last accessed may, 2025].

23. Barnoya J, Glantz SA. Cardiovascular effects of secondhand smoke: nearly as large as smoking. Circulation. 2005;111(20):2684-98.
24. Barua RS, Ambrose JA. Mechanisms of coronary thrombosis in cigarette smoke exposure. Arterioscler Thromb Vasc Biol. 2013;33(7):1460-7.
25. Mons U, Muezzinler A, Gellert C, Schöttker B, Abnet CC, Bobak M, et al. Impact of smoking and smoking cessation on cardiovascular events and mortality among older adults: meta-analysis of individual participant data from prospective cohort studies of the CHANCES consortium. BMJ. 2015;350:h1551.
26. Lee H, Son YJ. Influence of smoking status on risk of incident heart failure: a systematic review and meta-analysis of prospective cohort studies. Int J Environ Res Public Health. 2019;16(15):2697.
27. Roy A, Rawal I, Jabbour S, Prabhakaran D. Tobacco and cardiovascular disease: a summary of evidence. In: Prabhakaran D AS, Anand S, Gaziano TA, Mbanya JC, Wu Y, Nugent R (Eds). Cardiovascular, Respiratory, and Related Disorders, 3rd edition. Washington (DC): The International Bank for Reconstruction and Development/The World Bank; 2024.
28. Basu S, Glantz S, Bitton A, Millett C. The effect of tobacco control measures during a period of rising cardiovascular disease risk in India: a mathematical model of myocardial infarction and stroke. PLoS Med. 2013;10(7):e1001480.
29. Gupta S, Mal P, Bhadra D, Rajaa S, Goel S. Trend and determinants of tobacco use among Indian males over a 22-year period (1998-2021) using nationally representative data. PLoS One. 2024;19(10):e0308748.
30. Duong M, Rangarajan S, Zhang X, Killian K, Mony P, Swaminathan S, et al. Effects of bidi smoking on all-cause mortality and cardiorespiratory outcomes in men from south Asia: an observational community-based substudy of the Prospective Urban Rural Epidemiology Study (PURE). Lancet Glob Health. 2017;5(2):e168-76.
31. Rahman M, Fukui T. Bidi smoking and health. Public Health. 2000;114(2):123-7.
32. Suliankatchi Abdulkader R, Sinha DN, Jeyashree K, Rath R, Gupta PC, Kannan S, et al. Trends in tobacco consumption in India 1987-2016: impact of the World Health Organization Framework Convention on Tobacco Control. Int J Public Health. 2019;64(6):841-51.
33. Prasad DS, Kabir Z, Dash AK, Das BC. Smoking and cardiovascular health: a review of the epidemiology, pathogenesis, prevention and control of tobacco. Indian J Med Sci. 2009;63(11):520-33.
34. Mishra S, Joseph RA, Gupta PC, Pezzack B, Ram F, Sinha DN, et al. Trends in bidi and cigarette smoking in India from 1998 to 2015, by age, gender, and education. BMJ Glob Health. 2016;1(1):e000005.
35. Bhat SK. The cost of medicine. Ann Intern Med. 2003;139(1):74-5.
36. Bharathi B, Sahu KS, Pati S. Prevalence of smokeless tobacco use in India and its association with various occupations: A LASI study. Front Public Health. 2023;11:1005103.
37. Rawat R, Gouda J, Shekhar C. Smokeless tobacco use among adult males in India and selected states: assessment of education and occupation linkages. J Hum Behav Soc Environ. 2016;26:236-46.
38. Varkey B. Electronic cigarettes: the good, the bad and the unknown. Curr Opin Pulm Med. 2014;20(2):125-6.
39. Varkey B, Joshi M, Bartter T. Editorial: acute respiratory illness caused by vaping. Curr Opin Pulm Med. 2020;26(2):116-8.
40. John RM, Dauchy E. Trends in affordability of tobacco products before and after the transition to GST in India. Tob Control. 2021; 30(2):155-9.
41. US Surgeon General's Report. Smoking Cessation: US Surgeon General' report. U.S. Department of Health and Human Services. Atlanta, GA: U.S. Department of Health and Human Services, Centers for Disease Control and Prevention, National Center for Chronic Disease Prevention and Health Promotion, Office on Smoking and Health; 2020.
42. Yach D. WHO Framework Convention on Tobacco Control. Lancet. 2003;361(9357): 611-2.

43. GBD 2015. Tobacco Collaborators. Smoking prevalence and attributable disease burden in 195 countries and territories, 1990-2015: a systematic analysis from the Global Burden of Disease Study 2015. Lancet. 2017;389(10082):1885-906.
44. Collaborators GBDCoD. Global, regional, and national age-sex specific mortality for 264 causes of death, 1980-2016: a systematic analysis for the Global Burden of Disease Study 2016. Lancet. 2017;390(10100):1151-210.
45. Collaborators GBDM. Global, regional, and national age-sex-specific mortality and life expectancy, 1950-2017: a systematic analysis for the Global Burden of Disease Study 2017. Lancet. 2018;392(10159):1684-735.
46. Koh HK, Fiore MC. The Tobacco Industry and Harm Reduction. JAMA. 2022;328(20):2009-2010.
47. Siddiqi K, Husain S, Vidyasagaran A, Readshaw A, Mishu MP, Sheikh A. Global burden of disease due to smokeless tobacco consumption in adults: an updated analysis of data from 127 countries. BMC Med. 2020;18(1):222.
48. G. B. D. Risk Factors Collaborators. Global burden and strength of evidence for 88 risk factors in 204 countries and 811 subnational locations, 1990-2021: a systematic analysis for the Global Burden of Disease Study 2021. Lancet. 2024;403(10440):2162-203.
49. Schroeder SA, Koh HK. Tobacco control 50 years after the 1964 surgeon general's report. JAMA. 2014;311(2):141-3.

CHAPTER 5

Hypertension

■ INTRODUCTION

Hypertension (high blood pressure) is a pervasive global health threat that is often silent and often goes undetected. Despite causing nearly 8 million deaths annually from its complications such as cardiovascular diseases (CVDs) and kidney failure, hypertension is undiagnosed or inadequately controlled, more so in low- and middle-income countries (LMICs). Globally, fewer than one in four women and one in five men with hypertension achieve controlled levels.[1,2]

■ HISTORICAL ASPECTS

The invention of the cuff-based sphygmomanometer (Riva-Rocci, 1896) and Korotkoff's work on sounds during deflation (1905) enabled accurate blood pressure (BP) measurement. However, before World War II, and continuing on to the late 1940s, antihypertensive treatment modalities (among them thiocyanates, barbiturates, bismuth, and bromides) were ineffective or radical (pyrogen injections, sympathectomy, adrenalectomy, medical and surgical interventions). A large study by the Society of Actuaries (1934–1954) on the link between body build (height/weight), BP, and mortality rates found an association between hypertension and stroke and increased mortality rate.[1] However, this was not accepted and in fact was resisted by healthcare professionals[3,4] led by physician leaders like Paul Dudley White in the 1950s and Charles Friedberg (the author of the first textbook of cardiology in the US) in the 60s. The former, generally considered the father of Cardiology, stated "Hypertension may be an important compensatory mechanism which should not be tampered with, even where it is certain that we could control it." In 1950, the first edition of Harrison's Principles of Internal Medicine, reflected the prevalent belief that hypertension was not a disease and stated, "Those with chest pain or other overt signs of disease should have their hypertension treated; others should not."[4] In the 60s, during our medical student days in Kerala, the term "benign essential hypertension" was used for a condition, we now know is, neither benign nor essential.

Lesson from History

President Franklin D. Roosevelt's medical records are prototypical for the natural (i.e., untreated) history of hypertension. His BP readings were 162/98 mm Hg in 1937, 180/88 mm Hg in 1940, 188/105 mm Hg in 1941 (prescribed phenobarbital and massages). In March 1944, he was diagnosed with congestive heart failure and was treated with digitalis and low-salt rice diet and fruit juices. In 1944, he suffered "CV accidents" and in November, at the time of his reelection, his BP was 200/100 mm Hg. A few months later, before the historic Yalta Conference in February 1945, his BP was 260/150 mm Hg.[4] At the Yalta negotiations, Churchill's physician observed that the President appeared very ill. Did hypertension and CVD affect his thinking and decisions at the Yalta conference (potentially affecting the postwar political landscape)? A couple of months later, on April 12, 1945, at the age of 63, Roosevelt experienced a severe headache, lost consciousness (BP >300/190 mm Hg) and died of cerebral hemorrhage. It took time to recognize the devastating consequences of hypertension and the importance of controlling it. Slowly but surely, progress was made over the following decades.[4]

■ EVOLUTION OF THE DEFINITION

How to Define Hypertension?

The National High Blood Pressure Education Program (NHBPEP) launched in 1972, which later became the Joint National Committee (JNC), was instrumental in shaping our understanding of hypertension and how to manage it.[5] JNC's reports (1–7) between 1977 and 2008, provided evidence-based recommendations for diagnosis, guideline-directed medical therapy (GDMT), and prevention of hypertension. Notably, JNC 1 classified below 160/90 mm Hg as "normal" BP and this definition was accepted then by the World Health Organization (WHO) and most countries in the world. By extension a BP reading of 160/90 mm Hg and above was hypertension. Over the passage of time and cumulative evidence-based data the definition has progressively evolved.[6] The JNC's eventual successors, the American College of Cardiology (ACC) and American Heart Association (AHA) in 2017, classified 130/80 mm Hg and above as hypertension **(Table 1)** and categorized the stages of hypertension.[1]

TABLE 1: Classification of blood pressure (BP).

BP category	SBP	DBP
Normal	<120 mm Hg	and <80 mm Hg
Elevated	120–129 mm Hg	and <80 mm Hg
Hypertension		
Stage 1	130–139 mm Hg	or 80–89 mm Hg
Stage 2	≥140 mm Hg	or ≥90 mm Hg

Note: Individuals with systolic blood pressure (SBP) and diastolic blood pressure (DBP) in two categories should be designated to the higher BP category. BP reading used to classify is based on an average of ≥2 readings on ≥2 occasions.

The latest 2017 ACC/AHA guidelines have redefined normal BP as systolic blood pressure (SBP) <120 mm Hg and diastolic blood pressure (DBP) <80 mm Hg. Importantly, the guidelines made no adjustments for age even though it is known that the prevalence of hypertension increases with advancing age. For men the increase is threefold (from 28 to 80%) and sixfold in women (from 15 to 81%).[7] While BP under 120/80 mm Hg is normal per guidelines, research suggests that a Theoretical Minimum Risk Exposure Level (TMREL) that is SBP below 115 mm Hg could further reduce complications and mortality.[2,8]

■ ADVERSE HEALTH EFFECTS OF HYPERTENSION

Cardiovascular disease (CVD) encompasses cerebrovascular disease (leading to stroke), coronary artery disease (CAD and heart attack), and other disorders and is the leading cause of death and disability worldwide. An estimated 17.9 million people died from CVDs in 2019, representing 32% of all global deaths. Of these deaths, 85% were due to heart attack and stroke and most of these were in LMICs. Numerous studies have shown a graded association of hypertension and CVD—the higher the BP, the higher the risk of CVD.

A meta-analysis of 61 studies found a doubling in the risk of death from stroke, heart disease, or vascular disease with every 20 mm Hg increase in SBP or 10 mm Hg increase in DBP.[1] The increased CVD risk was observed across a broad age spectrum, from 30 years to >80 years of age.

Although the relative risk of CVD associated with higher SBP and DBP is smaller at older ages, the corresponding high BP-related increase in absolute risk is larger in older persons (>65 years) given the higher absolute risk of CVD at an older age.[1] Higher SBP has consistently been associated with increased CVD risk after adjustment for, or within strata of, DBP. In contrast, after consideration of SBP through adjustment or stratification, DBP has not been consistently associated with CVD risk. Patients with hypertension should be well informed on its long-term complications (particularly cardiovascular and renal systems) and be monitored, advised, and treated by a physician. Comorbid conditions and interlinked conditions such as diabetes, obesity, tobacco smoking, and high cholesterol commonly combine to create a potent mix that increases the risk of stroke and a heart attack.[1] In the Prospective Urban Rural Evaluation (PURE) study of all the risk factors for CVD, hypertension had the highest population attributable fraction (PAF), both globally (22.3%) and in India (14.3%)[9,10] (Chapter 3, **Figure 2**).

- Stroke is caused by bleeding (cerebral hemorrhage) or by a thrombus (ischemic). Elevated BP is common during acute ischemic stroke, occurring in up to 80% of the patients. BP often decreases spontaneously during the acute phase of ischemic stroke, as soon as 90 minutes after the onset of symptoms.
- *Heart disease (CAD):* >50% of deaths from stroke and CAD occur in those with hypertension.[1] As elaborated in Chapter 3, hypertension is a major risk factor for CAD.
- *Heart failure (HF):* Antecedent hypertension is present in 75% of patients with chronic HF. The risk of HF increases twofold when SBP >140 mm Hg and threefold when SBP >160 mm Hg.

Kidney Disease

Hypertension is the most common comorbidity (67–92%) in patients with chronic kidney disease (CKD), and its prevalence increases as kidney function declines.[1] Hypertension may occur as a result of kidney disease, but it is important to know that hypertension may also accelerate further kidney injury. Therefore, treatment of hypertension is important to prevent further functional decline. In 2012, hypertension accounted for 34% of incident end-stage renal disease (ESRD) cases in the US population.[1]

GLOBAL IMPACT OF HYPERTENSION

The global prevalence of hypertension has alarmingly doubled since 1990, to reach 1.3 billion adults in 2019. Even using a higher value of 140/90 mm Hg to define hypertension than the recommended American guidelines (2018), nearly one-third of the global population (without distinction between high- and low-income countries) had hypertension. Effectively controlling BP, markedly reduces the risk of CVD, the world's leading cause of death. Furthermore, 38% of deaths linked to high BP occur in adults under 70, emphasizing the need to act early.[2]

However, as **Table 2** documents hypertension is diagnosed and treated in just over

TABLE 2: Age-standardized prevalence, treatment, and control of blood pressure in selected countries.[2]							
	India	China	Canada	France	UK	US	World
Diagnosis	37%	52%	78%	65%	59%	80%	54%
Treatment	30%	39%	71%	52%	48%	70%	52%
Control	15%	16%	61%	28%	30%	48%	Women 25%, Men 20%
Deaths averted from achieving 50% control rate by 2050	4.6 M	10.3 M	52,000	155,000	137,000	1.2 M	76 M

(M: million; UK: United Kingdom; US: United States)

one-half of those affected. Adequate control is achieved in only 15% and 16% of those with hypertension in India and China, respectively. This is tragic as 120 million strokes, 79 million heart attacks, and 17 million cases of heart failure could be averted between 2024 and 2050 by controlling BP.

India can avert 4.6 million deaths by 2050 by increasing the control rate of hypertension to 50% (WHO goal 2023). Considering the proven increased risk of CVD caused by hypertension and that over 80% of adults with high BP have a 10-year atherosclerotic cardiovascular disease (ASCVD) risk of >7.5% that meet the standards for statin therapy by 2018 US guidelines.[2] Statin treatment for those who meet the standards would be hugely beneficial in reducing their risk for a major adverse cardiac events (MACE).

In the US, hypertension affects 122 million adults, with higher rates in African Americans and Hispanic Americans compared to Whites. The presence of multiple CVD risk factors in individuals with hypertension results in high absolute risks for CAD and stroke. For example, among US adults with hypertension, 42% had a 10-year CVD risk >20%, 41% had a risk of 10–20%, and only 18.4% had a risk <10%.[1] This level of high risk among individuals with hypertension justifies the use of statin therapy for most people with hypertension.

Though the prevalence of severe hypertension has been declining in the US over time, it is still of serious concern as approximately 12.3% of US adults with hypertension have an average SBP >160 mm Hg or average DBP >100 mm Hg. The risk of developing hypertension increases with advancing age. In normotensive 45-year-old persons the 40-year risk of developing hypertension (using 140/90 mm Hg as the cutoff) is 86% for whites and 93% for African Americans.[1]

In India, hypertension is the most important CVD risk factor with 1.63 million deaths and 33.9 million disability-adjusted life years (DALYs, the sum of the years of life lost due to premature mortality and the years lived with disability) in 2016. A large cross-sectional study involving eight states in India showed that 46% had hypertension, 42% had prehypertension, and only 12% had normal BP **(Fig. 1)**.[11] Studies have also found high rates of hypertension in children and teens, 10–19 years of age.[12]

These results highlight the pressing need in India to develop a comprehensive plan for early detection, intervention, and management of hypertension to prevent end-organ damage, morbidity, and mortality.[13-16] A few specific points to emphasize are:

- *Do not wait for symptoms:* Detect early and initiate treatment as treatment

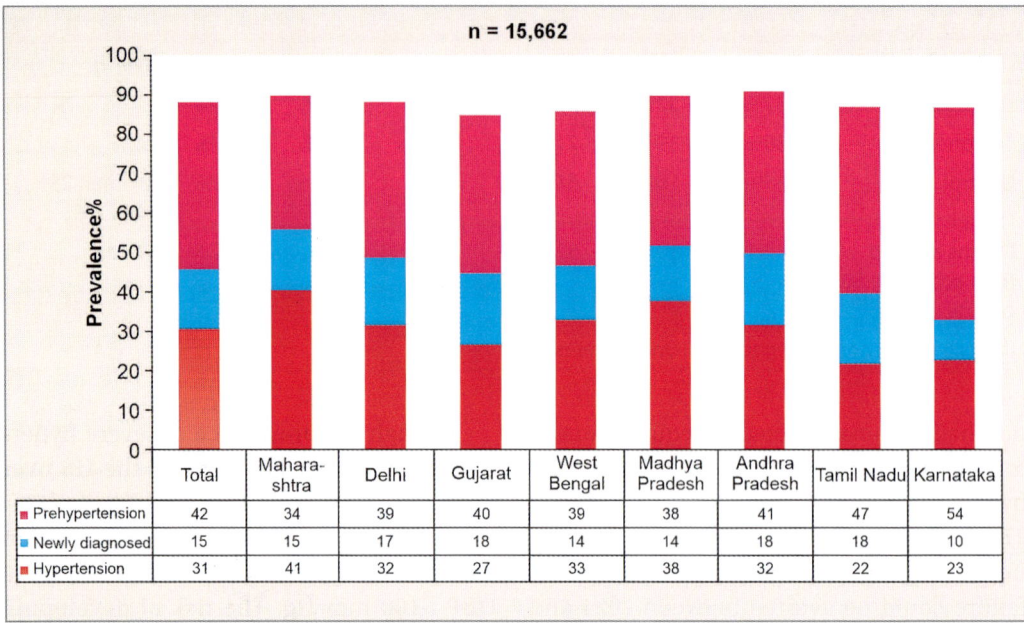

Fig. 1: Prevalence of known hypertension, newly detected hypertension, and prehypertension [systolic blood pressure (BP) 120–139 mm Hg or a diastolic BP 80–89 mm Hg] in India. Only 12% of Indian adults had BP <120/80 mm Hg).[11]

markedly reduces long-term health risks by preventing or minimizing end-organ damage.

- *Treatment is lifelong:* As hypertension is a chronic condition, do not expect a quick fix. Stopping medication after reaching the target BP, as may be practiced in India, is a common mistake. Adherence to prescribed medication(s), lifestyle changes and periodic monitoring are required. Hypertension requires ongoing management, including regular monitoring, medication adherence, and healthy lifestyle changes, and calls for a collaborative physician-patient relationship.[17]
- Hypertension is a silent threat to health and more so after a stroke. After a stroke, it is imperative to bring BP down to normal levels and to maintain it at normal range to curtail the damage and to reduce the risk for further strokes.[18]

DIAGNOSIS AND TREATMENT

Accurate ascertainment of BP as normal, hypertension stage 1 and 2 depends on proper measurement technique with a validated device. Issues related to BP measurements and instructions to ensure accurate readings are shown in **Table 3**.

A treatment plan for hypertension should be based on the stage of the disease as shown in **Table 1**.

Stage 1 Hypertension

A healthy lifestyle is the cornerstone of prevention and treating stage 1 hypertension **(Table 4)**. Antihypertensive medication needs to be considered if BP remains elevated or continues to rise.

TABLE 3: Strategies to ensure accuracy of blood pressure measurements.[1]	
Using oscillometric devices	These devices can automatically perform multiple BP measurements in one sitting; such devices have largely replaced manual auscultation
Using validated devices	Advisable to use devices certified by a third-party organization, like the Association for the Advancement of Medical Instrumentation (AAMI), e.g., Omron
Measure BP in a sitting position	When you measure your BP, you should be sitting on a comfortable chair with your back supported and your feet flat on the floor. Your arm should be at heart level
Measure BP at the same time each day	It is best to measure your BP at the same time each day, ideally first thing in the morning. This will help to ensure that your BP readings are consistent
Take multiple BP measurements	It is best to take two or three BP measurements in a row and average the results. This will help to reduce the chances of inaccurate reading
Avoid talking or moving during BP measurement	Talking or moving can affect your BP readings. It is important to stay still and quiet while your BP is being measured
Using the correct cuff size*	• The standard adult BP cuff is 30 cm long and 16 cm wide • The large adult is 36 cm long; the extra-large is 42 cm • The small adult is 22 cm long and 12 cm wide • The ideal cuff bladder length is ≥80% of patient's arm circumference • The ideal cuff width is ≥40% of patient's arm circumference

*The cuff size is crucial for accurate blood pressure readings. Ideally, the bladder should encircle at least 80% of the upper arm, with a width of 40% of the arm's circumference. Using an incorrect size significantly impacts readings. For instance, a small cuff on someone needing a regular size can inflate readings by 3 mm Hg, while a large cuff on someone requiring an extra-large one can cause a 10 mm Hg overestimation.

Restricting sodium (salt) in the diet is an essential part of hypertension control. Though the guideline recommends a daily intake of sodium not >2,300 mg, too many people far exceed that amount. In Western countries, processed foods are the main culprit, while in Asian countries it is often the heavy salting during cooking. Public health initiatives should target reducing sodium content in common foods such as breads, cereals, processed meats, and dairy.[19-22] Replacing table salt with a potassium-rich substitute can lower stroke risk, other major cardiovascular events, and even death rates. This is an affordable option for LMICs. However, people with kidney disease should consult with their doctor before using a potassium-rich substitute.[19,23,24]

Stage 2 Hypertension

Stage 2 hypertension requires a combined approach of lifestyle changes and medication(s) for effective BP control. Antihypertensive drugs have come a long way from rauwolfia and hydralazine to lifesaving hydrochlorothiazide in the 1950s, and then on to very effective medications such as angiotensin converting enzyme (ACE) inhibitors, angiotensin receptor blockers (ARBs), β-blockers, and calcium channel blockers. ARBs offer comparable BP control to ACE inhibitors but with less side effects (cough, leg swelling). Even seemingly resistant cases of hypertension can be managed with the right combination of medications. **Table 5** lists the approaches to achieve

TABLE 4: Diet and other lifestyle modifications in controlling hypertension.[1,25]

Vegetables	Load up on leafy greens and colorful veggies! Many vegetables such as spinach, broccoli, sweet potatoes, zucchini, cucumbers, mushrooms, and leafy greens are rich in potassium, magnesium, and nitrates, all nutrients that can help lower blood pressure (BP)
Beans and lentils	Beans and lentils are a powerhouse of potassium, a mineral that can help regulate BP
Lower-fat dairy products	Low-fat dairy such as milk, yogurt, and cheese are BP friendly. These foods offer calcium, potassium, and nutrients that can help keep your pressure in check
Nuts and seeds	Snack smart for heart health! Nuts and seeds such as almonds, walnuts, and pistachios are potassium powerhouses that can help control blood pressure. Choose unsalted varieties to maximize the benefits
Fish	Salmon, cod, tuna, halibut, and mackerel are all excellent choices for a blood pressure-lowering diet because they are packed with omega-3 fatty acids
Whole grains	Go whole for your heart! Whole grains such as wheat bread, brown rice, quinoa, and oats are rich in fiber, which can help lower blood pressure
Weight reduction	Lowers BP up to 5–20 mm Hg per 10 kg weight loss
Sodium restriction	Lowers BP 2–8 mm Hg
Physical activity	Lowers BP by 4–9 mm Hg
Moderation of alcohol	Alcoholic drinks (10–14 g of alcohol) increase SBP. Abstinence from alcohol can lower SBP up to 5 mm Hg among heavy alcohol users (four drinks per day)

TABLE 5: Optimizing blood pressure control in stage 2 hypertension.[1,26,27]

Initiating treatment	An inexpensive, once-daily generic medication (on top of a healthy lifestyle) with close monitoring of blood pressure (BP), can significantly improve medication adherence and achieve blood pressure control
Adding a new medication class	Adding medication from a different class is often better than increasing the dose of the current one. Delaying aggressive treatment raises health risks
Needing multiple classes of medications	While most hypertensive patients need multiple medications for optimal BP control, 40% of patients with uncontrolled BP receive less than two medications. This treatment gap, undertreatment, is a major missed opportunity to prevent serious complications
Poor BP control in India	Only 15% of persons with hypertension have controlled BP, with a significant urban-rural divide (20% vs. 10%). This falls far short of developed countries such as the US and Canada, where control rates reach 78–80%
Fixed dose combination (FDC) medications	Single-pills with fixed combinations of blood pressure medications (FDCs) are underused, even though they boost adherence and blood pressure control. This is particularly beneficial for those who struggle with taking multiple pills

BP control. Single pill with a fixed-dose combination of medications is easier for the patient and improves medication adherence.[26]

CONTROL OF HYPERTENSION PROGRESS IN WESTERN COUNTRIES, BUT LAGGING IN INDIA

We have come a long way from the 1940s in our understanding of hypertension, its deleterious effects, and the adverse outcomes of untreated hypertension that we can now unequivocally state that elevated BP is a major cardiovascular risk factor and that treating hypertension reduces morbidity and mortality of CVD. A recent large study confirms the power of treatment: A 20 mm Hg reduction in SBP resulted in significant reductions in the risk of stroke (52%), heart failure (52%), MACE (40%), CAD (32%), and CVD deaths (20%).[2,28]

The WHO's target of over 50% controlled hypertension rate globally remains a distant dream. Developed countries fare better than developing countries in this regard but social factors and economic factors continue to be barriers, especially in racial and ethnic minorities. In India, only 15% of hypertensive patients (10% in rural and 20% in urban areas) have controlled BP and this dismal figure with all its implications for morbidity and mortality[2,29] cries out for action on multiple fronts on the various contributors that include:[29]

- *Social determinants of health:* Poverty, limited healthcare access, and unhealthy lifestyles.
- *Clinical inertia:* Physician hesitancy to start or change medications and suboptimal treatment strategies.
- *Lack of national guidelines:* Inconsistent hypertension diagnosis and management.
- *Limited awareness:* Many with hypertension do not understand the risks of uncontrolled hypertension or the importance of adherence.
- *Medication affordability:* Treatment costs pose an imposing barrier for a sizable number of people.

A recent systematic review and meta-analysis of several studies from 2001 to 2020[30] confirmed poor control rates of hypertension in India. The pooled hypertension control rate was 17.5% [95% confidence interval (CI): 14.3–20.6%]—with a significant increase over the years, reaching 22.5% (95% CI: 16.9–28.0%) in 2016–2020. Subgroup analysis showed poorer control rates in males and rural populations than in females and urban populations. Although the control rate has improved over the decades, substantial differences were noted between regions (the southern states of Tamil Nadu and Kerala fared better than others).

Hypertension control is strongly influenced by healthcare system factors, patient factors such as lifestyle risk factors, and social determinants of health, and physician adherence to treatment guidelines. In a recent observational, cross-sectional, prospective prescription analysis of prescriptions for 4,723 newly diagnosed hypertension patients found that in 1,364 (29%), with a cardiovascular risk profile that would call for a dual medication, received only monotherapy.[31] Besides, for more focused research and actions to improve the current national program, India needs to develop and evaluate sustainable, community-based strategies and programs to improve detection and control of hypertension.[30]

KEY TAKEAWAYS

- Hypertension is a global healthcare crisis, doubling since 1990 to 1.3 billion cases (140/90 mm Hg) and causes millions of deaths annually (an estimated 1.6 million deaths in India alone).
- Uncontrolled hypertension causes CVD such as stroke, heart attack, and heart failure, etc. It is also a major cause of CKD and kidney failure.
- Only a quarter of women and even fewer men (20%) have their BP under control using the WHO criteria, and even lower by the 2017 ACC/AHA criteria. Thus, there is a critical gap in controlling this major health risk.
- Current guidelines define normal BP as systolic blood pressure (SBP) <120 mm Hg and diastolic blood pressure (DBP). Elevated BP is defined as (SBP) >120–129 mm Hg and DBP <80 mm Hg.
- Stage 1 hypertension is defined as SBP >130–139 mm Hg and DBP 80–89 mm Hg. Stage 1 hypertension can be treated with lifestyle modifications **(Table 4)** and monitored.
- Stage 2 hypertension is defined as SBP >140 mm Hg or DBP ≥90 mm Hg requiring anti-hypertensive medications on top of lifestyle modifications to bring it down to BP <130/80 mm Hg. Diuretics, ACE inhibitors/ARBs, β-blockers, and calcium channel blockers, are the mainstays of BP control. The strategy is to combine medications based on severity and concomitant disease (diabetes, CKD, heart failure, etc.) tailored to the patient.
- >80% of adults with high BP have a 10-year ASCVD risk of >10%, well above the 7.5% that meet the standards for statin therapy by 2018 US guidelines. Statin treatment for the large number of people who meet the standards would be hugely beneficial in reducing their risk for a MACE.
- Hypertension control rate is very suboptimal in India at 15%—rural 10% and urban 20%, well below the WHO goal of at least 50%. In comparison, Canada and the US have achieved BP control rates of >60%. A recent systematic review from India shows some degree of promise with an overall BP control rate of 22.5%. An estimated 4.6 million deaths by 2050 can be averted if India can meet the WHO goal of control of hypertension in 50% of those affected.

REFERENCES

1. Whelton PK, Carey RM, Aronow WS, Casey DE Jr, Collins KJ, Dennison Himmelfarb C, et al. 2017 ACC/AHA/AAPA/ABC/ACPM/AGS/APhA/ASH/ASPC/NMA/PCNA Guideline for the prevention, detection, evaluation, and management of high blood pressure in adults: A report of the American College of Cardiology/American Heart Association Task Force on Clinical Practice Guidelines. J Am Coll Cardiol. 2018;71(19):e127-e248.
2. World Health Organization. Global Report on Hypertension: the race against a silent Killer. Geneva, Switzerland: World Heart Federation; 2023.
3. Moser M. Historical perspectives on the management of hypertension. J Clin Hypertens (Greenwich). 2006;8(8 Suppl 2):15-20; quiz 39.
4. Moser M. Seven decades of progress. J Clin Hypertens (Greenwich). 2007;9(5):310-3.
5. Kotchen TA. Developing hypertension guidelines: an evolving process. Am J Hypertens. 2014;27(6):765-72.
6. Chobanian AV, Bakris GL, Black HR, Cushman WC, Green LA, Izzo JL Jr, et al. The Seventh Report of the Joint National Committee on prevention, detection, evaluation, and treatment of high blood pressure: the JNC 7 report. JAMA. 2003;289(19):2560-72.
7. Tsao CW, Aday AW, Almarzooq ZI, Anderson CAM, Arora P, Avery CL, et al. Heart disease and stroke statistics-2023 update: a report from the american heart association. Circulation. 2023;147(8):e93-e621.
8. Forouzanfar MH, Liu P, Roth GA, Ng M, Biryukov S, Marczak L, et al. Global burden of hypertension and systolic blood pressure of at least 110 to 115 mm Hg, 1990-2015. JAMA. 2017;317(2):165-82.
9. Yusuf S, Joseph P, Rangarajan S, Islam S, Mente A, Hystad P, et al. Modifiable risk factors, cardiovascular disease, and mortality in 155 722 individuals from 21 high-income, middle-income, and low-income countries (PURE): a prospective cohort study. Lancet. 2020;395(10226):795-808.

10. Sharma S, Gaur K, Gupta R. Trends in epidemiology of dyslipidemias in India. Indian Heart J. 2024;76(Suppl 1):S20-8.
11. Joshi SR, Saboo B, Vadivale M, Dani SI, Mithal A, Kaul U, et al. Prevalence of diagnosed and undiagnosed diabetes and hypertension in India-Results from the Screening India's Twin Epidemic (SITE) study. Diabetes Technol Ther. 2012;14(1):8-15.
12. Vasudevan A, Thomas T, Kurpad A, Sachdev HS. Prevalence of and factors associated with high blood pressure among adolescents in India. JAMA Netw Open. 2022; 5(10):e2239282.
13. Gupta R, Gupta VP, Prakash H, Agrawal A, Sharma KK, Deedwania PC. 25-Year trends in hypertension prevalence, awareness, treatment, and control in an Indian urban population: Jaipur Heart Watch. Indian Heart J. 2018;70(6):802-7.
14. Gupta R, Gaur K, CV SR. Emerging trends in hypertension epidemiology in India. J Hum Hypertens. 2019;33(8):575-87.
15. Joseph P, Kutty VR, Mohan V, Kumar R, Mony P, Vijayakumar K, et al. Cardiovascular disease, mortality, and their associations with modifiable risk factors in a multi-national South Asia cohort: a PURE substudy. Eur Heart J. 2022;43(30):2831-40.
16. Jose AP, Prabhakaran D. World Hypertension Day: Contemporary issues faced in India. Indian J Med Res. 2019;149(5):567-70.
17. Blood Pressure Lowering Treatment Trialists C. Pharmacological blood pressure lowering for primary and secondary prevention of cardiovascular disease across different levels of blood pressure: an individual participant-level data meta-analysis. Lancet. 2021; 397(10285):1625-36.
18. Lin Q, Ye T, Ye P, Borghi C, Cro S, Damasceno A, et al. Hypertension in stroke survivors and associations with national premature stroke mortality: data for 2.5 million participants from multinational screening campaigns. Lancet Glob Health. 2022;10(8):e1141-9.
19. Bhat S, Marklund M, Henry ME, Appel LJ, Croft KD, Neal B, et al. A systematic review of the sources of dietary salt around the world. Adv Nutr. 2020;11(3):677-86.
20. Mente A, O'Donnell M, Rangarajan S, Dagenais G, Lear S, McQueen M, et al. Associations of urinary sodium excretion with cardiovascular events in individuals with and without hypertension: a pooled analysis of data from four studies. Lancet. 2016;388(10043):465-75.
21. Aburto NJ, Hanson S, Gutierrez H, Hooper L, Elliott P, Cappuccio FP. Effect of increased potassium intake on cardiovascular risk factors and disease: systematic review and meta-analyses. BMJ. 2013;346:f1378.
22. Aburto NJ, Ziolkovska A, Hooper L, Elliott P, Cappuccio FP, Meerpohl JJ. Effect of lower sodium intake on health: systematic review and meta-analyses. BMJ. 2013;346:f1326.
23. Neal B, Wu Y, Feng X, Zhang R, Zhang Y, Shi J, et al. Effect of salt substitution on cardiovascular events and death. N Engl J Med. 2021;385(12):1067-77.
24. Marklund M, Singh G, Greer R, Cudhea F, Matsushita K, Micha R, et al. Estimated population wide benefits and risks in China of lowering sodium through potassium enriched salt substitution: modelling study. BMJ. 2020;369:m824.
25. World Health Organization. (1997). Tobacco or Health: First Global Status Report. [online] Available fromhttps://iris.who.int/handle/10665/41922 [Last accessed May, 2025].
26. Chen R, Suchard MA, Krumholz HM, Schuemie MJ, Shea S, Duke J, et al. Comparative First-Line Effectiveness and Safety of ACE (Angiotensin-Converting Enzyme) Inhibitors and Angiotensin Receptor Blockers: A Multinational Cohort Study. Hypertension. 2021;78(3):591-603.
27. The EMPA-KIDNEY Collaborative Group; Herrington WG, Staplin N, Wanner C, Green JB, Hauske SJ, Emberson JR, et al. Empagliflozin in patients with chronic kidney disease. N Engl J Med. 2023;388(2):117-27.
28. Blood Pressure Lowering Treatment Trialists C. Age-stratified and blood-pressure-stratified effects of blood-pressure-lowering pharmacotherapy for the prevention of cardiovascular disease and death: an individual

participant-level data meta-analysis. Lancet. 2021;398(10305):1053-64.
29. Collaboration NCDRF. Worldwide trends in hypertension prevalence and progress in treatment and control from 1990 to 2019: a pooled analysis of 1201 population-representative studies with 104 million participants. Lancet. 2021;398(10304):957-80.
30. Koya SF, Pilakkadavath Z, Chandran P, Wilson T, Kuriakose S, Akbar SK, et al. Hypertension control rate in India: systematic review and meta-analysis of population-level non-interventional studies, 2001-2022. Lancet Reg Health Southeast Asia. 2023;9:100113.
31. Alexander T, Hiremath JS, Swahney JPS, Chandra S, Jain P, Chandra P, et al. Identifying drug prescription in newly diagnosed hypertension patients in India. J Clin Hypertension. 2025;27:e14963.

CHAPTER 6

Diabetes Mellitus

INTRODUCTION

Diabetes mellitus (DM) is a heterogeneous metabolic disease, characterized by hyperglycemia (increased blood sugar level).[1] The most common type of DM is type 2 [type 2 diabetes (T2D)] and ~463 million adults aged 20–79 years worldwide are affected by it, which is projected to increase to 578 million people by 2030 across the world.[2] This increasing prevalence is largely related to economic development, urbanization, and change in life habits.

Hyperglycemia affects the structure and function of blood vessels (micro and macro) leading to multiple end-organ damage such as eyes (retinopathy), kidneys (nephropathy), and nerves (peripheral and autonomic neuropathy). The major cause of morbidity and mortality in patients with diabetes is cardiovascular diseases (CVDs) that include coronary artery disease (CAD), cerebrovascular disease, and peripheral artery disease (PAD) that cause heart attacks, heart failure, strokes, diabetic ischemic ulcers. Diabetic kidney disease (DKD) is a major complication of diabetes and almost invariably is associated with other CVDs.[1]

DIABETES IN INDIANS IN INDIA AND ABROAD

India is second only to China in the largest number of people with DM. This number is projected to increase 31% from 2019 to reach 101 million by 2030 **(Table 1)**, and disturbingly over one-half of these cases would remain undiagnosed.[3] The vulnerability to DM extends to Indian Americans (Asian Indians) whose risk of developing diabetes is nearly three times higher compared to the Whites and Chinese populations **(Fig. 1)**.[4] As visceral fat storage, even at normal weights is a suspect factor, international guidelines recommend earlier diabetes screening for Asian Americans (including Indians) at a body mass index (BMI) of 23.[5-8]

TABLE 1: Top five countries burdened by diabetes in 2019 and projected numbers for 2030 (International Diabetes Federation).[2]

Rank	Country	2019	2030
1	China	116.4 million	140.5 million
2	India	77.0 million	101.0 million
3	United States	31.0 million	34.4 million
4	Pakistan	19.4 million	26.2 million
5	Brazil	16.8 million	21.5 million

Epidemiological Insights

A recent large-scale study (ICMR-INDIAB) revealed the magnitude of diabetes in India, with over 11% of the population affected, exceeding 10% in most urban areas, and with a widely varying prevalence between states **(Fig. 2)**.[9]

Of greater concern is that 15% of Indians are prediabetic, harbinger of a surge in diabetes cases. This increase in diabetes,

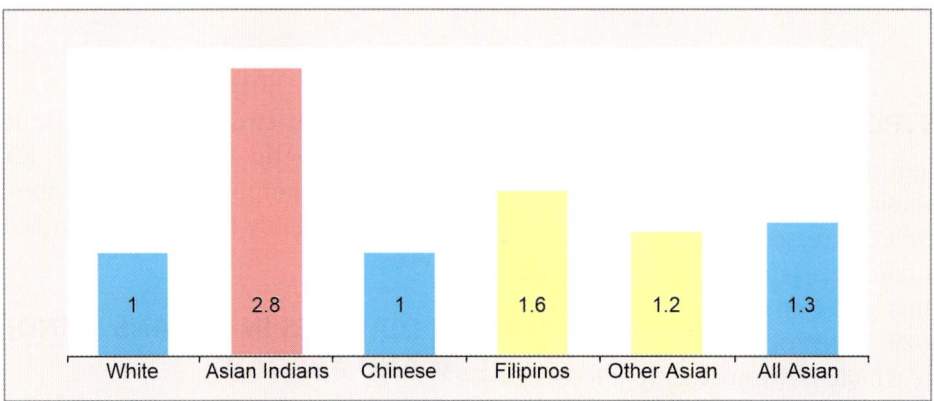

Fig. 1: Relative Risk of Diabetes for Indian Americans and Asian Americans compared to Whites [fully adjusted for age, sex, body mass index (BMI), education, income, smoking, alcohol use, and physical activity].
Source: Adapted from Lee et al.[4]

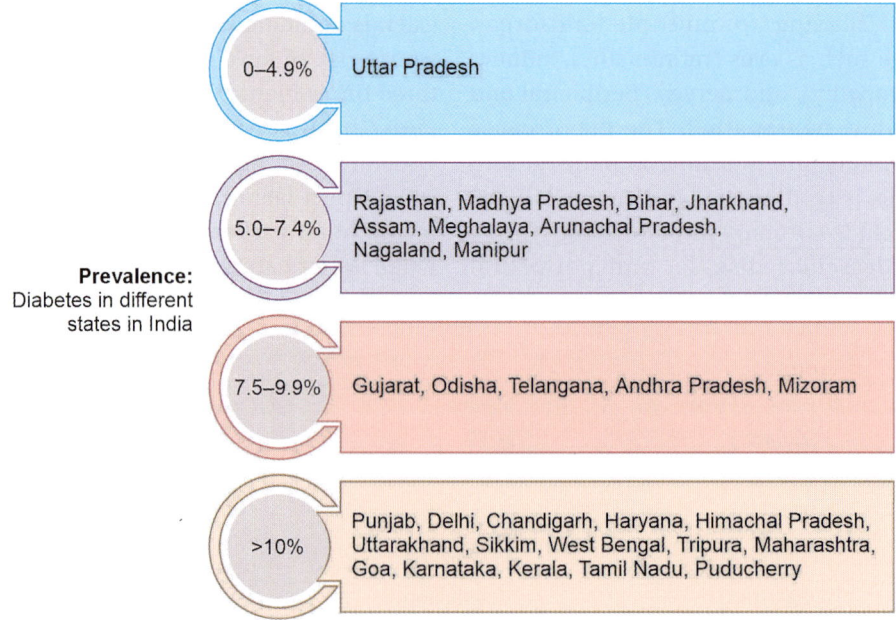

Fig. 2: Differences in the prevalence of diabetes in different states in India.[9]

a major public health issue, is not confined to DM but extends to chronic illnesses like hypertension (35.5%), obesity (28.6%), abdominal obesity (40%), and dyslipidemia (81%).[9]

Besides the fact that the increase in DM is related to economic development, urbanization, and change in life habits in the fast developing countries, Indians have other contributing factors. Some of the known factors include the propensity for visceral fat storage, suboptimal insulin secretion, and increased gestational diabetes (GDM).[10] Indians have a phenotype of lower insulin secretion, about one-half to one-third of insulin secretion compared to that of Pima Indians in the US.[11]

Indian women have a high risk (16–62%) of GDM compared to other ethnicities. Risk factors for GDM in Indian women include being overweight or obese (BMI >23), high blood pressure (BP), family history of diabetes, older maternal age (>25 years), and an unhealthy diet. Cultural factors like "eating for two" and lower activity levels may be contributing factors. Early detection is essential to avoid complications and providing relevant information about GDM and culturally sensitive resources is a priority.[12]

Kerala Diabetes Prevention Program (KDPP)

KDPP provided valuable data on the prevalence of factors associated with diabetes and prediabetes **(Table 2)**, in Kerala, a small southern state with a high degree of epidemiological transition. More than two-thirds had prediabetes and 71% were obese or overweight (BMI >23 kg/m^2). The mean cholesterol level and LDL-C level in Kerala was higher than the rest of India and the US (parenthetically, although LDL-C was >130 in two-thirds of participants, only 2% received statin therapy).[13] The KDPP identified a surprising risk factor—"normal-weight obesity", where individuals have a healthy weight (BMI) but high body fat percentage. While long-term results are pending, these findings suggest a potential rise in diabetes and heart disease in Kerala, aligning with studies that show a high risk of CVD in the state.[14,15]

DIABETES AND CARDIOVASCULAR DISEASES

As was mentioned in the introductory segment, DM affects multiple systems in the body. While diabetic nephropathy and

TABLE 2: The prevalence of risk factors in Kerala Diabetes Prevention Program (n = 1,007 individuals).[13]

Normal glucose tolerance	31%
Family history of diabetes	48%
Prediabetes	69%
Overweight/obesity	71%
Dyslipidemia	85%
Mean cholesterol	221 mg/dL
Mean LDL-C	148 mg/dL
LDL-C >130 mg/dL	67%
Mean triglycerides	210 mg/dL
Triglycerides >150 mg/dL	21%
Lipid-lowering therapy	2%
Hypertension	22%
Current tobacco use	34% (men)
Current alcohol use	39% (men)
No leisure time exercise	98%
No daily intake of fruit and vegetables	79%

Overweight is defined as BMI >23 and <25
Obesity defined as BMI >25
(BMI: body mass index; LDL-C: low-density lipoprotein cholesterol)

retinopathy may lead to end-stage renal disease and blindness, CVD is the major cause of mortality in patients with DM.[16] Several risk factors—hypertension, obesity, dyslipidemia—may be comorbid in patients with DM. Insulin resistance is an important factor in mediating atherothrombotic complications. Diabetes accounts for 5% of the population attributable fraction (PAF) for CVD in the global population but is higher at 10% in Indians (Chapter 3, **Figure 2**). The risk for CVD is doubled by diabetes not solely from high blood sugar but also, to a large extent, from the concomitant risk factors mentioned earlier.[17]

South Asians, particularly those living in high-income countries, have a higher risk for CVD than their White counterparts. This difference is more pronounced in South Asians with T2D, who have a higher rate of CVD and mortality and this is from a complex interplay of multiple factors. The possible factors include a genetic predisposition to abdominal adiposity and insulin resistance, lifestyle factors such as dietary habits and lower physical activity levels, and socioeconomic factors like limitations to healthcare access and health literacy. Earlier onset of both diabetes and CVD, coupled with a clustering of risk factors like hypertension and dyslipidemia, further widens the difference between the two populations. A multipronged approach involving increased awareness, early detection programs, lifestyle interventions, and culturally sensitive healthcare strategies is needed to reduce the CVD burden in the South Asian population.[18-22]

Basic Pathogenetic Mechanisms

Cholesterol, in particular low-density lipoprotein cholesterol (LDL-C), is a major contributor to atherosclerosis (Chapter 7). Diabetic dyslipidemia is characterized by high triglycerides (TG), low high-density lipoprotein (HDL), high non-HDL cholesterol (NHDL-C) and high apolipoprotein B.[23,24] Modified LDL-C containing ApoB retained in the arterial intima draws in macrophages that take up the modified LDL-C and differentiate into foam cells. These foam cells release cytokines that bring in more immune cells. Overproduction of reactive oxygen species (ROS) as a result of altered glucose metabolism and formation of advanced glycation end products further amplifies this process by activating nuclear factor κB (NFκB) and other proinflammatory pathways. In combination with endothelial cell insulin resistance, these changes cause endothelial dysfunction manifesting itself by increased expression of adhesion molecules and other changes. Further, leukocytes accumulate in the intima and vascular smooth muscle cells proliferate; the latter is a major source of extracellular matrix in the atherosclerotic plaque and its fibrous cap (Chapter 2).[17-25]

Consequences

Hyperglycemia promotes the development of CVD through advanced glycation end products, mentioned earlier, and oxidative stress among other factors. Insulin resistance promotes macrovascular abnormalities through formation of atheromatous plaques, diastolic dysfunction, and ventricular hypertrophy.[18] Both insulin resistance and hyperglycemia promote CAD, stroke, cerebrovascular disease, PAD, and heart failure. In relation to CVD, each of these disease states carries significant risk, and the combination of metabolic syndrome with diabetes increases CVD risk nearly fivefold[6] and South Asians are particularly impacted. CVD risk from diabetes has been found to be significantly higher in women. In a study of 5 million people with diabetes, CVD was

58% higher in women than men and deaths were higher (13%) too.[26] One explanation offered for this finding is that menopause strips women of their natural protection against atherosclerosis. Uncontrolled diabetes worsens these complications: A 1% increase in HbA1c (glycated hemoglobin or A1C) linked to a 40% rise in cardiovascular mortality and a 30% increase in all-cause mortality.[17] Conversely, good blood sugar control through improved treatment adherence can significantly reduce this risk.

Benefits of Control

A British study reported the benefits of adherence to optimal levels of five factors: No tobacco smoking, total cholesterol (TC) <160 mg/dL, TG <150 mg/dL, systolic blood pressure (SBP) <130 mm Hg, and average A1C <7%.[16] Those with optimal control of all five factors had only a 21% higher CVD risk than those without diabetes.[27] Every 1% reduction in HbA1c is associated with reduction in risk of 21% for any endpoint related to diabetes, 21% for diabetes-related deaths, 14% for myocardial infarction, 12% for stroke, 16% for heart failure, 43% for amputation or death from peripheral vascular disease, 37% for microvascular complications, 31% for retinopathy, and 33% for nephropathy.[18,19,28]

Diabetes increases the risk of death and/or recurrent heart attacks, within the first year after a heart attack. This heightened risk can be reduced with statin therapy (Chapter 13) that lowers LDL-C and TG. However, only a third of patients with diabetes receive statin before a heart attack and it goes up to only 66% after a heart attack.[17] This is a missed opportunity for preventative care as statin use, particularly high-intensity statin therapy in high-risk patients improves outcomes.[17,29]

■ DIAGNOSIS

Criteria for the diagnosis of diabetes has been streamlined and made easier for the physician and less cumbersome for the patient. Diagnosis requires one of the following three criteria:[17]
1. A fasting blood sugar (≥126 mg/dL) *or*
2. A 2-hour glucose tolerance >200 mg/dL *or*
3. HbA1c ≥6.5%

Prediabetes

Prediabetes is diagnosed when the fasting blood sugar is between 100 and 125 mg/dL or a 2-hour glucose tolerance is 140–199 mg/dL, *or* HbA1c (5.7–6.4%). In the absence of effective intervention prediabetes, progresses to full-blown diabetes at annual rates of 5–15% and likely even higher among Indians.[17]

Gestational Diabetes

Gestational diabetes increases risk to both mother and child. GDM increases the susceptibility to cardiovascular disease in women. The criteria to diagnose GDM are two or more blood sugar readings that exceed the following thresholds:
- *Fasting:* >92 mg/dL (5.1 mmol/L)
- *1 hour:* >180 mg/dL (10.0 mmol/L)
- *2 hours:* >153 mg/dL (8.5 mmol/L)

Proper management, a safe delivery and importantly of GDM allows for a healthy pregnancy and reduces the risk of developing T2D.[17]

■ TREATMENT

Nonpharmacologic Management

Lifestyle Changes

Lifestyle changes are the foundation of T2D management. This includes:[17]
- *Quit smoking:* Reduces risk of CVD and PAD and for overall health

- *Reduce calorie intake:* A 700-calorie deficit and a 7% weight loss can improve blood sugar management.
- *Caution with very low-carb diets:* Monitor closely if considering a very low-carb diet, as it might increase unhealthy fats and LDL-C levels (Chapters 15 and 16).[29]
- *Eat a balanced diet:* Prioritize fruits, vegetables, and whole grains to promote healthy blood sugar levels.
- *Regular exercise:* Engaging in at least 150 minutes of moderate-intensity exercise per week is vital.

Understanding Glycemic Index

Glycemic index (GI) ranks carbohydrate-containing foods based on their blood sugar-raising effect compared to a reference food (usually glucose). GI ranks foods (0–100) based on their blood sugar impact compared to pure glucose. Low-GI champions, like whole grains and legumes, release sugars slowly, preventing spikes and hypoglycemia. Conversely, high glycemic food causes not only hyperglycemia but also rebounds hypoglycemia **(Fig. 3)**.

Some important and easy to remember facts on GI are:[31]
- *Carbohydrate complexity:* Simple carbohydrates (white bread, white rice, potatoes, root vegetables, etc.) raise sugar faster than complex ones (whole grains).
- *Processing:* Processed foods generally have a higher GI than whole foods.
- *Ripeness:* Ripe fruits tend to have a higher GI than unripe ones.
- *Fiber content:* Fiber slows sugar absorption, so high-fiber foods have a lower GI.
- *Cooking method:* Steaming or grilling preserves fiber, leading to a lower GI compared to boiling or mashing.

Glycemic load (GL) takes it a step further by combining both GI and the amount of carbohydrate and is calculated by multiplying the GI of the food by the amount of carbohydrate in a serving, and then dividing by 100. Tables by Atkinson and colleagues[30] on the GI and GL of a variety of foods are helpful in making informed choices to control diabetes. An examples is choice between a low GL (0–10) food like lentils compared to a high GL food (20+) like bagel. Both may have

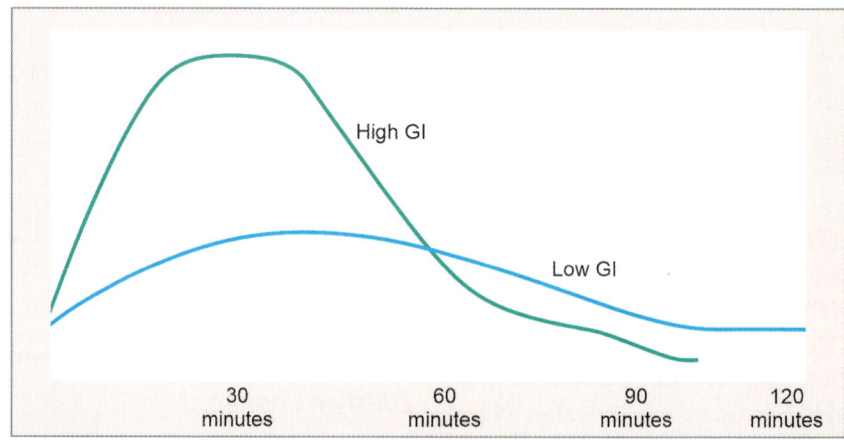

Fig. 3: The vertical axis represents blood glucose levels and the horizontal axis the time after intake of the same amount of carbohydrate but with different glycemic index (GI). Note the absence of a blood sugar spike with low GI food.
Source: VA Office of Patient Centered Care and Cultural Transformation.

comparable GI, but the bagel's larger portion size packs a bigger blood sugar punch. GL is classified as follows: Low: 0–10; medium: 11–19; high: 20 or more. People with or at risk of diabetes should avoid high GL.[31-33]

Continuous Glucose Monitoring

Continuous glucose monitoring (CGM) is a transformative advance in diabetes care because of its ease of use and accuracy. As the technology allows real-time insights into blood sugar levels, trends, and direction, patients can fine-tune their diet, exercise, and insulin dosing while reducing the risks of hypoglycemia and hyperglycemia. CGM is very useful in improving A1C.[34] Target blood sugar range: 70–180 mg/dL (the range is tighter 63–140 mg/dL in pregnancy). The goal is to maximize the time of blood sugar within the target range.

- *High:* 181–250 mg/dL
- *Very high:* >250 mg/dL
- *Low:* 54–69 mg/dL
- *Very low:* <54 mg/dL

Pharmacologic Management

Medication(s) may be necessary alongside lifestyle changes for optimal diabetes management, as recommended by American Diabetes Association (ADA) and American College of Cardiology (ACC). Medication when needed is not to be considered a failure. This combined approach can significantly reduce the risk of major adverse cardiovascular events (MACE) by over 50% in diabetic adults.[17] A detailed discussion of the ever-expanding list of medications available is beyond the scope of this chapter. The commonly used medications are listed below with brief notations.

Metformin is commonly used as it is safe (hypoglycemia is rare). It may lower vitamin B_{12} levels, so monitoring is recommended.[17]

Sulfonylureas and alpha-glucosidase inhibitors are falling out of favor in the US for DM management because of risk of hypoglycemia and the availability of better drugs.[3]

Thiazolidinediones (TZDs) improve insulin sensitivity and control blood sugar with only a minimal risk of hypoglycemia. Weight gain, fluid buildup, and a potential risk for heart failure limit their use.

Colesevelam, though it lowers blood sugar without causing hypoglycemia and reduces LDL-C, its effectiveness is modest. Constipation, indigestion, and potential for raised triglycerides limits its usefulness.

Dipeptidyl peptidase-4 (DP-4) inhibitors (gliptins) promote natural insulin release while lowering glucagon, resulting in improved blood sugar control with a minimal risk of low blood sugar. They provide modest A1C reduction and can be combined with other medications for enhanced glycemic control.

Insulin: Globally, 72 million rely on insulin (9 million T1D and 63 million T2D).[29,35] Advances like pens, pumps, and CGMs are making insulin use easier and more effective. Dosage should be adjusted regularly to achieve the desired glycemic targets while minimizing the risk of hypoglycemia compared to older formulations.

Hypoglycemia or low blood sugar <70 mg/dL is a serious medical urgency for people with diabetes. Recognize the warning signs like sweating, dizziness, palpitation, and confusion. Act immediately by consuming 15 g of fast-acting carbohydrates (glucose tabs, gels, or drinks) and avoiding high-fat foods. Repeat this after 15 minutes if symptoms persist. Insulin users should always have glucagon on hand for severe episodes. Train a family member to administer glucagon in case you are unable to do so yourself.

Early action is crucial to prevent serious complications.[17]

Two new classes of medications, sodium–glucose cotransporter-2 (SGLT2) inhibitors and glucagon-like peptide-1 receptor agonists (GLP-1 RAs) offer superior and multifaceted advantages as detailed below.[36]

Sodium–glucose cotransporter-2 inhibitors like dapagliflozin and empagliflozin offer significant cardiorenal benefits that go beyond lowering blood sugar and A1C. They reduce the risk of heart attack (by up to 35%), heart failure (by up to 39%), and kidney failure (by up to 44%) and slow the progression of kidney disease by 30–40%. Other positive attributes are low risk of hypoglycemia, lowering of BP, and reduced risk of gout flare-up. SGLT2 inhibitors remove excess sugar through urine and often lead to a modest weight loss.[17,30,37-40] A slight increase in genital yeast infections, manageable mostly by good hygiene practice, has been noted. Overall, the benefit–risk ratio is very favorable for SGLT2 inhibitor drugs. However, the cost of this class of drugs, currently ~1,400 dollars/month in the US, limits its wider use.

Glucagon-like peptide-1 agonists **(Table 3)** effectively control blood sugar by mimicking a gut hormone.

They significantly reduce heart-related deaths, strokes, and overall mortality (10–13%) independent of blood sugar control. Additionally, they provide kidney protection, improve cholesterol control, and are generally safe to use as side effects are minimal. As a cautionary note, avoid combining GLP-1 agonists with DP-4 inhibitors (gliptins) because of overlapping mechanisms of action.[17,40-43] Caution should be exercised in using GLP-1 agonists in patients with gastroparesis or severe gastroesophageal reflux disease.

COMPREHENSIVE MANAGEMENT BEYOND CONTROL OF HIGH BLOOD SUGAR

Diabetes seldom occurs in isolation but is often accompanied by CVD risk factors

TABLE 3: Use of glucagon-like peptide-1 receptor agonists (GLP-1 RAs).[17,40-43]

Guideline recommendations	The 2025 guidelines support combining GLP-1 agonists and SGLT2 inhibitors for T2DM in patients struggling with blood sugar control as a must prior to insulin
Advantages over insulin	GLP-1 RAs provide several significant advantages over insulin in managing T2D including superior blood sugar control without hypoglycemia. Convenient prefilled pens make them an attractive alternative to insulin's mixing and measuring routine
Cardiovascular benefits	GLP-1 RAs reduce major adverse cardiac events (MACE) by 10–15%. One of them, semaglutide, with a remarkable 20% MACE reduction, was approved by the Food and Drug Administration (FDA) for CVD prevention in high-risk patients
Renal protection	GLP-1 RAs show promise in moderate to advanced diabetic kidney disease (DKD) and are of potential benefit even with very low kidney function [estimated glomerular filtration rate (eGFR) down to 15 mL/min/1.73 m^2]
Weight loss	GLP-1 agonists promote significant weight loss by reducing appetite and slowing down digestion, leading to decreased calorie intake. FDA approved them for treating obesity (BMI ≥30 kg/m^2) or overweight (BMI ≥25 kg/m^2) with associated conditions like diabetes, high blood pressure, or high cholesterol

(BMI: body mass index; T2D: type 2 diabetes; SGLT2: sodium–glucose cotransporter-2; T2DM: type 2 diabetes mellitus)

like hypertension, hypercholesterolemia/dyslipidemia (abnormal lipids), and obesity. Therefore, in addition to blood sugar control, all CVD risk factors need to be controlled to prevent adverse outcomes. A comprehensive approach that addresses all the CVD risk factors is essential. Present management plans often lack this comprehensive approach. Studies show that only 17.3% of T2D patients reached the ABC (A1C, BP, cholesterol) or "trifecta of care"—control of HbA1c, BP, and LDL-C in the US[16] and only 8% in India.[44]

Some conditions and aspects that are underappreciated, underrecognized, and therefore untreated deserve further comments. People with diabetes are at least twice as likely to develop heart failure and so adults with diabetes should be screened with a blood test that measures natriuretic peptides [B-type natriuretic peptide (BNP) or N-terminal pro-BNP (NT-proBNP)]. This allows for timely intervention to prevent or delay the progression of heart failure.[17] Young adults with T2D are at increased risk for early CAD and may benefit from early statin therapy to lower cholesterol. Moderate-intensity statins are recommended for those without existing heart disease, while high-intensity statins are recommended (Chapter 13) for those with heart disease or have additional CVD risk factors. Semaglutide and tirzepatide that control blood sugar and are cardioprotective are the preferred drugs to treat diabetic patients who are overweight or obese as they aid in weight loss too. Both SGLT2 inhibitors and GLP-1 receptor agonists are effective in reducing cardiovascular risk in people with diabetes. Recent research suggests that combining these two drug classes may offer even greater benefits for both heart and kidney and reduce cardiovascular and kidney complications.[17]

DIABETIC KIDNEY DISEASE (DIABETIC NEPHROPATHY)

Diabetic kidney disease is the leading cause of chronic kidney disease (CKD) and end-stage kidney disease globally. The common features of CKD are proteinuria, elevated BP, and fall in kidney function. The process to CKD is a slow and progressive one and often goes unrecognized. Estimated glomerular filtration rate (eGFR) using serum creatinine is the standard method of determining kidney function and the course of kidney disease. DKD affects about 25–40% of adults with diabetes in the US and those with end-stage kidney disease may require hemodialysis and may be transplant candidates. Besides kidney failure, patients with DKD are prone to suffer heart failure, heart attacks, strokes, and death. The leading cause of mortality in patients with DKD is a MACE. The management of DKD is challenging but newer drugs are improving the outlook.[45-47] **Table 4** distills the measures for optimal treatment of DKD.

DIABETES CONTROL IN INDIA

The prevalence of diabetes in India is 11% and prediabetes 15% with higher rates in urban India. A markedly higher prevalence rate was reported in Kerala, as more than two-thirds of the 1,007 individuals tested had prediabetes.[13] Control of blood glucose in those with diabetes in Kerala—a state with the highest epidemiological transition and known for good medical care—was only 15% compared to 26% for India as a whole.[48] With the forgoing data as a backdrop there are efforts underway to diabetes control and care. Particularly notable is IMPACT India, an initiative to bring together all the like-minded partners in diabetes care to reduce the diabetes burden in India by a three-pronged approach: Education of healthcare providers (HCPs), increasing awareness

TABLE 4: Optimizing cardiovascular health in diabetic kidney disease (DKD).[17]

Angiotensin-converting enzyme (ACE) inhibitors and angiotensin receptor blockers (ARBs)	ACE inhibitors and ARBs improve outcomes for patients with T2D, hypertension, and CKD by lowering blood pressure and protecting heart health
SGLT2 inhibitors	SGLT2 inhibitors are highly recommended for patients with T2D and CKD. They lower blood sugar, fight inflammation, and dramatically slow kidney disease progression
GLP-1 agonists	GLP-1RA is combined with an SGLT2 inhibitor when patients with T2D need additional blood sugar control
Finerenone	Finerenone, a mineralocorticoid receptor antagonist (MRA) is a promising treatment for DKD patients with heart failure, as it reduces albuminuria, fights inflammation, and prevents tissue scarring (fibrosis). It is suitable for patients with GFR above 25 mL/min/1.73 m^2 and significant albuminuria (>30 mg/g)
Combination therapy	Combining ACE inhibitors/ARBs, SGLT2 inhibitors, GLP-1RAs, and MRAs offers the potential to dramatically improve kidney and heart health in DKD patients
Hyperkalemia	ACE inhibitors, ARBs, and MRAs can sometimes worsen kidney function in patients with existing kidney dysfunction (eGFR <45 mL/min/1.73 m^2), potentially limiting their dosage and effectiveness in managing heart failure and CKD
Cardiovascular–kidney–metabolic (CKM) syndrome	Kidney function is vital for maintaining a healthy heart. When kidneys decline, the risk of CVD increases dramatically. Recognizing this crucial link, the American Heart Association identifies CKM syndrome and its progression from stage 0 to stage 4 (Chapter 12)

(CKD: chronic kidney disease; CVD: cardiovascular disease; eGFR: estimated glomerular filtration rate; GLP-1RA: glucagon-like peptide-1 receptor agonist; SGLT2: sodium–glucose cotransporter 2; T2D: type 2 diabetes)

among society, and encouraging patients to timely monitor and control their diabetes.[18] At baseline (January 2018 to June 2018), the database (2.39 million) revealed an HbA1c of 8.56%, 74% of the patients had HbA1c >7%, and fasting blood sugar of 172 mg/dL. The IMPACT India program aims to positively impact diabetes care in India by achieving at least 1% HbA1c reduction in 1,000 days.[18] This would be a highly desirable outcome as every 1% increase in the HbA1c level in persons living with diabetes is likely associated with an approximately 40% increase in CVD mortality and a 30% increase in all-cause mortality.[19]

In the US, diabetes is a costly disease, about one-quarter of US healthcare spending is for diabetes care and nearly half of the costs stem from CVD complications. India, for instance, spent an average of $209 per patient with diabetes in 2017. The use of medications like SGLT2 inhibitors, GLP-1RAs, and finerenone is likely to further escalate treatment costs.[49]

ENCOURAGING TRENDS IN DIABETES

South Asian immigrants in western countries (high-income countries) with diabetes had higher rates of CVD and fare worse than their White counterparts.[20] However, newer studies show a positive change with reduced mortality rates in South Asians living in high-income countries (Canada, US, and the UK, etc.) due to improvement in CVD management.[50-54]

A large Canadian study of patients with newly diagnosed diabetes (15,066 South Asian, 17,754 Chinese, and 244,017 Whites) found that though South Asians led in incidence, their mortality was 31% lower than of the White patients.[55] The rate of heart attack, stroke, and heart failure was also similar or lower in the Chinese and Indians than in Whites. This encouraging trend is likely due to several factors—increased awareness of CVD risk in South Asians leading to earlier diagnosis and better blood sugar control, a comprehensive management with the use of cardioprotective medications like angiotensin-converting enzyme (ACE) inhibitors/angiotensin receptor blockers (ARBs), SGLT2 inhibitors, GLP-1 agonists, and improved management of BP and cholesterol.

These trends in diabetes among South Asians in western countries should be encouraging to those in South Asia who grapple with poor control of diabetes and its health consequences. The reported rates of diabetes awareness in South Asia is 50%, glycemic control is 26%, and CKD awareness is 10% to <15%.[56] Underdiagnosis and undertreatment result in higher rates of myocardial infarction and stroke with adverse outcomes.

■ KEY TAKEAWAYS

- There is a surge in diabetes worldwide and more so in fast developing countries like China and India. By the year 2030, India is projected to have more than 100 million with diabetes. Without concerted efforts more than one-half of those affected would remain undiagnosed.
- Diabetes affects multiple systems in the body that lead to end-organ damage, causing morbidity. Atherosclerotic cardiovascular disease (ASCVD) from atherosclerosis is the major cause of mortality and insulin resistance is an important factor in mediating atherothrombotic complications. CKD is a major cause of morbidity in diabetes as a large percentage (>25%) of patients develop DKD.
- Diagnostic criteria have been simplified and standardized for diabetes, prediabetes, and GDM.
- Indian women have a propensity (20–62% of pregnancies) to develop GDM that adversely impacts both mother and child. Preexisting conditions like prediabetes, high BP, overweight (BMI >23) and age over 25 raise the risk of GDM.
- Understanding GI and GL and using them to make healthy choices in diet is of great benefit in controlling blood sugar.
- New drugs, SGLT2s and GLP agonists, are game changers in T2D care. These drugs go beyond blood sugar control, offering double-duty protection for heart and kidneys. They reduce hospitalizations for heart failure and cardiovascular mortality. These drugs combined with others slow kidney function decline and heart complication in patients with DKD.
- The importance of control of blood sugar cannot be overstressed to prevent vascular damage and its consequences to kidneys, heart, peripheral arteries, and other organs.
- Every 1% reduction in HbA1c is associated with reduction in risk of 21% for any endpoint related to diabetes, 21% for deaths related to diabetes, 14% for heart attack, 12% for stroke, 16% for heart failure, 43% for amputation or death from PAD, 37% for microvascular complications, 31% for retinopathy, and 33% for nephropathy.[17-19,28]
- Management of patients with diabetes should be comprehensive and not just the control of blood sugar. All the cardiovascular risk factors need to be evaluated and treated as CVD is the major cause of mortality and morbidity.
- Despite its importance, the disappointing reality is that only a meager 7% of patients with diabetes achieve the optimal trifecta of care (control of blood sugar, BP, and cholesterol) in India and this deficiency contributes to high ASCVD morbidity and mortality.

REFERENCES

1. Banday MZ, Sameer AS, Nissar S. Pathophysiology of diabetes: an overview. Avicenna J Med. 2020;10(4):174-88.
2. Saeedi P, Petersohn I, Salpea P, Malanda B, Karuranga S, Unwin N, et al.; IDF Diabetes Atlas Committee. Global and regional diabetes prevalence estimates for 2019 and projections for 2030 and 2045: Results from the International Diabetes Federation Diabetes Atlas, 9th edition. Diabetes Res Clin Pract. 2019;157:107843.
3. Joseph JJ, Deedwania P, Acharya T, Aguilar D, Bhatt DL, Chyun DA, et al.; American Heart Association Diabetes Committee of the Council on Lifestyle and Cardiometabolic Health; Council on Arteriosclerosis, Thrombosis and Vascular Biology; Council on Clinical Cardiology; and Council on Hypertension. Comprehensive Management of Cardiovascular Risk Factors for Adults With Type 2 Diabetes: A Scientific Statement From the American Heart Association. Circulation. 2022;145(9):e722-e759.
4. Lee JW, Brancati FL, Yeh HC. Trends in the Prevalence of Type 2 Diabetes in Asians Versus Whites: Results from the United States National Health Interview Survey, 1997-2008. Diabetes Care. 2011;34(2):353-7.
5. Echouffo-Tcheugui JB, Perreault L, Ji L, Dagogo-Jack S. Diagnosis and management of prediabetes: a review. JAMA. 2023;329(14):1206-16.
6. Kwan TW, Wong SS, Hong Y, Kanaya AM, Khan SS, Hayman LL, et al.; American Heart Association Council on Epidemiology and Prevention; Council on Lifestyle and Cardiometabolic Health; Council on Arteriosclerosis, Thrombosis and Vascular Biology; Council on Clinical Cardiology; Council on Cardiovascular and Stroke Nursing; and Council on Genomic and Precision Medicine. Epidemiology of Diabetes and Atherosclerotic Cardiovascular Disease Among Asian American Adults: Implications, Management, and Future Directions: A Scientific Statement From the American Heart Association. Circulation. 2023;148(1):74-94.
7. Sattar N, Rawshani A, Franzén S, Rawshani A, Svensson AM, Rosengren A, et al. Age at Diagnosis of Type 2 Diabetes Mellitus and Associations With Cardiovascular and Mortality Risks. Circulation. 2019;139(19):2228-37.
8. Kanaya AM, Herrington D, Vittinghoff E, Ewing SK, Liu K, Blaha MJ, et al. Understanding the high prevalence of diabetes in U.S. south Asians compared with four racial/ethnic groups: the MASALA and MESA studies. Diabetes Care. 2014;37(6):1621-8.
9. Anjana RM, Unnikrishnan R, Deepa M, Pradeepa R, Tandon N, Das AK, et al.; ICMR-INDIAB Collaborative Study Group. Metabolic non-communicable disease health report of India: the ICMR-INDIAB national cross-sectional study (ICMR-INDIAB-17). Lancet Diabetes Endocrinol. 2023;11(7):474-89.
10. Gupta R, Guptha S, Gupta VP, Agrawal A, Gaur K, Deedwania PC. Twenty-year trends in cardiovascular risk factors in India and influence of educational status. Eur J Prev Cardiol. 2012;19(6):1258-71.
11. Narayan KM. Type 2 Diabetes: Why We Are Winning the Battle but Losing the War? 2015 Kelly West Award Lecture. Diabetes Care. 2016;39(5):653-63.
12. Bandyopadhyay M. Gestational diabetes mellitus: a qualitative study of lived experiences of South Asian immigrant women and perspectives of their health care providers in Melbourne, Australia. BMC Pregnancy Childbirth. 2021;21(1):500.
13. Sathish T, Oldenburg B, Tapp RJ, Shaw JE, Wolfe R, Sajitha B, et al. Baseline characteristics of participants in the Kerala Diabetes Prevention Program: a cluster randomized controlled trial of lifestyle intervention in Asian Indians. Diabet Med. 2017;34(5):647-53.
14. Haregu T, Lekha TR, Jasper S, Kapoor N, Sathish T, Panniyammakal J, et al. The long-term effects of Kerala Diabetes Prevention Program on diabetes incidence and cardiometabolic risk: a study protocol. BMC Public Health. 2023;23(1):539.

15. Geldsetzer P, Manne-Goehler J, Theilmann M, Davies JI, Awasthi A, Danaei G, et al. Geographic and sociodemographic variation of cardiovascular disease risk in India: a cross-sectional study of 797,540 adults. PLoS Med. 2018;15(6):e1002581.
16. Morrish NJ, Wang SL, Stevens LK, Fuller JH, Keen H. Mortality and causes of death in the WHO Multinational Study of Vascular Disease in Diabetes. Diabetologia. 2001; 44 Suppl 2:S14-21.
17. American Diabetes Association Professional Practice Committee. Cardiovascular Disease and Risk Management: Standards of Care in Diabetes—2025. Diabetes Care. 2025; 48(Supplement_1):S207-S238.
18. Das AK, Mohan V, Joshi S, Shah S, Zargar AH, Kalra S, et al. IMPACT India: A Novel Approach for Optimum Diabetes Care. J Diabetology. 2021;12:239-45.
19. Khaw KT, Wareham N, Bingham S, Luben R, Welch A, Day N. Association of hemoglobin A1c with cardiovascular disease and mortality in adults: the European prospective investigation into cancer in Norfolk. Ann Intern Med. 2004;141(6):413-20.
20. Mather HM, Chaturvedi N, Fuller JH. Mortality and morbidity from diabetes in South Asians and Europeans: 11-year follow-up of the Southall Diabetes Survey, London, UK. Diabet Med. 1998;15(1):53-9.
21. Bellary S, O'Hare JP, Raymond NT, Mughal S, Hanif WM, Jones A, et al. Premature cardiovascular events and mortality in south Asians with type 2 diabetes in the United Kingdom Asian Diabetes Study—effect of ethnicity on risk. Curr Med Res Opin. 2010; 26(8):1873-9.
22. Stratton IM, Adler AI, Neil HA, Matthews DR, Manley SE, Cull CA, et al. Association of glycaemia with macrovascular and microvascular complications of type 2 diabetes (UKPDS 35): prospective observational study. BMJ. 2000;321(7258): 405-12.
23. Muilwijk M, Ho F, Waddell H, Sillars A, Welsh P, Iliodromiti S, et al. Contribution of type 2 diabetes to all-cause mortality, cardiovascular disease incidence and cancer incidence in white Europeans and South Asians: findings from the UK Biobank population-based cohort study. BMJ Open Diabetes Res Care. 2019;7(1):e000765.
24. Tillin T, Sattar N, Godsland IF, Hughes AD, Chaturvedi N, Forouhi NG. Ethnicity-specific obesity cut-points in the development of Type 2 diabetes—a prospective study including three ethnic groups in the United Kingdom. Diabet Med. 2015;32(2):226-34.
25. Tillin T, Hughes AD, Mayet J, Whincup P, Sattar N, Forouhi NG, et al. The relationship between metabolic risk factors and incident cardiovascular disease in Europeans, South Asians, and African Caribbeans: SABRE (Southall and Brent Revisited)—a prospective population-based study. J Am Coll Cardiol. 2013;61(17):1777-86.
26. Sniderman A, Langlois M, Cobbaert C. Update on apolipoprotein B. Curr Opin Lipidol. 2021;32(4):226-30.
27. Rask-Madsen C, King GL. Vascular complications of diabetes: mechanisms of injury and protective factors. Cell Metab. 2013; 17(1):20-33.
28. Wang Y, O'Neil A, Jiao Y, Wang L, Huang J, Lan Y, et al. Sex differences in the association between diabetes and risk of cardiovascular disease, cancer, and all-cause and cause-specific mortality: a systematic review and meta-analysis of 5,162,654 participants. BMC Med. 2019;17(1):136.
29. Das SR, Everett BM, Birtcher KK, Brown JM, Januzzi JL Jr, Kalyani RR, et al. 2020 Expert Consensus Decision Pathway on Novel Therapies for Cardiovascular Risk Reduction in Patients With Type 2 Diabetes: A Report of the American College of Cardiology Solution Set Oversight Committee. J Am Coll Cardiol. 2020;76(9):1117-45.
30. Atkinson FS, Foster-Powell K, Brand-Miller JC. International tables of glycemic index and glycemic load values: 2008. Diabetes Care. 2008;31(12):2281-3.
31. Battelino T, Danne T, Bergenstal RM, Amiel SA, Beck R, Biester T, et al. Clinical Targets for Continuous Glucose Monitoring

Data Interpretation: Recommendations From the International Consensus on Time in Range. Diabetes Care. 2019;42(8):1593-603.
32. ElSayed NA, Aleppo G, Aroda VR, Bannuru RR, Brown FM, Bruemmer D, et al.; on behalf of the American Diabetes Association. 1. Improving Care and Promoting Health in Populations: Standards of Care in Diabetes-2023. Diabetes Care. 2023;46(Supplement_1): S10-S18.
33. Russell-Jones D, Bawlchhim Z. Discovery of insulin 100 years on. Postgrad Med J. 2023;99(1173):661-8.
34. Davies MJ, Aroda VR, Collins BS, Gabbay RA, Green J, Maruthur NM, et al. Management of Hyperglycemia in Type 2 Diabetes, 2022. A Consensus Report by the American Diabetes Association (ADA) and the European Association for the Study of Diabetes (EASD). Diabetes Care. 2022;45(11):2753-86.
35. Handelsman Y, Anderson JE, Bakris GL, Ballantyne CM, Beckman JA, Bhatt DL, et al. DCRM Multispecialty Practice Recommendations for the management of diabetes, cardiorenal, and metabolic diseases. J Diabetes Complications. 2022;36(2): 108101.
36. Ali MU, Mancini GBJ, Fitzpatrick-Lewis D, Lewis R, Jovkovic M, Zieroth S, et al. The effectiveness of sodium-glucose cotransporter 2 inhibitors and glucagon-like peptide-1 receptor agonists on cardiorenal outcomes: systematic review and meta-analysis. Can J Cardiol. 2022;38(8):1201-10.
37. Jain V, Qamar A, Matsushita K, Vaduganathan M, Ashley KE, Khan MS, et al. Impact of Diabetes on Outcomes in Patients Hospitalized With Acute Myocardial Infarction: Insights From the Atherosclerosis Risk in Communities Study Community Surveillance. J Am Heart Assoc. 2023;12(10):e028923.
38. Morales J, Handelsman Y. Cardiovascular Outcomes in Patients With Diabetes and Kidney Disease: JACC Review Topic of the Week. J Am Coll Cardiol. 2023;82(2):161-70.
39. Berg DD, Kolkailah AA, Sarraju A, Kerchberger AM, Eljalby M, McGuire DK. Interpreting Absolute and Relative Risk Reduction in the Context of Recent Cardiovascular Outcome Trials in Patients with Type 2 Diabetes. Curr Diab Rep. 2021; 21(11):45.
40. Davies MJ, D'Alessio DA, Fradkin J, Kernan WN, Mathieu C, Mingrone G, et al. Management of Hyperglycemia in Type 2 Diabetes, 2018. A Consensus Report by the American Diabetes Association (ADA) and the European Association for the Study of Diabetes (EASD). Diabetes Care. 2018;41(12):2669-701.
41. Bethel MA, Patel RA, Merrill P, Lokhnygina Y, Buse JB, Mentz RJ, et al.; EXSCEL Study Group. Cardiovascular outcomes with glucagon-like peptide-1 receptor agonists in patients with type 2 diabetes: a meta-analysis. Lancet Diabetes Endocrinol. 2018; 6(2):105-13.
42. Zelniker TA, Wiviott SD, Raz I, Im K, Goodrich EL, Furtado RHM, et al. Comparison of the Effects of Glucagon-Like Peptide Receptor Agonists and Sodium-Glucose Cotransporter 2 Inhibitors for Prevention of Major Adverse Cardiovascular and Renal Outcomes in Type 2 Diabetes Mellitus. Circulation. 2019;139(17):2022-31.
43. Caparrotta TM, Templeton JB, Clay TA, Wild SH, Reynolds RM, Webb DJ, et al. Glucagon-Like Peptide 1 Receptor Agonist (GLP1RA) Exposure and Outcomes in Type 2 Diabetes: A Systematic Review of Population-Based Observational Studies. Diabetes Ther. 2021;12(4):969-89.
44. Andary R, Fan W, Wong ND. Control of Cardiovascular Risk Factors Among US Adults With Type 2 Diabetes With and Without Cardiovascular Disease. Am J Cardiol. 2019;124(4):522-7.
45. Anjana RM, Unnikrishnan R, Deepa M, Venkatesan U, Pradeepa R, Joshi S, et al.; ICMR-INDIAB collaborators. Achievement of guideline recommended diabetes treatment targets and health habits in people with self-reported diabetes in India (ICMR-INDIAB-13): a national cross-sectional study. Lancet Diabetes Endocrinol. 2022;10(6): 430-41.

46. Agarwal R, Filippatos G, Pitt B, Anker SD, Rossing P, Joseph A, et al.; FIDELIO-DKD and FIGARO-DKD investigators. Cardiovascular and kidney outcomes with finerenone in patients with type 2 diabetes and chronic kidney disease: the FIDELITY pooled analysis. Eur Heart J. 2022;43(6):474-84.
47. Bakris GL, Agarwal R, Anker SD, Pitt B, Ruilope LM, Rossing P, et al. Effect of Finerenone on Chronic Kidney Disease Outcomes in Type 2 Diabetes. N Engl J Med. 2020;383(23):2219-29.
48. Pitt B, Filippatos G, Agarwal R, Anker SD, Bakris GL, Rossing P, et al.; FIGARO-DKD Investigators. Cardiovascular Events with Finerenone in Kidney Disease and Type 2 Diabetes. N Engl J Med. 2021;385(24):2252-63.
49. Sathyanath S, Kundapur R, Deepthi R, Poojary SN, Rai S, Modi B, et al. An economic evaluation of diabetes mellitus in India: a systematic review. Diabetes Metab Syndr. 2022;16(11):102641.
50. Johns E, Sattar N. Cardiovascular and Mortality Risks in Migrant South Asians with Type 2 Diabetes: Are We Winning the Battle? Curr Diab Rep. 2017;17(10):100.
51. Khan NA, Grubisic M, Hemmelgarn B, Humphries K, King KM, Quan H. Outcomes after acute myocardial infarction in South Asian, Chinese, and white patients. Circulation. 2010;122(16):1570-7.
52. Shah BR, Victor JC, Chiu M, Tu JV, Anand SS, Austin PC, et al. Cardiovascular complications and mortality after diabetes diagnosis for South Asian and Chinese patients: a population-based cohort study. Diabetes Care. 2013;36(9):2670-6.
53. Sattar N, Gill JM. Type 2 diabetes in migrant south Asians: mechanisms, mitigation, and management. Lancet Diabetes Endocrinol. 2015;3(12):1004-16.
54. Wright AK, Kontopantelis E, Emsley R, Buchan I, Sattar N, Rutter MK, et al. Life Expectancy and Cause-Specific Mortality in Type 2 Diabetes: A Population-Based Cohort Study Quantifying Relationships in Ethnic Subgroups. Diabetes Care. 2017;40(3):338-45.
55. Khan NA, Wang H, Anand S, Jin Y, Campbell NR, Pilote L, et al. Ethnicity and sex affect diabetes incidence and outcomes. Diabetes Care. 2011;34(1):96-101.
56. Misra A. Prevention of diabetes: countless opportunities and clear challenges. Am J Lifestyle Med. 2018;12(1):25-9.

CHAPTER 7

Cholesterol and Heart Disease

"Cholesterol is the most highly decorated small molecule in biology. Thirteen Nobel Prizes have been awarded to scientists who devoted major parts of their careers to cholesterol. Ever since it was isolated from gallstones in 1784, cholesterol has exerted an almost hypnotic fascination for scientists from the most diverse areas of science and medicine.... Cholesterol is a Janus-faced molecule. The very property that makes it useful in cell membranes, namely its absolute insolubility in water, also makes it lethal."
—Michael Brown and Joseph Goldstein Nobel Lectures (1985)

■ INTRODUCTION

A personal anecdote from the time of my (EAE) cardiology fellowship would serve as a good start for this chapter as it is quite instructive in the evolution of our knowledge on cholesterol and heart disease and when and how to intervene in hypercholesterolemia. The year was 1975, and my total cholesterol (TC) was 320 mg/dL; this number hardly raised an eyebrow on the senior cardiologist I consulted. This was partly due to the loose definition of hypercholesterolemia (~330 mg/dL) and mostly due to the lack of effective medications (bile acid-binding agents became available in 1984). The lack of action could not have been due to lack of awareness as much was already known about cholesterol and heart disease. The first half of the century can be called the era of cholesterol as there were incrementally marked advances as shown in **Box 1**.[1]

The second half of the century can be rightly considered the era of low-density lipoprotein cholesterol (LDL-C) as it was identified as a risk factor for coronary artery

> **BOX 1:** The era of cholesterol.
> - 1910—Cholesterol found in human atherosclerotic plaques
> - 1913—High-cholesterol diet causes atherosclerosis in rabbits
> - 1919—Heart attacks recognized clinically
> - 1933—Feedback inhibition of cholesterol synthesis demonstrated
> - 1938—Familial hypercholesterolemia (FH) described
> - 1950—Cholesterol biosynthetic pathway elucidated
> - 1951—High-fat diets raise plasma cholesterol
> - 1953—Risk factor concept advanced

disease (CAD) in 1955 and in 1973 LDL receptor was discovered. Though the statin class of drugs were discovered in 1976, lovastatin, the first drug of its class, gained approval only in 1987. This ushered through an era of effective treatment that improved cardiovascular morbidity and mortality. Besides treatment advances, the approach to the preventive aspects of heart disease are also evolving. Emerging research shows that plaque buildup continues at LDL-C levels, as low as 60–70 mg/dL and that the theoretical minimum risk LDL range is now believed to be a mere 25–50 mg/dL.[2] As we move forward, we must be flexible to reassess our approaches and be open to new frontiers in the fight against heart disease.[3]

A plethora of scientific studies implicate cholesterol-carrying LDL-C as the instigator of atherosclerotic plaques and high dietary fat as a major cause of pathologically elevated LDL levels.[4] The correlation between high LDL levels and heart attacks is one of the tightest correlations in all of medicine. Though the primacy of LDL-C in causing cardiovascular diseases (CVDs) that include heart disease, stroke, and peripheral arterial disease (PAD) is undisputed, there are also other atherogenic lipoproteins. The first step toward better understanding of lipoproteins and their actions is to know their definitions **(Table 1)**.[5-8]

TABLE 1: Lipids and lipoproteins: Terminology and classification.[5-8]	
Lipids (fats)	Lipids are hydrophobic molecules vital for the body and require protein carriers (lipoproteins) to travel through our blood's watery environment. The major types of fats, cholesterol and triglycerides, rely on these lipoproteins for transport and function
Cholesterol or total cholesterol (TC)	Cholesterol is an essential building block to form cell walls and provides key support to the production of hormones—testosterone, estrogen, cortisol
Triglycerides (TG)	These fats function as the body's primary energy reserves, stored in fat cells and released into the bloodstream for fuel. They even provide some thermal insulation
Chylomicrons	Dietary fat is converted to TG in the intestines and packaged into chylomicrons, the largest lipoproteins. These "fat shuttles" TG from the gut to the liver and tissues for energy storage
Lipoproteins	Lipoproteins are particles that transport lipids (TC and TG) in the bloodstream. These lipoproteins vary in composition and function. Lipoproteins other than high-density lipoprotein (HDL) are atherogenic
VLDL [remnant cholesterol (RC)]	Very low-density lipoprotein (VLDL), now termed remnant cholesterol, transports fats through the bloodstream. VLDL is the largest and least dense of the lipoproteins. It is produced in the liver and transports TG to other tissues in the body
IDL	Intermediate-density lipoprotein (IDL) is formed when VLDL loses some of its TG. It can be further processed into LDL or be removed from the bloodstream by the liver
LDL	Low-density lipoprotein (LDL) is often referred to as "bad" cholesterol as it contributes to the buildup of plaque in the arteries, a condition called atherosclerosis. This buildup of plaque narrows the arteries and increases the risk of heart attack and stroke
Lipoprotein(a) [Lp(a)]	Most atherogenic of all lipoproteins (Chapter 8)
HDL	HDL is often referred to as "good" cholesterol as it helps to remove cholesterol from the arteries and transport it back to the liver. High HDL levels were considered protective against heart disease and stroke

ATHEROGENIC LIPOPROTEINS: FOCUS ON LOW-DENSITY LIPOPROTEIN CHOLESTEROL

As depicted in **Flowchart 1**, the atherogenic lipoproteins are very low-density lipoprotein (VLDL) [remnant cholesterol (RC)], intermediate-density lipoprotein (IDL), LDL, and lipoprotein(a) [Lp(a)]. These have in common apolipoprotein B (ApoB) particles that are drivers of atherosclerosis and diseases of the cardiovascular system (CAD, stroke, and PAD). Among these lipoproteins, LDL-C is the dominant player with the strongest evidence for its causative role in heart disease as noted below.[9,10]

Low-density lipoprotein cholesterol is not only an essential factor in the pathogenesis of atherosclerosis and CAD; the disease process is "dose-related" by LDL-C level and the cumulated years lived with high LDL-C. In individuals with hyperlipidemia [defined as non-high-density lipoprotein cholesterol (NHDL-C) ≥160 mg/dL or LDL-C >130 mg/dL] the prevalence of CAD by age 50 increased with the duration of exposure, even when accounting for other risk factors. Here is a breakdown of the CAD rates:[11]

- *No hyperlipidemia:* 4.4% risk
- *1–10 years of exposure:* Risk nearly doubles to 8.1%
- *11–20 years of exposure:* Risk quadruples to 16.5%
- Persons with a rare gene mutation that causes ultra-low LDL-C (15 mg/dL) throughout their lives experience no atherosclerosis (plaque buildup in arteries) and no negative side effects because of ultra-low LDL-C.[12]
- Individuals with genetic mutations greatly benefit by reducing their LDL-C as there is a 54% reduction in heart attacks and strokes per 40 mg/dL reduction in LDL-C.[13] This dwarfs the 25% decrease achieved through statin therapy in randomized controlled trials, per 40 mg reduction pointing to the power of lowering LDL-C earlier in life.[6]
- LDL-C <60 mg/dL arrests the progression of plaque and keeping LDL-C potentially below 40 mg/dL, might offer even greater benefits.[14]
- The landmark Scandinavian Simvastatin Survival study (4S trial 1994) dramatically reduced cardiovascular and all-cause mortality through aggressive LDL-C reduction. In the US, the significant decline in LDL-C over the past 30 years is credited as a major factor in the dramatic 70% decrease in cardiovascular mortality, surpassing the impact of any other intervention.

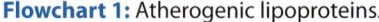

Flowchart 1: Atherogenic lipoproteins.

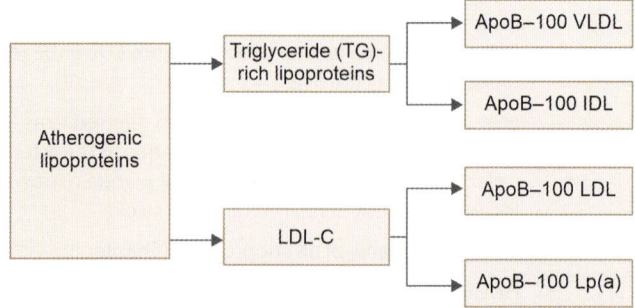

[ApoB: apolipoprotein B; IDL: intermediate-density lipoprotein; LDL-C: low-density lipoprotein cholesterol; Lp(a): lipoprotein(a); VLDL: very low-density lipoprotein]

- The ongoing Coronary Artery Risk Development in Young Adults (CARDIA) study reveals that heart disease risk rises as LDL-C levels increase. Compared to those with LDL-C 70 mg/dL, nearly individuals with LDL-C >160 mg/dL have six times higher risk **(Fig. 1)**[15] and cements the need for stricter cholesterol control for optimal cardiovascular health. These findings have led to revised guidelines with more stringent lipid targets (<70 mg/dL).[6]

Low-density Lipoprotein Score

Low-density lipoprotein score, a quantitative method, is a significant forward step in understanding an individual's risk of heart disease. By factoring in both LDL-C levels in mg/dL (before treatment) and age, the LDL score estimates an individual's cumulative exposure to LDL-C, potentially reflecting the total burden of plaque buildup (both calcified and noncalcified) in their arteries. The calculation of LDL score is similar to "pack-years" (cigarettes smoked × years smoked) used in smokers. Example: A person with an LDL-C of 125 mg/dL would have an LDL score of 5,000 at age 40 (125 × 40) and 10,000 at age 80. **Figure 2** illustrates the scores with different levels of LDL-C over time.[16]

A higher LDL score indicates greater LDL-C exposure over time, translating to a higher risk of plaque buildup and heart disease. Just as quitting smoking after many decades of smoking cannot fully erase the damage to lungs and heart, lowering LDL-C later in life may not fully mitigate the risks associated with a high LDL score. Different LDL-C score thresholds indicate varying risk levels, which allow targeted preventive measures **(Table 2)**.

Atherogenic Dyslipidemia

Atherogenic dyslipidemia is characterized by high triglycerides (TG), high RC, high ApoB, moderately increased LDL-C, and low HDL-C levels and is generally associated with prediabetes or diabetes in Indians.[6,7] The high cardiovascular risk associated with

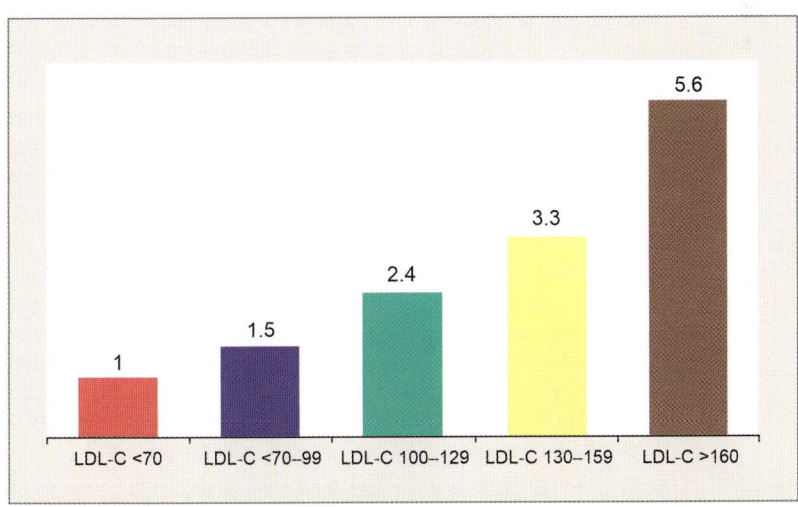

Fig. 1: Increasing atherosclerotic cardiovascular disease (ASCVD) risk with increasing low-density lipoprotein cholesterol (LDL-C) in 3,258 Black and White youths measured 20 years earlier in the Coronary Artery Risk Development in Young Adults (CARDIA) study.
Source: Pletcher et al.[15]

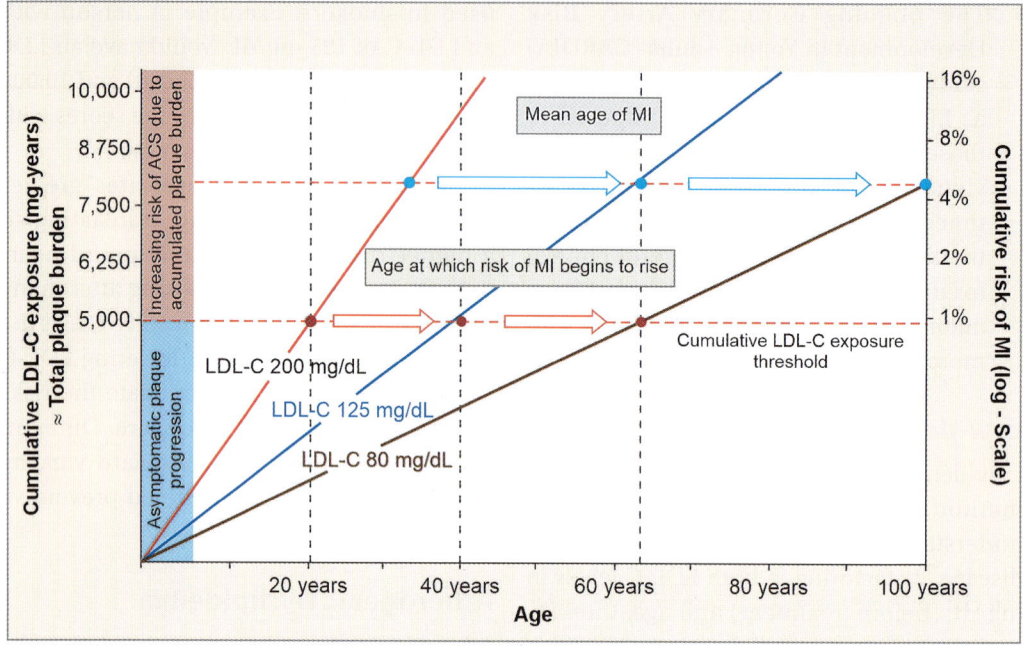

Fig. 2: Age at which one reaches low-density lipoprotein (LDL) score of 5,000 and 8,000 mg-years at different levels of LDL cholesterol (LDL-C). (MI: myocardial infarction)
Source: Reproduced with permission from Ference et al.[16]

TABLE 2: Low-density lipoprotein cholesterol (LDL-C) score and its implications.[16]	
<5,000 mg-years	Heart attacks rarely occur solely due to coronary plaque volume at this LDL score except with high lipoprotein(a), established risk factors, risk-enhancing factors, or a combination of these
5,000 mg-years	Signifies transition from low 1% annual risk to an exponentially higher risk of 16% by 10,000 **(Fig. 3)**. An individual with LDL-C 125 mg reaches this level at age 40 (125 × 40) whereas an individual with a lower LDL-C of 80 mg/dL would reach the same 5,000 LDL score, 22 years later at age 62.5
8,000 mg-years	The increased risk of heart attack at this score is further amplified with additional risk factors. An individual with LDL 125 mg/dL would reach this score by age 64. This LDL score assumes great importance as most heart attacks are correlated with this score. Individuals falling into this category should have their Coronary Artery Calcium (CAC) score measured to further intensity and refine lifestyle changes and lipid-lowering therapy. The CAC integrates the effects of both lipid and nonlipid factors. Those with CAC score >300 should follow the prevention guidelines detailed in later chapters
10,000 mg-years	Score of 10,000 indicates a markedly increased risk (16% per year) of heart disease. A comprehensive approach—prevention and treatment—including aggressive lipid-lowering therapy should be started without further delay (should have been undertaken earlier). Maintaining LDL-C <50 mg/dL may be required if CAC score >500

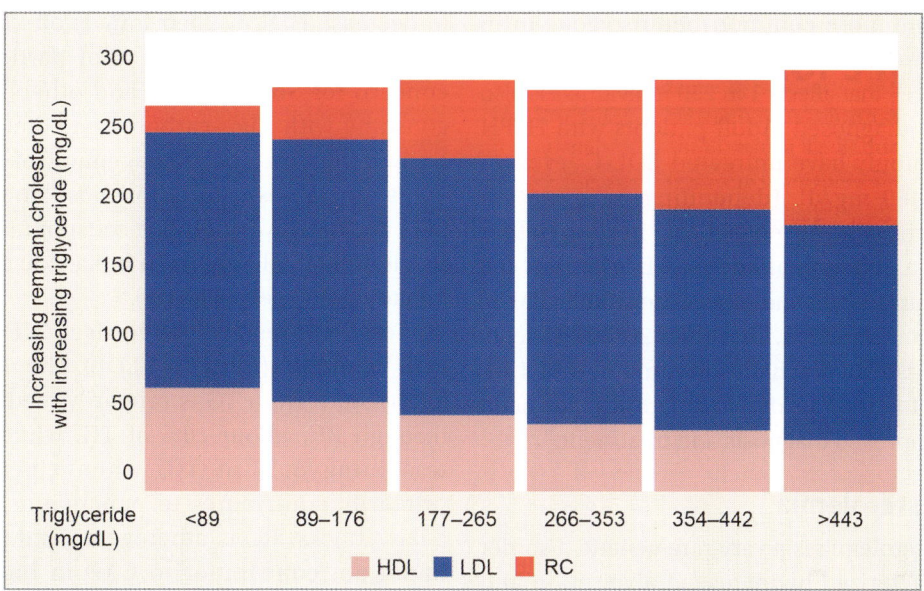

Fig. 3: The inverse relationship between remnant cholesterol (RC) and low-density lipoprotein cholesterol (LDL-C) and high-density lipoprotein cholesterol (HDL-C) is schematically represented.
Source: Adapted from Chapman et al.[27]

this dyslipidemia stems from its high ApoB content—a protein that plays a major role in transporting artery-clogging cholesterol.[7]

Dysbetalipoproteinemia or Type III Hyperlipoproteinemia

Dysbetalipoproteinemia (DBL) or type III hyperlipoproteinemia is a rare (1 in 5,000–10,000 individuals), but serious genetic disorder, characterized by high TG and cholesterol, markedly increases the risk of early CVD. A defective *ApoE* gene hinders the body's ability to clear RC, leading to harmful cholesterol deposits (xanthomas) and clogged arteries. People with DBL face a 5–10 times greater risk of premature CVD, making early diagnosis and treatment essential.[17,18]

Familial Hypercholesterolemia

Familial Hypercholesterolemia is a genetic disorder that leads to very high LDL-C levels that is more common in Ashkenazi Jews, some Lebanese groups, and French Canadians.[19] The rare homozygous form [homozygous familial hypercholesterolemia (HoFH)], inherited from both parents affecting one in 250,000, causes LDL-C levels to markedly rise (450–1,100 mg/dL), and if untreated, leads to very early (mean age 12 years) atherosclerotic cardiovascular disease (ASCVD) events and deaths (mean age 18 years).[20,21] Physical examination may show cholesterol deposits in the skin (hands, elbows, knees, around the eyes), thickening of tendons (Achilles and hand), and a gray ring around the iris of the eye (corneal arcus). Sadly, this condition often goes undiagnosed in low- and middle-income countries (LMICs). Compared to high-income countries, LMICs face a quadruple burden of higher LDL-C, underdiagnosis, lower treatment rates, and earlier heart attacks that call for concerted corrective action.[22,23]

The more common heterozygous form [heterozygous familial hypercholesterolemia (HeFH)] that affects 1 in 250 individuals is also underdiagnosed. Adult patients with HeFH commonly have untreated LDL-C levels of 190–450 mg/dL (depending on mutation severity and other factors) in association with a 50% risk of an ASCVD event by age 50 years in men and 65 years in women if they remain untreated. Less than 25% of patients with HeFH reach the recommended LDL target (<100 mg/dL), highlighting the need for improved diagnosis and treatment.[20,22-24]

Sitosterolemia

Sitosterolemia is a very rare genetic disorder characterized by increased absorption and decreased excretion of dietary plant sterols (phytosterols), which results in accumulation in blood and tissues. Manifestations range from xanthomas (fatty deposits under the skin), high coronary artery calcium score on radiographic imaging to premature CVD and acute myocardial infarction (AMI), and the need for coronary bypass surgery at a very young age <40 years.[25,26] Treatment calls for restriction of cholesterol and especially plant sterols in diet. Corn oil, rapeseed oil, sesame oil, rice oil, sesame seeds, peanuts, soybeans, and avocado are rich in plant sterols while vegetables and fruits such as potato, carrot, and apple have less plant sterols. Bile acid sequestrants and ezetimibe are the drugs used to reduce sterol absorption and promote excretion.[25,26]

High Triglycerides and Remnant Cholesterol

Triglycerides harbor RC, a sneaky culprit that constitutes 20% of the total TG, that independently increases heart disease risk while lowering both the LDL-C level and HDL-C **(Fig. 3)**. While elevated TG are known to decrease HDL-C, their impact on LDL-C is often overlooked. This is of particular concern for South Asians and others who consume with high-carbohydrate diets.[27,28] Early detection and management of high TG is crucial, especially for those on diets high on carbohydrates. The consumption of rice is several fold higher in India (630 g/day intake vs. Europe's 18 g/day).[28]

Total cholesterol comprises HDL-C, LDL-C, and RC (formerly VLDL). The risk of heart attack from TG is primarily mediated through RC, about 20% of TG, while the remaining 80% of TG, when elevated, primarily contributes to pancreatitis, not heart attacks. RC is atherogenic and is an important contributor to CAD in Indians who have high TG and is correlated with both prematurity and severity of CAD.[7]

The hidden danger posed by RC that may be overlooked can be brought to light by the following example: An individual with a normal TG level of 150 mg/dL has a normal RC level of 30 mg/dL. However, when TG increases by 200–350 mg/dL, RC increases by 40 mg/L to reach 70 mg/dL. This increase in RC is accompanied by a proportional decrease in LDL-C and HDL-C, creating a misleading impression of well-controlled LDL-C. Therefore, NHDL-C, which includes both LDL-C and RC, is a better predictor of cardiovascular risk when TG levels are elevated.

NON-HIGH-DENSITY LIPOPROTEIN-CHOLESTEROL: RELIABLE MEASURE TO ASSESS CARDIOVASCULAR DISEASE RISK

Non-HDL-C is calculated by subtracting HDL-C from TC. This simple, cost-effective test captures both LDL-C and RC, acting as a powerful predictor of heart disease. While Western nations have been successful in lowering NHDL-C, Asian countries face challenges due to dietary habits and limited statin access. In LMICs, economic growth at a fast pace has led to unhealthy dietary shifts contributing to rising NHDL-C and increased CVD deaths. Advantages of NHDL-C measurement are:[7]

- NHDL-C accounts for both LDL-C and RC, providing a more accurate risk assessment.
- NHDL-C can be done without fasting and without incurring additional expense.
- Depending on the TG level, NHDL-C is generally 25–36 mg higher than the LDL-C.
- The American Heart Association (AHA), in 2022, redefined the optimal lipid metric as NHDL-C 130 mg/dL; this level corresponds to LDL-C 100 mg/dL and TC 170 mg/dL (adjusted down from 200 mg/dL).
- NHDL-C of <100 mg/dL is a more appropriate target for Indians without CVD and 70–85 mg/dl for those with CAD; these levels should be achieved early and sustained over many decades.[29]

APOB TEST: A MORE PRECISE PREDICTOR OF CARDIOVASCULAR DISEASE RISK

Future guidelines may place more emphasis on ApoB test, as newer evidence suggests that it is a more accurate indicator of CVD risk than NHDL-C, TC, or LDL-C. Further points to note are:[30-35]

- Besides directly quantifying harmful cholesterol particles, ApoB measurement when TG is ≥200 mg/dL helps to determine the atherogenicity of high TG.
- Even very high TG (>500 mg/dL) may not indicate elevated CAD risk if ApoB remains low.
- High NHDL-C without elevated ApoB may not signal increased CVD risk, while high ApoB with normal NHDL-C does.
- Lp(a) is an independent ASCVD risk factor, even with normal ApoB. Its high atherogenic potential (6.6 × more than LDL-C per particle) makes Lp(a) an important factor in pathogenesis and in risk assessment (Chapter 8).

Apolipoprotein B test in Indians may offer some advantages over other tests as a predictor of risk of AMI especially among Indians whose TG levels, on average are 40 mg/dL higher than Whites.[36] The lipoprotein and ApoB profiles are different in Indians than Whites. A recent analysis involving data of 4,244 adults from Delhi, India, and 11,778 from the United States compared the lipids and ApoB among participants from India and the US. This study found that TC, NHDL-C, and LDL-C were higher among Americans, whereas TG, and ApoB were higher among Indians. The mean LDL-C (mg/dL) was 112 versus 105 and ApoB (mg/dL) 89 versus 95 in Americans and Indians, respectively.[31]

HIGH-DENSITY LIPOPROTEIN CHOLESTEROL: IS IT STILL "GOOD CHOLESTEROL"?

Our understanding of HDL-C has evolved. Though it was considered "good cholesterol" and a marker of good cardiovascular health, recent research paints a more complex picture.[37-41] Clinical trials to raise HDL-C level have failed to show any benefit. High HDL-C does not always indicate a lower risk for heart disease and heart attacks. In fact, some individuals who are genetically predisposed to high HDL-C may have an increased risk of heart attack. In the UK Biobank study (500,000 participants) HDL-C level above

80 mg/dL was associated with nearly double the risk of cardiovascular mortality and all-cause mortality.[37,38] Very high HDL may also be from chronic alcoholism or dysfunctional HDL that can contribute to heart disease. The present evidence points to a U-shaped relationship between HDL and mortality. Both very high and very low levels of HDL-C are associated with increased risk and based on our current knowledge the desired level of HDL-C for cardiovascular health is between 58 and 77 mg/dL.[37,38] HDL-C is no longer a treatment target and treatment strategies should be personalized to address each patient's unique risk profile.

INDIA'S CHOLESTEROL CHALLENGE

While national data on the epidemiology of dyslipidemia in different parts of the country and lipid profiles in India are limited, a recent large-scale study has provided valuable insights in these areas.[42,43] Importantly the prevalence of dyslipidemia varies widely among states **(Table 3)**.[42] One half or nearly one-half of subjects from Kerala and Goa had high cholesterol and high LDL-C whereas in Assam and Jharkhand it was 5–8%.[42] The high prevalence of dyslipidemia in Kerala and Goa aligns with the high rates of heart disease and heart attacks in these states and cries out for further studies to find answers as to why this is happening. Intriguingly, an Indian Council of Medical Research (ICMR) study showed that TC levels are 30–40 mg/dL higher in both rural and urban Kerala compared to the rest of India.[43,44] Though the reasons for consistently high TC in Kerala and Goa require further investigation, a possible link to high consumption of coconut is suggested.

Table 4 provides further information on lipid profile with breakdown on the population studied: Urban, rural, male, female. Overall mean values are provided and for comparison values from the US population are also provided. Important to note are the bottom two rows that show that LDL >130 mg/dL and TC >200 mg/dL in 21% and 24%, respectively. A word of caution needs to be added in comparing these numbers

TABLE 3: Epidemiology: Prevalence of dyslipidemia and their variance among select Indian states (n = 113,043).

States	TC >200 mg/dL	LDL-C >130 mg/dL	TG >150 mg/dL	HDL <40—M/<50—F
Kerala	50%	52%	33%	68%
Goa	46%	47%	32%	69%
Rajasthan	37%	35%	23%	52%
Gujarat	18%	16%	30%	56%
Karnataka	17%	12%	42%	71%
Andhra Pradesh	22%	18%	39%	64%
Tamil Nadu	22%	20%	33%	71%
Assam	8%	5%	28%	71%
Jharkhand	5%	3%	27%	75%

(F: female; HDL: high-density lipoprotein; LDL-C: low-density lipoprotein cholesterol; M: male; TC: total cholesterol; TG: triglycerides)
Source: Sharma et al.[42]

TABLE 4: Lipid profile in India compared to the US.[43-45]

	Urban (33,357)	Rural (79,506)	Male (M) (52,602)	Female (F) (60,441)	Overall (113,043)	US overall NA
TC (mg/dL)	175	167	169	170	170	189
TG (mg/dL)	149	136	153	128	140	M/F 108/85
LDL (mg/dL)	104	99	99	103	101	110
HDL (mg/dL/L)	41	41	40	42	41	M/F 49/59
LDL >130 mg/dL	24%	20%	17%	22%	21%	32%
TC >200 mg/dL	27%	22%	23%	25%	24%	33%

(HDL: high-density lipoprotein; LDL: low-density lipoprotein cholesterol; TC: total cholesterol; TG: triglycerides)

to those in the US. Though the numbers are higher in the US, one should not be sanguine as Indians have a multiplicity of factors (many known and some still being researched) that raise their risk for heart disease.

A previous cross-sectional study reported that almost one half of all Indians, both genders, had LDL-C exceeding 100 mg/dL. Concerningly, 50–60% of Indians with existing heart disease have LDL-C levels above 100 mg/dL, with 70% exceeding 170 mg/dL.[44,45]

Cholesterol Levels in the United States

The past 60 years have brought a wave of positive change in cholesterol levels in Americans. TC has seen a dramatic decline, dropping from an average of 222 mg/dL in the early 1960s to 190 mg/dL by 2018.[46,47] This positive trend extends to LDL-C and TG as well. The decline in cholesterol levels is a result of a multipronged approach, increased public health awareness, dietary changes, and the wider use of statin medications. Interestingly, despite having the highest obesity rates in the US, Black Americans show a more favorable lipid profile than the Whites, with a higher HDL level and lower NHDL-C (114 mg/dL).[47] There is room for further improvement as about 8% of adults in the US still had LDL-C exceeding 160 mg/dL in 2020.

CHOLESTEROL SCREENING AND LIPID TESTING

Universal cholesterol screening is now recommended in the US, starting between ages 9 and 11 years and again between 17 and 21 years.[48] According to the 2018 cholesterol guidelines, adults with normal cholesterol level are advised follow-up tests every 5 years.[6] These recommendations can be adapted for India as well: Start cholesterol screening at age 10 with follow-up checks every 5 years. More frequent testing is appropriate for those with abnormal results. Testing at an earlier age (2–5 years) is suggested for children with a family history of premature heart disease. The key takeaway is not to wait until midlife to get the first cholesterol screening. TC measurement is a screening test and may suffice to make treatment decisions but further lipid testing (also called lipoproteins or lipid panel or lipid profile) is needed if TC is ≥140 mg/mL for Indians).[49] Lipid testing is vital to assess heart disease risk in both children and adults as emphasized in the National Lipid Association (NLA) guidelines.[50] Notably, elevated LDL-C and NHDL-C levels in childhood and adolescence are associated

TABLE 5: Desired lipoprotein levels for Americans and Indians.[49,50,52]

	United States population	Indian population
Non-high-density cholesterol (NHDL-C)	130 mg/dL	100 mg/dL
Low-density lipoprotein cholesterol (LDL-C)	100 mg/dL	70 mg/dL
Total cholesterol	170 mg/dL	140 mg/dL
Triglycerides	150 mg/dL	150 mg/dL
Apolipoprotein B	80–100 mg/dL	65–80 mg/dL
High-density lipoprotein (HDL-C)	No longer a target	No longer a target

with mid-life subclinical atherosclerosis and clinical events, in a dose-dependent fashion independent of other risk factors.[50]

CHOLESTEROL AND LIPOPROTEIN IN INDIANS: DESIRED LEVELS

The AHA recently lowered its ideal NHDL-C target to 130 mg/dL, which corresponds to an LDL-C of 100 mg/dL.[51] Lp(a) and ApoB enrich LDL-C and increase their atherogenicity (plaque formation capability). Recognizing the occurrence of AMI at a lower LDL-C in Indians it is not only reasonable but appropriate to set a lower target of 70 mg/dL **(Table 5)**.

Current evidence indicates that atheromatous plaques may continue to accumulate even at a low LDL-C of 70 mg/dL and halting the progression requires an LDL-C of ≤60 mg/dL (below current official recommendations). Further impetus to aggressively lower LDL-C with lipid-lowering drugs comes from a study of patients who have had a heart attack that found that patients who achieved a LDL-C level of 24 mg/dL had regression of plaque volume and other objective benefits.[53] We will elaborate on this new area of aggressive treatment and how newer technologies are aiding in our assessment of coronary arteries on our chapters on statins and non-statins (Chapters 13 and 14).

■ KEY TAKEAWAYS

- Cholesterol-carrying atherogenic lipoproteins—VLDL (RC), IDL, LDL, and Lp(a)—are the instigators and drivers of plaque formation and ASCVDs.
- Among the atherogenic lipoproteins, LDL-C has the dominant role in causing ASCVD and is an essential factor in genesis of heart disease and heart attacks (AMI). High LDL-C level has a strong correlation with heart attacks.
- LDL score is a quantitative method (level × years) useful in CV risk assessment as plaque formation is "dose-related". Similar to quitting smoking early to avoid lung damage, controlling LDL-C early is required to prevent heart disease and heart attacks.
- Elevated TG requires scrutiny as it hides RC that increases CV risk.
- NHDL-C calculated by subtracting HDL from TC is a simple measure that is cost-effective and is a good predictor of heart disease. NHDL-C offers a more complete picture of heart disease risk than LDL-C alone. It also includes RC and ApoB.
- ApoB level is a superior predictor of CVD risk but ApoB test is not widely used and not covered by most insurance companies in the US. Indians have a different lipid profile (higher TG and ApoB) than Americans.
- There is marked regional variability in dyslipidemia in India. Total and LDL-C are high in ~50% of people tested in Kerala and Goa. This profile aligns with the high rate of heart attacks and heart diseases found in these states.
- HDL-C is no longer a treatment target and treatment strategies should be personalized to address each patient's unique risk profile.

- Universal cholesterol screenings are recommended in the US at early ages of 9–11 years and at ages 17 and 21 years. Testing at an even earlier age between 2 and 5 years is suggested for children with a family history of premature heart disease. Similar recommendations would be very appropriate for India.
- For Indians the desired lipoproteins levels are NHDL-C <100 mg/dL and LDL-C <70 mg/dL. These are 30 mg lower than that recommended for Americans. The lower target is due to increased and early heart attack risks in Indians at a lower level of atherogenic lipoproteins.
- New research points to marked benefits (including plaque volume regression and increase in blood flow) by aggressive lipid-lowering treatment to lower LDL-C to a level below than the currently recommended one (Chapter 13).
- Lifestyle modifications, especially diet and exercise, are essential steps to reduce CVDs (Chapters 16 and 17) and major adverse cardiac events (Chapters 11 and 12).

REFERENCES

1. Goldstein JL, Brown MS. A century of cholesterol and coronaries: from plaques to genes to statins. Cell. 2015;161(1):161-72.
2. Fernández-Friera L, Fuster V, López-Melgar B, Oliva B, García-Ruiz JM, Mendiguren J, et al. Normal LDL-cholesterol levels are associated with subclinical atherosclerosis in the absence of risk factors. J Am Coll Cardiol. 2017;70(24):2979-91.
3. Enas EA, Kuruvilla A. Retracing the heroic steps from lipid hypothesis to aggressive treatment of blood cholesterol: A revolution in preventive cardiology. In: Chopra HK (Ed). Textbook of Cardiology. New Delhi: Jaypee Brothers Medical Publishers; 2012. pp. 180-94.
4. Ference BA, Ginsberg HN, Graham I, Ray KK, Packard CJ, Bruckert E, et al. Low-density lipoproteins cause atherosclerotic cardiovascular disease. 1. Evidence from genetic, epidemiologic, and clinical studies. A consensus statement from the European Atherosclerosis Society Consensus Panel. Eur Heart J. 2017;38(32):2459-72.
5. NCD Risk Factor Collaboration (NCD-RisC). National trends in total cholesterol obscure heterogeneous changes in HDL and non-HDL cholesterol and total-to-HDL cholesterol ratio: a pooled analysis of 458 population-based studies in Asian and Western countries. Int J Epidemiol. 2020; 49(1):173-92.
6. Grundy SM, Stone NJ, Bailey AL, Beam C, Birtcher KK, Blumenthal RS, et al. 2018 AHA/ACC/AACVPR/AAPA/ABC/ACPM/ADA/AGS/APhA/ASPC/NLA/PCNA Guideline on the Management of Blood Cholesterol: Executive Summary: A Report of the American College of Cardiology/American Heart Association Task Force on Clinical Practice Guidelines. J Am Coll Cardiol. 2019;73(24):3168-209.
7. Enas EA, Chacko V, Pazhoor SG, Chennikkara H, Devarapalli HP. Dyslipidemia in South Asian patients. Curr Atheroscler Rep. 2007; 9(5):367-74.
8. Ference BA, Kastelein JJP, Catapano AL. Lipids and Lipoproteins in 2020. JAMA. 2020;324(6):595-6.
9. Ray KK, Ference B, Séverin T, Blom D, Nicholls SJ, Shiba MH, et al. World Heart Federation Cholesterol Roadmap 2022. Glob Heart. 2022;
10. Goldstein JL, Brown MS. The LDL receptor. Arterioscler Thromb Vasc Biol. 2009;29(4): 431-8.
11. Navar-Boggan AM, Peterson ED, D'Agostino RB Sr, Neely B, Sniderman AD, Pencina MJ. Hyperlipidemia in early adulthood increases long-term risk of coronary artery disease. Circulation. 2015;131:451-8.
12. Ferdinand KC, Nasser SA. PCSK9 Inhibition: discovery, current evidence, and potential effects on LDL-C and Lp(a). Cardiovasc Drugs Ther. 2015;29(3):295-308.
13. Ference BA, Yoo W, Alesh I, Mahajan N, Mirowska KK, Mewada A, et al. Effect of long-term exposure to lower low-density lipoprotein cholesterol beginning early in life on the risk of coronary artery disease: a Mendelian randomization analysis. J Am Coll Cardiol. 2012;60:2631-9.

14. Ibanez B, Fernández-Ortiz A, Fernández-Friera L, García-Lunar I, Andrés V, Fuster V. Progression of Early Subclinical Atherosclerosis (PESA) Study: JACC Focus Seminar 7/8. J Am Coll Cardiol. 2021;78(2):156-79.
15. Pletcher MJ, Bibbins-Domingo K, Liu K, Sidney S, Lin F, Vittinghoff E, et al. Nonoptimal lipids commonly present in young adults and coronary calcium later in life: the CARDIA (Coronary Artery Risk Development in Young Adults) study. Ann Intern Med. 2010;153(3):137-46.
16. Ference BA, Graham I, Tokgozoglu L, Catapano AL. Impact of Lipids on Cardiovascular Health: JACC Health Promotion Series. J Am Coll Cardiol. 2018;72(10):1141-56.
17. Hopkins PN, Brinton EA, Nanjee MN. Hyperlipoproteinemia type 3: the forgotten phenotype. Curr Atheroscler Rep. 2014;16(9):440.
18. Paquette M, Bernard S, Blank D, Paré G, Baass A. A simplified diagnosis algorithm for dysbetalipoproteinemia. J Clin Lipidol. 2020;14(4):431-7.
19. Beheshti SO, Madsen CM, Varbo A, Nordestgaard BG. Worldwide Prevalence of Familial Hypercholesterolemia: Meta-Analyses of 11 Million Subjects. J Am Coll Cardiol. 2020;75(20):2553-66.
20. Raal FJ, Pilcher GJ, Panz VR, van Deventer HE, Brice BC, Blom DJ, et al. Reduction in mortality in subjects with homozygous familial hypercholesterolemia associated with advances in lipid-lowering therapy. Circulation. 2011;124(20):2202-7.
21. Goldstein JL, Hobbs H, Brown M. Familial hypercholestrolemia. In: Scriver CR (Ed). Metabolic and Molecular Bases of Inherited Disease, 7th edition. New York: McGraw-Hill; 1995. pp. 1981-2030.
22. Tromp TR, Hartgers ML, Hovingh GK, Vallejo-Vaz AJ, Ray KK, Soran H, et al.; Homozygous Familial Hypercholesterolaemia International Clinical Collaborators. Worldwide experience of homozygous familial hypercholesterolaemia: retrospective cohort study. Lancet. 2022;399(10326):719-28.
23. Khera AV, Won HH, Peloso GM, Lawson KS, Bartz TM, Deng X, et al. Diagnostic Yield and Clinical Utility of Sequencing Familial Hypercholesterolemia Genes in Patients With Severe Hypercholesterolemia. J Am Coll Cardiol. 2016;67(22):2578-89.
24. Kawamura R, Saiki H, Tada H, Hata A. Acute myocardial infarction in a 25-year-old woman with sitosterolemia. J Clin Lipidol. 2018;12(1):246-9.
25. Salen G, Horak I, Rothkopf M, Cohen JL, Speck J, Tint GS, et al. Lethal atherosclerosis associated with abnormal plasma and tissue sterol composition in sitosterolemia with xanthomatosis. J Lipid Res. 1985;26(9):1126-33.
26. Kolovou G, Voudris V, Drogari E, Palatianos G, Cokkinos DV. Coronary bypass grafts in a young girl with sitosterolemia. Eur Heart J. 1996;17(6):965-6.
27. Chapman MJ, Ginsberg HN, Amarenco P, Andreotti F, Borén J, Catapano AL, et al.; European Atherosclerosis Society Consensus Panel. Triglyceride-rich lipoproteins and high-density lipoprotein cholesterol in patients at high risk of cardiovascular disease: evidence and guidance for management. Eur Heart J. 2011;32(11):1345-61.
28. Enas EA, Senthilkumar A, Chennikkara H, Bjurlin MA. Prudent diet and preventive nutrition from pediatrics to geriatrics: current knowledge and practical recommendations. Indian Heart J. 2023;55:310-38.
29. Enas EA, Varkey B. Management of dyslipidemia in Indians: Implications of cholesterol guidelines and practical applications. In: Rao G (Ed). Clinical Handbook of Coronary Artery Disease, 1st edition. Bombay: Jaypee Brothers Medical Publishers; 2020.
30. Schubert J, Leosdottir M, Lindahl B, Westerbergh J, Melhus H, Modica A, et al. Intensive early and sustained lowering of non-high-density lipoprotein cholesterol after myocardial infarction and prognosis: the SWEDEHEART registry. Eur Heart J. 2024;45(39):4204-15.
31. Singh K, Thanassoulis G, Dufresne L, Nguyen A, Gupta R, Narayan KV, et al. A Comparison of Lipids and apoB in Asian Indians and Americans. Glob Heart. 2021;16(1):7.

32. Singh K, Prabhakaran D. Apolipoprotein B—An ideal biomarker for atherosclerosis? Indian Heart J. 2024;76 Suppl 1(Suppl 1): S121-S129.
33. Sniderman AD, Thanassoulis G, Glavinovic T, Navar AM, Pencina M, Catapano A, et al. Apolipoprotein B Particles and Cardiovascular Disease: A Narrative Review. JAMA Cardiol. 2019;4(12):1287-95.
34. Marston NA, Giugliano RP, Melloni GEM, Park JG, Morrill V, Blazing MA, et al. Association of Apolipoprotein B-Containing Lipoproteins and Risk of Myocardial Infarction in Individuals With and Without Atherosclerosis: Distinguishing Between Particle Concentration, Type, and Content. JAMA Cardiol. 2022;7(3):250-6.
35. Khan SU, Khan MU, Valavoor S, Khan MS, Okunrintemi V, Mamas MA, et al. Association of lowering apolipoprotein B with cardiovascular outcomes across various lipid-lowering therapies: systematic review and meta-analysis of trials. Eur J Prev Cardiol. 2020;27(12):1255-68.
36. Soffer DE, Marston NA, Maki KC, Jacobson TA, Bittner VA, Peña JM, et al. Role of apolipoprotein B in the clinical management of cardiovascular risk in adults: An Expert Clinical Consensus from the National Lipid Association. J Clin Lipidol. 2024;18(5): e647-e663.
37. Liu C, Dhindsa D, Almuwaqqat Z, Sun YV, Quyyumi AA. Very High High-Density Lipoprotein Cholesterol Levels and Cardiovascular Mortality. Am J Cardiol. 2022;167: 43-53.
38. Liu C, Dhindsa D, Almuwaqqat Z, Ko YA, Mehta A, Alkhoder AA, et al. Association Between High-Density Lipoprotein Cholesterol Levels and Adverse Cardiovascular Outcomes in High-risk Populations. JAMA Cardiol. 2022;7(7):672-80.
39. Madsen CM, Nordestgaard BG. Is it time for new thinking about high-density lipoprotein? Arterioscler Thromb Vasc Biol. 2018;38(3):484-6.
40. Madsen CM, Varbo A, Nordestgaard BG. Extreme high high-density lipoprotein cholesterol is paradoxically associated with high mortality in men and women: two prospective cohort studies. Eur Heart J. 2017;38(32):2478-86.
41. Mamede I, Braga MAP, Martins OC, Franchini AEO, Silveira Filho RB, Santos MCF. Association between very high HDL-C levels and mortality: a systematic review and meta-analysis. J Clin Lipidol. 2024;18(5): e701-e709.
42. Sharma S, Gaur K, Gupta R. Trends in epidemiology of dyslipidemias in India. Indian Heart J. 2024;76 Suppl 1:S20-S28.
43. Shah B, Mathur P. Surveillance of cardiovascular disease risk factors in India: the need & scope. Indian J Med Res. 2010;132: 634-42.
44. Thankappan KR, Shah B, Mathur P, Sarma PS, Srinivas G, Mini GK, et al. Risk factor profile for chronic non-communicable diseases: results of a community-based study in Kerala, India. Indian J Med Res. 2010;131:53-63.
45. Guptha S, Gupta R, Deedwania P, Bhansali A, Maheshwari A, Gupta A, et al. Cholesterol lipoproteins and prevalence of dyslipidemias in urban Asian Indians: a cross sectional study. Indian Heart J. 2014;66(3):280-8.
46. Aggarwal R, Bhatt DL, Rodriguez F, Yeh RW, Wadhera RK. Trends in Lipid Concentrations and Lipid Control Among US Adults, 2007-2018. JAMA. 2022;328(8):737-45.
47. Sayed A, Navar AM, Slipczuk L, Ballantyne CM, Samad Z, Lavie CJ, et al. Prevalence, Awareness, and Treatment of Elevated LDL Cholesterol in US Adults, 1999-2020. JAMA Cardiol. 2023;8(12):1185-7.
48. Daniels SR; U.S. Department of Health and Human Services; National Heart Lung and Blood Institute. (2012). Expert Panel on Integrated Guidelines for Cardiovascular Health and Risk Reduction in Children and Adolescents: Full Report. [online] Available from http://www.nhlbi.nih.gov/guidelines/ cvd_ped/index.htm [Last accessed May 2025].
49. Enas EA, Varkey B, Gupta R. Expanding statin use for prevention of ASCVD in Indians: reasoned and simplified proposals. Indian Heart J. 2020;72(2):65-9.

50. Wilson PWF, Jacobson TA, Martin SS, Jackson EJ, Le NA, Davidson MH, et al. Lipid measurements in the management of cardiovascular diseases: Practical recommendations, a scientific statement from the national lipid association writing group. J Clin Lipidol. 2021;15(5):629-48.
51. Lloyd-Jones DM, Larson MG, Leip EP, Beiser A, D'Agostino RB, Kannel WB, et al. Lifetime risk of developing congestive heart failure. The Framingham Heart Study. Circulation. 2002;106:3068-72.
52. Enas EA. Ethnicity and Cardiovascular Disease. In: Kapadia S (Ed). Textbook of Interventional Cardiology: A Global Perspective. New Delhi: Jaypee Brothers Medical Publishers; 2017.
53. Biccirè FG, Häner J, Losdat S, Ueki Y, Shibutani H, Otsuka T, et al. Concomitant Coronary Atheroma Regression and Stabilization in Response to Lipid-Lowering Therapy. J Am Coll Cardiol. 2023;82(18):1737-47.

CHAPTER 8

Lipoprotein(a): Underrecognized Heritable Risk Factor for Heart Disease

INTRODUCTION

Lipoprotein(a) [Lp(a)] is a genetically determined risk factor for atherosclerotic cardiovascular disease (ASCVD) that affects a large number (~1.5 billion) of people worldwide and is often overlooked in clinical practice.[1] Deficits in understanding the atherogenic properties of Lp(a) and standardized guidelines for assessment and management contribute to this oversight. We are in full agreement with Nathan Wong's forthright statement *"The failure to screen and identify those with Lp(a)-associated risk represents a missed opportunity to address this risk, not only with our existing repertoire of treatments, but hopefully in the future with promising therapies in development targeting Lp(a)."*[2] Previously we have extensively reviewed the topic of Lp(a).[3,4] Our aim, in this chapter, is to provide our readers up-to-date clinically focused information on Lp(a) that can be readily applied to practice.

Lipoprotein(a) is a lipoprotein that carries cholesterol, triglycerides, phospholipids, cholesterol esters, and apolipoproteins and each one of these has disease-causing risk.[5] Lp(a) is atherogenic (causes atherosclerosis) and is the most potent of the four atherogenic lipoproteins [~6-fold more atherogenic than low-density lipoprotein cholesterol (LDL-C)].[6] Lp(a) has apolipoprotein(a) covalently linked to an apolipoprotein(apo) B-containing lipoprotein. Both these apolipoproteins contribute to atherosclerosis. Lp(a) is not only atherogenic but also prothrombotic, pro-inflammatory, and pro-calcific.[7] The expression of apo(a) component is controlled by the *LPA* gene and thus 90% of Lp(a) level is genetically predetermined.[8,9]

Genetic Determination of Lp(a)

Lp(a) levels are determined at the time conception by the Lp(a) gene (*LPA*) passed on to a child from one of the parents with this gene. The children, siblings, and parents of each person with the *LPA* gene has a 50% chance of inheriting it.[10,11] The *LPA* gene located on chromosome 6q26-q27 is the major gene locus for Lp(a) concentrations and this gene is one of the strongest monogenic risk factors for coronary artery disease (CAD). Cloning and sequencing of LPA reveal an extensive structural homology with the plasminogen gene.[12] Genetic variants including a highly polymorphic copy number variation of the so-called kringle IV-2 (KIV-2) repeats at this locus have a pronounced influence on Lp(a) concentrations **(Figs. 1 and 2B)**.[3]

Prevalence of Lp(a)

Prevalence of Lp(a) globally and in the US is shown on **Table 1 and Figure 2A**. One in five individuals worldwide (~1.5 billion) are estimated to have high Lp(a) of ≥100–125 nmol/L (~50 mg/dL).[13] Prevalence is ~3 times higher than diabetes and ~60 times higher than familial hypercholesterolemia (FH).[14-16]

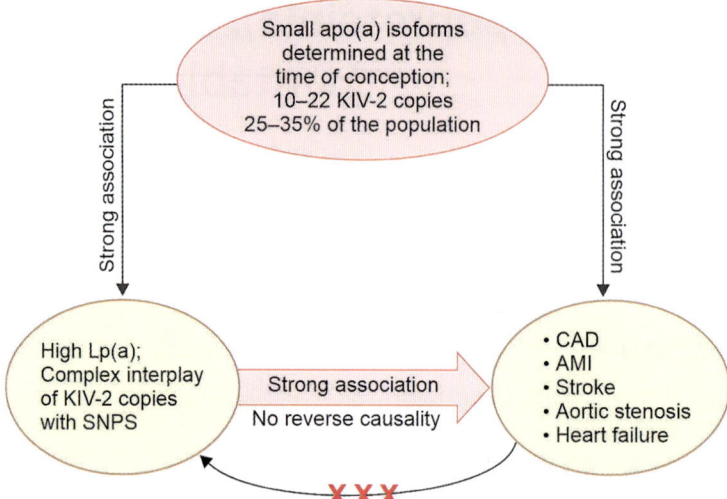

Fig. 1: Small Lipoprotein(a) [Lp(a)] isoforms (10–22 KIV copies) determined at the time of conception determine the Lp(a) level, which in turn determines the cardiovascular phenotypic expression. (AMI: acute myocardial infarction; CAD: coronary artery disease; SNPS: single nucleotide polymorphisms)
Source: Enas EA, Varkey B, Dharmarajan TS, Pare G, Bahl VK. Lipoprotein(a): An independent, genetic, and causal factor for cardiovascular disease and acute myocardial infarction. Indian Heart J. 2019;71(2):99-112.[3]

TABLE 1: Lipoprotein(a) [Lp(a)] distribution in the general population.

Lp(a) levels	>30 mg/dL	60 mg/dL	90 mg/dL	116 mg/dL	180 mg/dL
Prevalence	35%	20%	10%	5%	1%
Number global	2.45 billion	1.4 billion	700 million	38 million	8 million
United States	112 million	64 million	32 million	16 million	3 million

Source: Adapted from Tsimikas S, Stroes ESG. The dedicated "Lp(a) clinic": A concept whose time has arrived? Atherosclerosis. 2020;300:1-9.[16]

Ethnic Differences in Lp(a)

The prevalence of high Lp(a) levels >50 mg/dL varies from 10 to 30% depending on ancestry with South Asians having median Lp(a) level that is 60% higher than in Whites and double that of Chinese **(Fig. 3)**.[17]

Blacks (Africans and African Americans) have the highest Lp(a) level.[19-21] An unexplained observation is that the type of CVD may be different, as high Lp(a) in African Americans is linked more to peripheral artery disease (PAD) and abdominal aortic aneurysms,[19,21,22] while in Indians and Whites it is linked to heart disease.[20] In the INTERHERT Lp(a) study South Asians had highest risk of AMI from elevated Lp(a).[20]

HIGH LIPOPROTEIN(A) RISK OF ATHEROSCLEROTIC CARDIOVASCULAR DISEASE AND OTHER DISORDERS

Stability of Lp(a) Levels Over Time and Disease Associations

Unlike other risk factors that may change over time, genetically determined Lp(a)

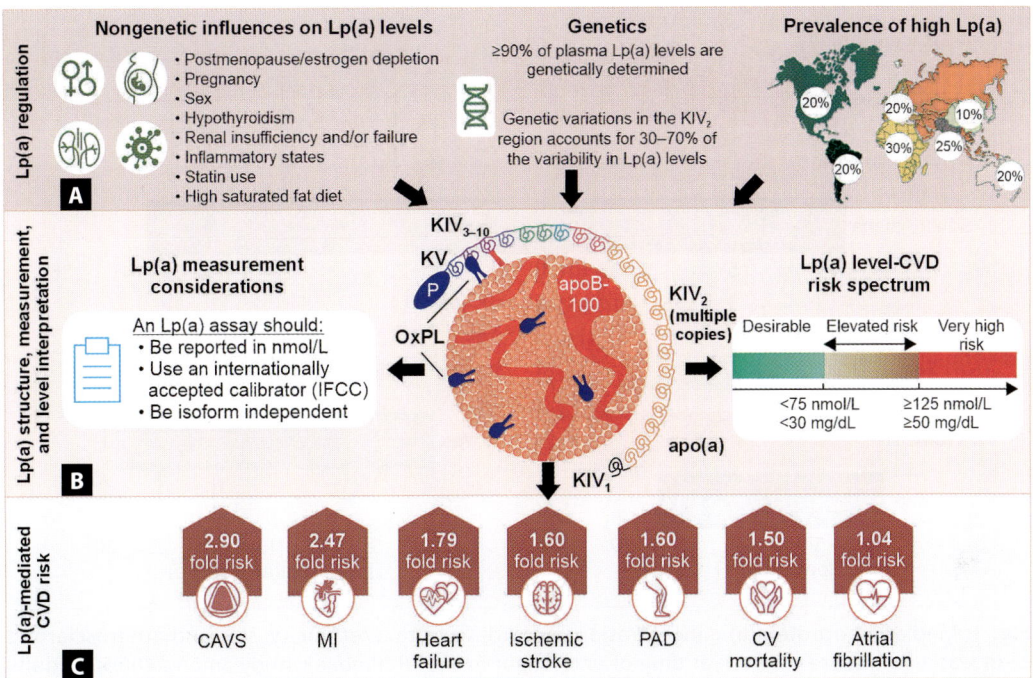

Figs. 2A to C: Overview of the structure, regulation, measurement considerations, and level interpretation of lipoprotein(a) [Lp(a)] and cardiovascular disease (CVD)-associated risk. (A) Listing of non-genetic and genetic factors that modulate Lp(a) levels. Lp(a) levels are primarily determined by variability in the *LPA* gene which codes for the apolipoprotein(a) [apo(a)] component of the particle. The prevalence of high Lp(a) levels ranges from 10 to 30% and varies depending on ancestry; (B) The Lp(a) particle comprises a single apolipoprotein B-100 (apoB-100) containing lipoprotein covalently associated with apo(a). Oxidized phospholipids (OxPLs) are covalently associated with apo(a), apoB-100 and the lipid core. Apo(a) consists of 10 kringle IV (KIV) domains, a single KV domain and an inactive, protease-like domain. Different apo(a) isoforms have different KIV2 copy numbers; (C) Adjusted hazard ratios for select CVD outcomes comparing participants in the top percentile of Lp(a) distribution.
Source: Reprinted with permission from Masson W, Barbagelata L, Oberti P, Falconi M, Lavalle-Cobo A, Corral P, et al. High lipoprotein(a) levels and mitral valve disease: A systematic review. Nutr Metab Cardiovasc Dis. 2023;33(5):925-33.[18]

remains relatively stable from childhood to adulthood and therefore the risk imparted by Lp(a) is lifelong. High Lp(a) levels are strongly associated with CAD, ischemic stroke **(Fig. 2C)** and other ASCVDs. In addition to ASCVDs, Lp(a) is suspected to play a role in various other diseases/disorders-mitral valve disease,[24] chronic kidney disease,[25-27] preeclampsia,[28] and low birth weight.[29] **Figure 2C** shows the strong association (2.90-fold risk) between high Lp(a) and calcific aortic valve stenosis (CAVS), the most prevalent form of valvular heart disease. The *LPA* gene is the only identified monogenic risk factor for CAVS.[29] Reciprocally, genetically lowered Lp(a) levels by one standard deviation lower risk of CAVS (37%) PAD (31%), CAD (29%), heart failure (17%), and stroke (13%).[30] Thus pharmacological lowering of plasma Lp(a) has the potential to positively alter the course of a range of atherosclerosis-related diseases.

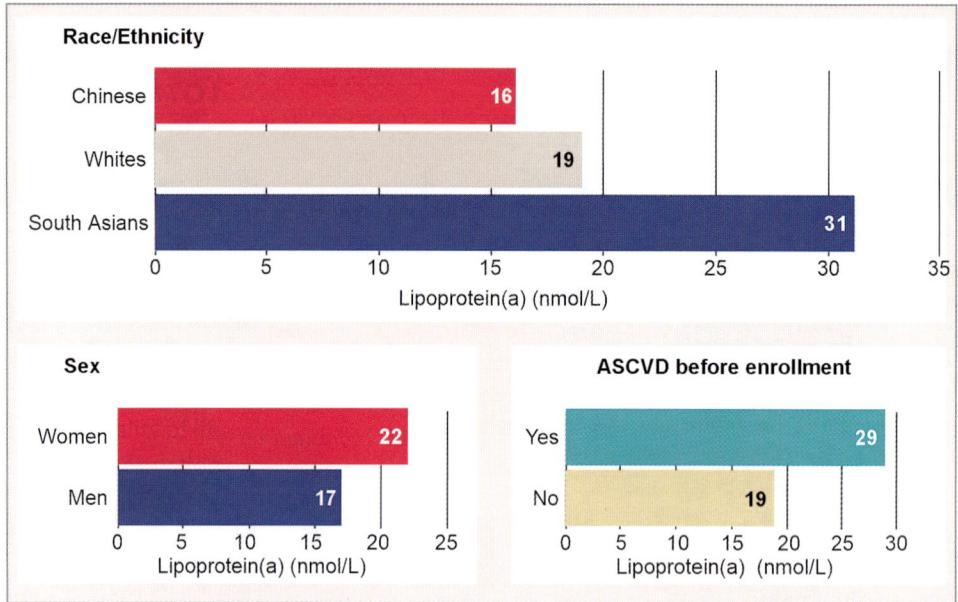

Fig. 3: Median lipoprotein(a) concentrations according to race/ethnicity, sex, and atherosclerotic cardiovascular disease (ASCVD) at time of enrollment in the UK Biobank study among 460,506 adults 40–69 years of age with a median follow-up of 11.2 years.
Source: Adapted from Patel AP, Wang M, Kartoun U, Ng K, Khera AV. Quantifying and Understanding the Higher Risk of Atherosclerotic Cardiovascular Disease Among South Asian Individuals: Results from the UK Biobank Prospective Cohort Study. Circulation. 2021;144(6):410-22.[23]

Heart disease (CAD) and heart attacks (AMIs): The properties of Lp(a) that increase the risk for coronary artery disease (CAD) and acute myocardial infarction (AMI) are listed in **Table 2**.

A recent study of Lp(a) and monocyte subsets in 60 patients with coronary atherosclerosis and in a control group of 30 apparently healthy persons showed that the patients had a significantly higher median monocytic percentage, higher Lp(a), and higher C-reactive protein values than the controls.[36] Among the patients, those with high Lp(a) had higher non-classical monocytes (31.5% vs. 20%) and the severity of coronary atherosclerosis was associated with both higher Lp(a) levels and non-classical monocytes. This provides a tie between monocytes and inflammation in high Lp(a) and leads the way to studies on cellular inflammation and possibly to strategies to slow atherosclerosis.

Elevated Lp(a) is a powerful risk factor for CVD, associated with both premature onset and severe manifestations such as heart attacks and strokes.[4] A recent meta-analysis of 14 (five prospective and nine retrospective) studies (series ranging from 350 to 18,544 patients) showed that elevated Lp(a) levels were significantly associated with increased risk of major adverse cardiovascular event (MACE), all-cause mortality, myocardial infarction, and revascularization in patients with ischemic heart disease.[37] **Table 3** lists the adverse impacts of high Lp(a) on CVD.

Effects on patients with known ASCVD: Now that the properties of Lp(a) and the impact

TABLE 2: Lipoprotein(a) [Lp(a)] increases the risk for coronary artery disease (CAD) and acute myocardial infarction (AMI).[20,31-35]

A lifelong risk	As it is genetically transmitted the risk from high Lp(a) is lifelong. A test done in childhood is valuable to assess long-term CV risk as the level remains mostly steady through adulthood. Only ≤10% of the level is non-genetically influenced and these conditions are shown in **Figure 2A**
Increasing threat along a continuum of Lp(a) levels	Even levels of seemingly low Lp(a), around 30 mg/dL, can pose a risk similar to that of low-density lipoprotein cholesterol (LDL-C) of around 130 mg/dL[30]
The higher the level, the higher the risk	Lp(a) risk increases with each rise in its level. Every 50 nmol/L (20 mg/dL) increase translates to an 11% greater chance of heart disease.[28] This makes especially high levels (>180 mg/dL) particularly risky[11] as their risk is similar to those with familial hypercholesterolemia (FH)
Atherogenesis	It promotes plaque buildup such as LDL-C but is much more potent. Lp(a) level in blood correlates with its accumulation in atherosclerotic plaque
Inflammation	It promotes inflammatory changes that accelerate pathological changes in the arterial wall
Accelerated progression	Accelerated progression of high-risk plaque (necrotic core) with increased risk of AMI[32-34]
Increased vulnerable coronary plaques and rapid progression demonstrated with computed tomography angiography (CTA) imaging	Prospective serial CTA imaging, with a 10-year scan interval has shown increased burden of high-risk, inflammatory, rupture prone, coronary plaques at baseline and rapid progression of plaque burden in patients with elevated Lp(a) levels compared with patients with low Lp(a)[33,34]

TABLE 3: Multidimensional impact of high lipoprotein(a) [Lp(a)] on coronary artery disease (CAD), acute myocardial infarction (AMI), and major adverse cardiovascular event (MACE).

Characteristics	*Comments*
Severity CAD	Individuals with elevated Lp(a) are more likely to experience multivessel disease, left main disease, or polyvascular disease[38-44]
Thrombus burden	Lp(a) has been linked to increased thrombus burden in culprit arteries, contributing to the risk of MI, and other cardiovascular events[44,45]
Acute coronary syndrome (ACS) in young and multivessel disease	A study of 1,021 patients with ACS in India reported elevated Lp(a) (≥50 mg/dL) in 34% of the patients (more were young). The study also showed a strong link between elevated Lp(a) and multivessel disease (40% vs. 26% single-vessel disease)[46]
Premature myocardial infarction	Lp(a) is consistently linked to an increased risk of early-onset MI.[47-49] Studies show that elevated Lp(a) detected before the age of 20 significantly increases the risk of major adverse cardiovascular event (MACE) before age 50[3,31,47,50,51]
Severity of AMI and recurrence of MI	Elevated Lp(a) is associated with larger MI events, resulting in heart failure and poor outcomes. Elevated Lp(a) is also associated with recurrent MACE, including MI, stroke, and cardiovascular death[43,52-54]

Contd...

Contd...

Characteristics	Comments
MI with nonobstructive coronary arteries (MINOCA)	Lp(a) has been implicated in the pathogenesis of MINOCA[55]
Premenopausal MI	Elevated Lp(a) is a risk factor for MI in premenopausal women[56,57]
Coronary revascularization	Both initial and repeat revascularization are more common in individuals with higher Lp(a).[50,58] Elevated Lp(a) levels have been linked to an increased risk of in-stent restenosis—a condition where the vessel re-narrows after a percutaneous coronary intervention (PCI). This is likely due to Lp(a)'s propensity to accumulate in areas of vascular injury, such as those caused by stent placement or coronary artery bypass graft (CABG) surgery.[59] This underscores the importance of considering Lp(a) levels in treatment decisions for PCI[59] as elevated Lp(a) can turn a successful procedure into a temporary fix[60,61]
Increased MACE	Increased risk of AMI[20,49,53,62] and stroke in young adults[63] and children[64]
Increased mortality	Elevated Lp(a) is associated with a worse long-term prognosis, including increased risk of cardiovascular death[65-68]

of high Lp(a) on cardiovascular diseases **(Tables 2 and 3)** have been explained, it is contextual to examine the effects of high Lp(a) level on those with prior ASCVD and compare them to those without known ASCVD. In two large cohort studies, Lp(a) levels were measured in 21,400 patients (62% had a history of ASCVD) between 2000 and 2019. Among those with no prior ASCVD, the absolute ASCVD risk for the top 10% was lower (26%) but a linear association was found between Lp(a) and cardiovascular events ($p < 0.001$). In contrast, among those with prior ASCVD, the absolute ASCVD events were higher (93%) ($p < 0.001$) and plateaued at Lp(a) levels between 150 and 200 nmol/L.[69]

IMPORTANCE OF LIPOPROTEIN(A) MEASUREMENT IN PATIENT MANAGEMENT

A standard lipid profile test does not include Lp(a) and normal levels of LDL-C and triglyceride (TG) do not rule out the possibility of a high Lp(a). Several national organizations and specialty associations now recommend Lp(a) measurement at least once in each adult person's lifetime.[5,8,70,71] This consensus guidance for a Lp(a) test is particularly important in understanding that CVD events may occur in the absence of traditional risk factors.[72] In such situations and in premature CVD, the physician can target modifiable lifestyle factors more intensively and can more readily increase the patient's understanding and active involvement in his or her care.

A recent observational analysis of participants from the Multiethnic Study of Atherosclerosis (MESA), followed for a median of 13.4 years, demonstrated that CVD risk in a primary prevention setting significantly increased with high Lp(a), even when LDL-C levels are optimal.[73,74] Lp(a) is now recognized as a risk-enhancing factor for CVDs and measuring Lp(a) levels is recommended for a comprehensive CVD risk assessment.[75]

Recent studies have shown that the risk of a MACE with Lp(a) >30 mg/dL and LDL-C

>130 mg/dL is comparable, each increasing the risk two-fold and to four-fold when both Lp(a) and LDL-C are elevated.[31]

While traditional risk factors such as high LDL-C, blood pressure, and diabetes increase the baseline risk for ASCVD events, Lp(a) significantly amplifies it. This was well demonstrated in a study **(Fig. 4)** that showed a significantly increased risk of MACEs in individuals with both high Lp(a) levels and high baseline risk compared to those with low baseline risk (43.1% vs. 8.6%).[5] The figure also shows (text in red) that as Lp(a) level increases the risk of ASCVD events also rises.

In a large, pooled cohort of 27,756 persons without previous ASCVD, from five prospective studies in the United States, the risk of ASCVD from diabetes (odds ratio 1.42) increased significantly when associated with elevated Lp(a) (odds ratio 1.92).[65] This report, because of its magnitude and prospective design, supersedes other reports with some variance and establishes the additive risk of diabetes and high Lp(a)–both of concern and importance to Indians. Therefore Lp(a) level should be measured and optimal goal-directed management of all traditional risk factors is of importance to all and is of the highest priority in Indians who are at a high risk for MACE.

As listed on **Tables 2 and 3** and further explained in the text, high Lp(a) has a multi-dimensional impact on CAD, AMI, and MACE. Many studies have also linked high Lp(a) to premature onset of CAD and to severe disease. Thus, as we have stated in our previous publications,[3,4,20,76] there is ample ground to suspect that high Lp(a) has more than a contributory role, likely a causal role, in

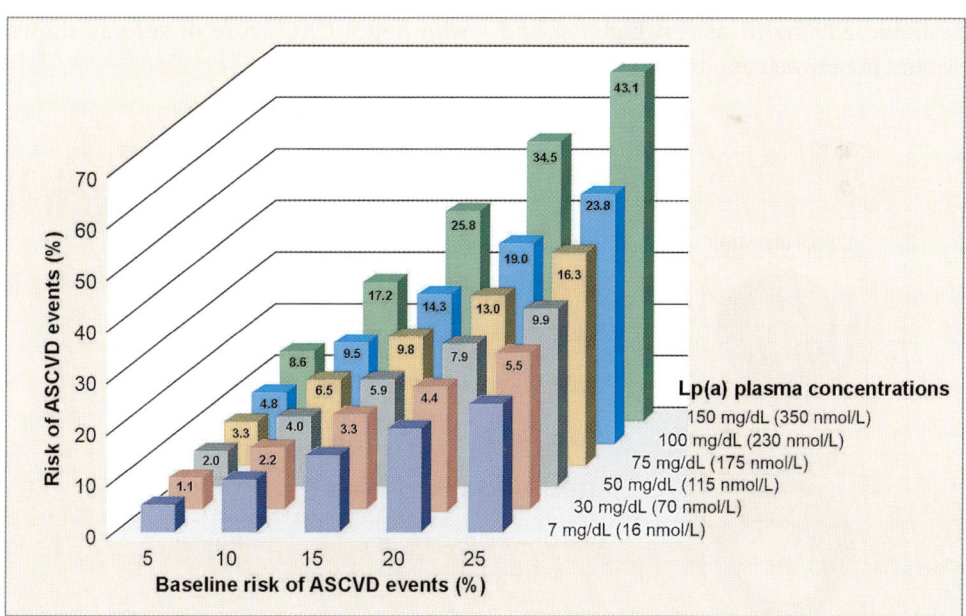

Fig. 4: Synergistic risk of varying baseline atherosclerotic cardiovascular disease (ASCVD) risk and Lp(a) levels.
Source: Reproduced with permission from Kronenberg F, Mora S, Stroes ESG, Ference BA, Arsenault BJ, Berglund L, et al. Lipoprotein(a) in atherosclerotic cardiovascular disease and aortic stenosis: a European Atherosclerosis Society consensus statement. Eur Heart J. 2022;43(39):3925-46.[5]

premature and severe CAD in Indians who have no or only scanty traditional risk factors.

LIPOPROTEIN(A): WHAT IS THE THRESHOLD VALUE FOR INCREASED CARDIOVASCULAR DISEASE RISK?

It is recommended that Lp(a) be tested by an isoform insensitive assay and the result be reported in nmol/L though the older and familiar version of milligrams per deciliter (mg/dL) continues to be used. The UK Biobank data showed that there is not a single threshold that signifies CVD risk from elevated Lp(a). "The continuous gradient of risk with increased Lp(a) implies that clinical decision-making should be influenced by the degree of Lp(a) elevation and the patient's other risk factors, not the mere presence of elevated Lp(a)."[8] The same concept is graphically depicted in **(Fig. 2B)**: <30 mg/dL as desirable, ≥50 mg/dL as very high risk and the values in between as elevated risk.

ACTIONABLE PLANS FOR THOSE AT RISK

Risk Calculators

The measured level of Lp(a) can be incorporated into the ACC/AHA 10-year predicted risk assessment to get the patient's risk category and to implement mitigation interventions appropriate for that category. Thus, it was observed that ASCVD was 11% higher for each 50 nmol/L increment of Lp(a);[18,19] the 10-year risk estimate for a patient with an Lp(a) of 200 nmol/L is 1.52-fold higher than modeled in ACC/AHA pooled cohort equation.[8]

Coronary Artery Calcium (CAC) Score

A CAC score of ≥100 and high Lp(a) level in the upper quintile in asymptomatic people was associated with ~5-fold increase in CVD risk compared to those in the lower quintiles who had a CAC score of zero as shown in **Figure 5**.[77]

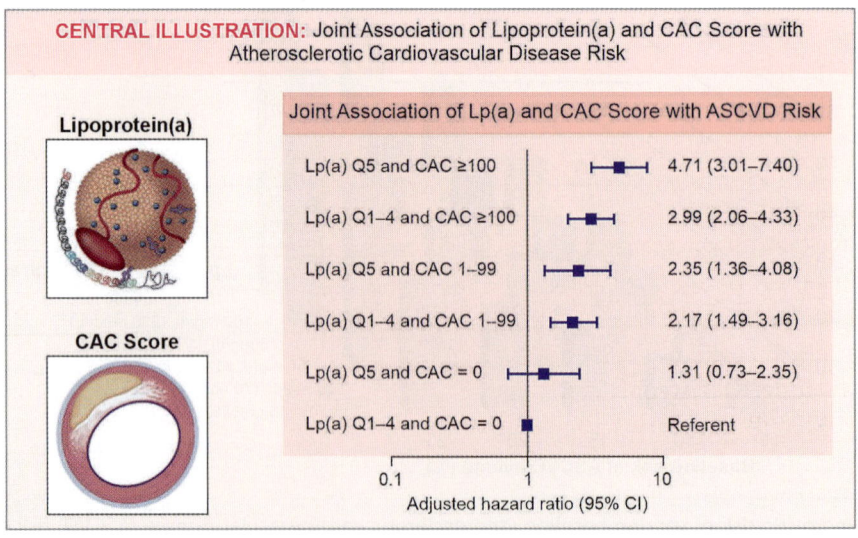

Fig. 5: Joint association of lipoprotein(a) [Lp(a)] and coronary artery calcium (CAC) score.
Source: Reproduced with permission Mehta A, Vasquez N, Ayers CR, Patel J, Hooda A, Khera A, et al. Independent Association of Lipoprotein(a) and Coronary Artery Calcification with Atherosclerotic Cardiovascular Risk. J Am Coll Cardiol. 2022;79(8):757-68.[75]

MANAGEMENT: GENERAL MEASURES

Cascade screening identifies family members with the same genetic condition as the patient. Cascade testing for high Lp(a) in relatives of a person with high Lp(a) can identify others with high Lp(a). This is particularly indicated and effective when the person has both elevated Lp(a) and FH. High Lp(a) is often found in persons with FH and increases their risk for cardiovascular adverse events ~5-fold.[68,78,79] Early identification enables lifestyle modifications and appropriate medications and early interventions.

Lifestyle modifications are essential in managing all CVDs and target modifiable risk factors by following "Life's Essential 8"— healthy diet, physical activity, healthy weight, healthy sleep, avoidance of tobacco smoking, healthy levels of blood lipids, blood glucose, and blood pressure. Though these steps do not lower Lp(a) they have a salutary effect in improving outcomes.[80]

Lipoprotein apheresis is the only currently Food and Drug Administration (FDA)-approved modality to reduce Lp(a) by removing apo B and apo A containing lipoproteins. Lipoprotein apheresis is effective in acutely lowering Lp(a) by ~70% and ~35% time averaged between bi-weekly treatment sessions.[81] Moriarty et al. reported a remarkable recovery of an 11-year-old boy with multiple thrombotic strokes due to high Lp(a) who underwent lipoprotein apheresis and made a full recovery with no stroke recurrence. Presently apheresis, a costly and cumbersome modality is indicated in very high-risk persons such as those with FH and high Lp(a), those with multiple risk factors and recurrent CVD events associated with high Lp(a).

Medications

Currently approved and available medications, primarily aim to reduce comorbidities and to reduce MACE. Medication management is best done by cardiologists, especially those with a focus on prevention and dyslipidemia management.

Statins are indicated in those with elevated non-high-density lipoprotein cholesterol (NHDL-C), though they do not reduce Lp(a) and may moderately increase Lp(a) level by 9-20%.[82] However, this should not dissuade the use of statins as their proven benefit of reducing MACE far outweighs the risk.[83]

Niacin can lower Lp(a) but has not shown any incremental benefit to statin in reducing MACE.[84] It is also associated with adverse effects.

Ezetimibe and *bempedoic acid* used in reducing LDL-C (Chapter 14) are not recommended in Lp(a) management. But they are to be considered to reduce MACE, if LDL-C remains above goals.[8]

Proprotein convertase subtilisin kexin 9 (PCSK9) inhibitors can lower Lp(a) and lower LDL-C but has not been approved for this indication by the FDA.[84-86]

Aspirin use in prophylaxis of cardiovascular events has fallen into disfavor. However, it is recommended in those with high Lp(a) as two separate trials have shown their efficacy in reducing cardiovascular events.[87-89]

MANAGEMENT: TARGETED SPECIFIC MEASURES

New Targeted Lp(a) Lowering Drugs

Antisense oligonucleotides (ASOs) are short, synthetic, single-stranded RNA or DNA molecules that can bind to specific RNA molecules and alter RNA.[90,91] Small interfering RNA (siRNA) is a type of RNA molecule that plays a crucial role in gene silencing.[92] It is a double-stranded RNA molecule that is processed from longer RNA transcripts. siRNA binds to specific messenger RNA (mRNA) molecules, leading to their degradation and preventing the translation of the corresponding gene into a protein. ASOs are injected subcutaneously and enter the liver, where they bind to the mRNA) of Lp(a) and disrupt protein translation. This prevents the production of apo(a) in the hepatocyte, which is the source of about 99% of plasma Lp(a).

Several new drugs are in various phases of clinical trials and hold promise that in 2025–2026 there would be effective drugs for reducing Lp(a). Among these drugs are muvalaplin, olpasiran, lepodisiran, pelacarsen, and zerlasiran.[91] Pelacarsen, an ASO medication, is on the late phase of a large scale, randomized, double-blind, placebo-controlled study (HORIZON trial) to determine cardiovascular outcomes and safety of the drug. In a phase 2 randomized clinical trial zerlasiran, another ASO drug that acts by gene silencing blocking production of a protein needed to make Lp(a), yielded very positive results. In a trial over the course of 36 weeks, zerlasiran reduced Lp(a) levels by >80% on average without major side effects.[92]

Another exciting new development is gene-editing technology such as clustered regularly interspersed short palindromic repeats (CRISPR) that can revolutionize the treatment of genetically inherited disorders. It is quite possible that gene-editing technology can target the *LPA* gene thereby "cure" the excessive production of Lp(a).[93]

■ KEY TAKEAWAYS

- High Lp(a), the most common genetic hyperlipidemia affects one in five people and increases the risk for ASCVD: CAD, ischemic stroke, and PAD.
- Indians have a high prevalence (25%) of high Lp(a) and also develop CAD at an early age and have increased mortality. India accounts for 30% of deaths from heart disease in people under 50 years of age in the world. High Lp(a) detected before 20 years of age increases the risk of major cardiovascular adverse events before age 50.
- ≥90% of Lp(a) is genetically determined. The *LPA* gene is one of the strongest monogenic risk factors for CAD.
- Lp(a) is the most potent of all atherogenic lipoproteins. It is also pro-inflammatory, pro-thrombotic and is associated with characteristics of "vulnerable" plaque.
- High Lp(a) increases the risk of heart attack (2.47-fold), ischemic stroke (1.60-fold), PAD (1.60-fold), and cardiovascular mortality 1.50-fold.
- High Lp(a) has multidimensional adverse impact on ASCVD (details on **Table 3**)—multivessel CAD, left main CAD, increased clot burden, early onset MI, and stroke in children and young adults.
- Lp(a) amplifies the ASCVD risk from well-established risk factors such as high LDL-C, high blood pressure, and high blood glucose.
- Lp(a) is recognized as a risk-enhancing factor for ASCVDs and measurement of Lp(a) is part of a comprehensive cardiovascular disease assessment. It is recommended that everyone should get a Lp(a) measurement at least once in their lifetime.
- Lp(a) level of <30 mg/dL is desirable, ≥50 mg/dL is high risk, and in between values are elevated risk. Risk stratification and clinical decision-making should use a continuous gradient of Lp(a) level and combine it with the patient's other risk factors.
- CAC score and Lp(a) level have a positive association. The combination of a CAC score of ≥100 and a high Lp(a) in the upper quintile is associated with a ~5-fold increase in ASCVD risk compared to CAC zero and Lp(a) in the lower quantiles.
- Currently lipoprotein apheresis is the only FDA-approved modality to reduce Lp(a). Statins are indicated in those with increased NHDL-C even though statins may moderately increase Lp(a) level as benefit outweighs

possible risk. Aspirin is recommended as prophylaxis against MACE. New drugs especially antisense oligonucleotides (ASOs) usher in a new era as early results of trials show that they are effective in lowering Lp(a).

■ REFERENCES

1. Reyes-Soffer G, Ginsberg HN, Berglund L, Duell PB, Heffron SP, Kamstrup PR, et al. Lipoprotein(a): A Genetically Determined, Causal, and Prevalent Risk Factor for Atherosclerotic Cardiovascular Disease: A Scientific Statement from the American Heart Association. Arterioscler Thromb Vasc Biol. 2022;42(1):e48-e60.
2. Wong ND. Lipoprotein(a): Ready for Prime Time? J Am Coll Cardiol. 2024;83(9): 887-9.
3. Enas EA, Varkey B, Dharmarajan TS, Pare G, Bahl VK. Lipoprotein(a): An independent, genetic, and causal factor for cardiovascular disease and acute myocardial infarction. Indian Heart J. 2019;71(2):99-112.
4. Enas EA, Varkey B, Dharmarajan TS, Pare G, Bahl VK. Lipoprotein(a): An underrecognized genetic risk factor for malignant coronary artery disease in young Indians. Indian Heart J. 2019;71(3):184-98.
5. Kronenberg F, Mora S, Stroes ESG, Ference BA, Arsenault BJ, Berglund L, et al. Lipoprotein(a) in atherosclerotic cardiovascular disease and aortic stenosis: a European Atherosclerosis Society consensus statement. Eur Heart J. 2022;43(39):3925-46.
6. Bjornson E, Adiels M, Taskinen MR, Burgess S, Chapman MJ, Packard CJ, et al. Lipoprotein(a) Is Markedly More Atherogenic Than LDL: An Apolipoprotein B-Based Genetic Analysis. J Am Coll Cardiol. 2024;83(3):385-95.
7. Marcovina SM. Lipoprotein(a): a genetically determined risk factor for cardiovascular disease. Crit Rev Clin Lab Sci. 2023:1-13.
8. Koschinsky ML, Bajaj A, Boffa MB, Dixon DL, Ferdinand KC, Gidding SS, et al. A focused update to the 2019 NLA scientific statement on use of lipoprotein(a) in clinical practice. J Clin Lipidol. 2024;18(3):e308-19.
9. Kronenberg F, Utermann G. Lipoprotein(a): resurrected by genetics. J Intern Med. 2013;273(1):6-30.
10. Wilcken DE, Wang XL, Greenwood J, Lynch J. Lipoprotein(a) and apolipoproteins B and A-1 in children and coronary vascular events in their grandparents. J Pediatr. 1993; 123(4):519-26.
11. McLean JW, Tomlinson JE, Kuang WJ, Eaton DL, Chen EY, Fless GM, et al. cDNA sequence of human apolipoprotein(a) is homologous to plasminogen. Nature. 1987; 330(6144):132-7.
12. Tsimikas S, Fazio S, Ferdinand KC, Ginsberg HN, Koschinsky ML, Marcovina SM, et al. NHLBI Working Group Recommendations to Reduce Lipoprotein(a)-Mediated Risk of Cardiovascular Disease and Aortic Stenosis. J Am Coll Cardiol. 2018;71(2):177-92.
13. Sun H, Saeedi P, Karuranga S, Pinkepank M, Ogurtsova K, Duncan BB, et al. IDF Diabetes Atlas: Global, regional and country-level diabetes prevalence estimates for 2021 and projections for 2045. Diabetes Res Clin Pract. 2022;183:109119.
14. Hu P, Dharmayat KI, Stevens CAT, Sharabiani MTA, Jones RS, Watts GF, et al. Prevalence of Familial Hypercholesterolemia Among the General Population and Patients with Atherosclerotic Cardiovascular Disease: A Systematic Review and Meta-Analysis. Circulation. 2020;141(22): 1742-59.
15. Nissen SE, Wolski K, Cho L, Nicholls SJ, Kastelein J, Leitersdorf E, et al. Lipoprotein(a) levels in a global population with established atherosclerotic cardiovascular disease. Open Heart. 2022;9(2):e002060.
16. Tsimikas S, Stroes ESG. The dedicated "Lp(a) clinic": A concept whose time has arrived? Atherosclerosis. 2020;300:1-9.
17. Patel AP, Wang M, Pirruccello JP, Ellinor PT, Ng K, Kathiresan S, et al. Lp(a) (Lipoprotein[a]) Concentrations and Incident Atherosclerotic Cardiovascular Disease: New Insights from a Large National Biobank. Arterioscler Thromb Vasc Biol. 2021;41(1): 465-74.

18. Masson W, Barbagelata L, Oberti P, Falconi M, Lavalle-Cobo A, Corral P, et al. High lipoprotein(a) levels and mitral valve disease: A systematic review. Nutr Metab Cardiovasc Dis. 2023;33(5):925-33.
19. Brandt EJ, Mani A, Spatz ES, Desai NR, Nasir K. Lipoprotein(a) levels and association with myocardial infarction and stroke in a nationally representative cross-sectional US cohort. J Clin Lipidol. 2020;14(5):695-706 e4.
20. Satterfield BA, Dikilitas O, Safarova MS, Clarke SL, Tcheandjieu C, Zhu X, et al. Associations of Genetically Predicted Lp(a) (Lipoprotein [a]) Levels with Cardiovascular Traits in Individuals of European and African Ancestry. Circ Genom Precis Med. 2021;14(4):e003354.
21. Pare G, Caku A, McQueen M, Anand SS, Enas E, Clarke R, et al. Lipoprotein(a) Levels and the Risk of Myocardial Infarction Among 7 Ethnic Groups. Circulation. 2019; 139(12):1472-82.
22. Reyes-Soffer G, Yeang C, Michos ED, Boatwright W, Ballantyne CM. High lipoprotein(a): Actionable strategies for risk assessment and mitigation. Am J Prev Cardiol. 2024;18:100651.
23. Patel AP, Wang M, Kartoun U, Ng K, Khera AV. Quantifying and Understanding the Higher Risk of Atherosclerotic Cardiovascular Disease Among South Asian Individuals: Results from the UK Biobank Prospective Cohort Study. Circulation. 2021;144(6): 410-22.
24. Bajaj A, Damrauer SM, Anderson AH, Xie D, Budoff MJ, Go AS, et al. Lipoprotein(a) and Risk of Myocardial Infarction and Death in Chronic Kidney Disease: Findings from the CRIC Study (Chronic Renal Insufficiency Cohort). Arterioscler Thromb Vasc Biol. 2017;37(10):1971-8.
25. Yun JS, Ahn YB, Song KH, Yoo KD, Park YM, Kim HW, et al. Lipoprotein(a) predicts a new onset of chronic kidney disease in people with Type 2 diabetes mellitus. Diabet Med. 2016;33(5):639-43.
26. Zhu Y, Chen S, Chen Z, Wang Y, Fu G, Zhang W. Causal effect of lipoprotein(a) level on chronic kidney disease of European ancestry: a two-sample Mendelian randomization study. Ren Fail. 2024;46(2):2383727.
27. Parvin S, Samsuddin L, Ali A, Chowdhury SA, Siddique I. Lipoprotein(a) level in preeclampsia patients. Bangladesh Med Res Counc Bull. 2010;36(3):97-9.
28. Rodriguez-Moran M, Guerrero-Romero F. Low birthweight and elevated levels of lipoprotein(a) in prepubertal children. J Paediatr Child Health. 2014;50(8):610-4.
29. Emdin CA, Khera AV, Natarajan P, Klarin D, Won HH, Peloso GM, et al. Phenotypic Characterization of Genetically Lowered Human Lipoprotein(a) Levels. J Am Coll Cardiol. 2016;68(25):2761-72.
30. Raitakari O, Kartiosuo N, Pahkala K, Hutri-Kähönen N, Bazzano LA, Chen W, et al. Lipoprotein(a) in Youth and Prediction of Major Cardiovascular Outcomes in Adulthood. Circulation. 2023;147(1):23-31.
31. Kaiser Y, Daghem M, Tzolos E, Meah MN, Doris MK, Moss AJ, et al. Association of Lipoprotein(a) With Atherosclerotic Plaque Progression. J Am Coll Cardiol. 2022;79(3):223-33.
32. Shui X, Wen Z, Chen Z, Xie X, Wu Y, Zheng B, et al. Elevated serum lipoprotein(a) is significantly associated with angiographic progression of coronary artery disease. Clin Cardiol. 2021;44(11):1551-9.
33. Nurmohamed NS, Gaillard EL, Malkasian S, de Groot RJ, Ibrahim S, Bom MJ, et al. Lipoprotein(a) and Long-Term Plaque Progression, Low-Density Plaque, and Pericoronary Inflammation. JAMA Cardiol. 2024;9(9):826-34.
34. Enas EA. Rapid angiographic progression of coronary artery disease in patients with elevated lipoprotein(a). Circulation. 1995;92(8):2353-4.
35. Kamel A, Farag NM, Allam E, Khaled M, Ismail DE. Expression of monocytes subsets in patients diagnosed with coronary atherosclerosis and their impact on disease severity. Cureus. 2024;16:e74670.
36. Hamid IH, Muppa N, Modi D, Sompalli S, Habib I, Chaudhari SS, et al. Effect of

Increased Level of Lipoprotein(a) on Cardiovascular Outcomes in Patients with Ischemic Heart Disease: A Systematic Review and Meta-Analysis. Cureus. 2024;16(10):e72776.
37. Rifai N, Ma J, Sacks FM, Ridker PM, Hernandez WJ, Stampfer MJ, et al. Apolipoprotein(a) size and lipoprotein(a) concentration and future risk of angina pectoris with evidence of severe coronary atherosclerosis in men: The Physicians' Health Study. Clin Chem. 2004;50(8): 1364-71.
38. Budde T, Fechtrup C, Bosenberg E, Vielhauer C, Enbergs A, Schulte H, et al. Plasma Lp(a) levels correlate with number, severity, and length-extension of coronary lesions in male patients undergoing coronary arteriography for clinically suspected coronary atherosclerosis. Arterioscler Thromb. 1994;14(11):1730-6.
39. Shi YP, Cao YX, Jin JL, Liu HH, Zhang HW, Guo YL, et al. Lipoprotein(a) as a predictor for the presence and severity of premature coronary artery disease: a cross-sectional analysis of 2433 patients. Coron Artery Dis. 2021;32(1):78-83.
40. Ashfaq F, Goel PK, Sethi R, Khan MI, Ali W, Idris MZ. Lipoprotein (a) Levels in Relation to Severity of Coronary Artery Disease in North Indian Patients. Heart Views. 2013; 14(1):12-6.
41. Leistner DM, Laguna-Fernandez A, Haghikia A, Abdelwahed YS, Schatz AS, Erbay A, et al. Impact of elevated lipoprotein(a) on coronary artery disease phenotype and severity. Eur J Prev Cardiol. 2024;31(7):856-65.
42. Ashfaq F, Goel PK, Moorthy N, Sethi R, Khan MI, Idris MZ. Lipoprotein(a) and SYNTAX Score Association with Severity of Coronary Artery Atherosclerosis in North India. Sultan Qaboos Univ Med J. 2012; 12(4):465-72.
43. Sankhesara DM, Lan NSR, Gilfillan P, Zounis E, Rajgopal S, Chan DC, et al. Lipoprotein(a) is associated with thrombus burden in culprit arteries of younger patients with ST-segment elevation myocardial infarction. Cardiology. 2023;148(2):98-102.
44. Koschinsky ML. Lipoprotein(a) and the link between atherosclerosis and thrombosis. Can J Cardiol. 2004;20 Suppl B:37B-43B.
45. Sawhney JPs, Kumar A, Tyagi K, Madan K. Prevalence of lipoprotein(a) in acute coronary syndrome and its association with severity of heart disease among patients admitted to a tertiary care hospital Atherosclerosis abstract number 167. 2023;379:117162.
46. Statescu C, Anghel L, Benchea LC, Tudurachi BS, Leonte A, Zăvoi A, et al. A Systematic Review on the Risk Modulators of Myocardial Infarction in the "Young"-Implications of Lipoprotein (a). Int J Mol Sci. 2023;24(6): 5927.
47. Loh WJ, Chang X, Aw TC, Phua SK, Low AF, Chan MY, et al. Lipoprotein(a) as predictor of coronary artery disease and myocardial infarction in a multi-ethnic Asian population. Atherosclerosis. 2022;349:160-5.
48. Kamstrup PR, Benn M, Tybjaerg-Hansen A, Nordestgaard BG. Extreme Lipoprotein(a) Levels and Risk of Myocardial Infarction in the General Population. The Copenhagen City Heart Study. Circulation. 2008;117(2): 176-84.
49. Wang Z, Xiao S, Liu N. Association of lipoprotein(a) with coronary severity in patients with new-onset acute myocardial infarction: A large cross-sectional study. Clin Chim Acta. 2023;540:117220.
50. Afshar M, Pilote L, Dufresne L, Engert JC, Thanassoulis G. Lipoprotein(a) Interactions with Low-Density Lipoprotein Cholesterol and Other Cardiovascular Risk Factors in Premature Acute Coronary Syndrome (ACS). J Am Heart Assoc. 2016;5(4):e003012.
51. Rigattieri S, Cristiano E, Tempestini F, Lo Monaco M, Cava F, Bongiovanni M, et al. Lipoprotein(a) and the risk of recurrent events in patients with acute myocardial infarction treated by percutaneous coronary intervention. Minerva Cardiol Angiol. 2023; 71(4):406-13.
52. Sumarjaya I, Nadha IKB, Lestari AAW. High Lipoprotein(a) Levels as a Predictor of Major Adverse Cardiovascular Events in Hospitalized-Acute Myocardial Infarction

53. Li N, Zhou J, Chen R, Zhao X, Li J, Zhou P, et al. Prognostic impacts of diabetes status and lipoprotein(a) levels in patients with ST-segment elevation myocardial infarction: a prospective cohort study. Cardiovasc Diabetol. 2023;22(1):151.
54. Kallmeyer A, Pello Lazaro AM, Blanco-Colio LM, Aceña Á, González-Lorenzo Ó, Tarín N, et al. Absence of High Lipoprotein(a) Levels Is an Independent Predictor of Acute Myocardial Infarction without Coronary Lesions. J Clin Med. 2023;12(3):960.
55. Gao S, Ma W, Huang S, Lin X, Yu M. Effect of Lipoprotein (a) Levels on Long-term Cardiovascular Outcomes in Patients with Myocardial Infarction with Nonobstructive Coronary Arteries. Am J Cardiol. 2021;152: 34-42.
56. Orth-Gomer K, Mittleman MA, Schenck-Gustafsson K, Wamala SP, Eriksson M, Belkic K, et al. Lipoprotein(a) as a determinant of coronary heart disease in young women. Circulation. 1997;95(2):329-34.
57. Enas EA. Lipoprotein(a) as a determinant of coronary heart disease in young women: a stronger risk factor than diabetes? Circulation. 1998;97(3):293-5.
58. Qin SY, Liu J, Jiang HX, Hu BL, Zhou Y, Olkkonen VM. Association between baseline lipoprotein(a) levels and restenosis after coronary stenting: meta-analysis of 9 cohort studies. Atherosclerosis. 2013;227(2): 360-6.
59. Yuan X, Han Y, Hu X, Jiang M, Feng H, Fang Y, et al. Lipoprotein (a) is related to In-Stent neoatherosclerosis incidence rate and plaque vulnerability: Optical Coherence Tomography Study. Int J Cardiovasc Imaging. 2023;39(2):275-84.
60. Yuan S, Li F, Zhang H, Zeng J, Su X, Qu J, et al. Impact of High Lipoprotein(a) on Long-Term Survival Following Coronary Artery Bypass Grafting. J Am Heart Assoc. 2024;13(3):e031322.
61. Kamstrup PR, Tybjaerg-Hansen A, Steffensen R, Nordestgaard BG. Genetically elevated lipoprotein(a) and increased risk of myocardial infarction. JAMA. 2009; 301(22):2331-9.
62. Christopher R, Kailasanatha KM, Nagaraja D, Tripathi M. Case-control study of serum lipoprotein(a) and apoprotein(a) A-I and B in stroke in the young. Acta Neurol Scand. 1996;94(2):127-30.
63. Moriarty PM, Tennant H, Sehar N, Denney L, Luna P, Perez-Marques F, et al. Case report of male child with elevated lipoprotein (a) leading to acute ischemic stroke. J Clin Apher. 2017;32(6):574-8.
64. Wong ND, Fan W, Hu X, Ballantyne C, Hoodgeveen RC, Tsai MY, et al. Lipoprotein(a) and Long-Term Cardiovascular Risk in a Multi-Ethnic Pooled Prospective Cohort. J Am Coll Cardiol. 2024;83(16):1511-25.
65. Dai K, Shiode N, Yoshii K, Kimura Y, Matsuo K, Jyuri Y, et al. Impact of Lipoprotein (a) on Long-Term Outcomes in Patients with Acute Myocardial Infarction. Circ J. 2023;87(10):1356-61.
66. Miñana G, Gil-Cayuela C, Bodi V, de la Espriella R, Valero E, Mollar A, et al. Lipoprotein(a) and long-term recurrent infarction after an episode of ST-segment elevation acute myocardial infarction. Coron Artery Dis. 2020;31(4):378-84.
67. Langsted A, Kamstrup PR, Nordestgaard BG. High lipoprotein(a) and high risk of mortality. Eur Heart J. 2019;40(33):2760-70.
68. Berman AN, Biery DW, Besser SA, Singh A, Shiyovich A, Weber BN, et al. Lipoprotein(a) and Major Adverse Cardiovascular Events in Patients with or Without Baseline Atherosclerotic Cardiovascular Disease. J Am Coll Cardiol. 2024;83(9):873-86.
69. Pearson GJ, Thanassoulis G, Anderson TJ, Barry AR, Couture P, Dayan N, et al. 2021 Canadian Cardiovascular Society Guidelines for the Management of Dyslipidemia for the Prevention of Cardiovascular Disease in Adults. Can J Cardiol. 2021;37(8): 1129-50.
70. Mach F, Baigent C, Catapano AL, Koskinas KC, Casula M, Badimon L, et al. 2019 ESC/EAS Guidelines for the management of

dyslipidaemias: lipid modification to reduce cardiovascular risk. Eur Heart J. 2020;41(1): 111-88.
71. Kronenberg F. Measuring lipoprotein(a): do it without ifs and buts. Eur J Prev Cardiol. 2022;29(5):766-8.
72. Rikhi R, Bhatia HS, Schaich CL, Ashburn N, Tsai MY, Michos ED, et al. Association of Lp(a) (Lipoprotein[a]) and Hypertension in Primary Prevention of Cardiovascular Disease: The MESA. Hypertension. 2023; 80(2):352-60.
73. Rikhi R, Hammoud A, Ashburn N, Snavely AC, Michos ED, Chevli P, et al. Relationship of low-density lipoprotein-cholesterol and lipoprotein(a) to cardiovascular risk: The Multi-Ethnic Study of Atherosclerosis (MESA). Atherosclerosis. 2022;363:102-8.
74. Grundy SM, Stone NJ, Bailey AL, Beam C, Birtcher KK, Blumenthal RS, et al. 2018 AHA/ACC/AACVPR/AAPA/ABC/ACPM/ADA/AGS/APhA/ASPC/NLA/PCNA Guideline on the Management of Blood Cholesterol: Executive Summary: A Report of the American College of Cardiology/American Heart Association Task Force on Clinical Practice Guidelines. J Am Coll Cardiol. 2019; 73(24):3168-209.
75. Mehta A, Vasquez N, Ayers CR, Patel J, Hooda A, Khera A, et al. Independent Association of Lipoprotein(a) and Coronary Artery Calcification with Atherosclerotic Cardiovascular Risk. J Am Coll Cardiol. 2022; 79(8):757-68.
76. Langsted A, Kamstrup PR, Benn M, Tybjaerg-Hansen A, Nordestgaard BG. High lipoprotein(a) as a possible cause of clinical familial hypercholesterolaemia: a prospective cohort study. Lancet Diabetes Endocrinol. 2016;4(7):577-87.
77. Alonso R, Andres E, Mata N, Fuentes-Jiménez F, Badimón L, López-Miranda J, et al. Lipoprotein(a) levels in familial hypercholesterolemia: an important predictor of cardiovascular disease independent of the type of LDL receptor mutation. J Am Coll Cardiol. 2014;63(19):1982-9.
78. Lloyd-Jones DM, Allen NB, Anderson CAM, Black T, Brewer LC, Foraker RE, et al. Life's Essential 8: Updating and Enhancing the American Heart Association's Construct of Cardiovascular Health: A Presidential Advisory from the American Heart Association. Circulation. 2022;146(5):e18-e43.
79. Schumann F, Kassner U, Spira D, Zimmermann FF, Bobbert T, Steinhagen-Thiessen E, et al. Long-term lipoprotein apheresis reduces cardiovascular events in high-risk patients with isolated lipoprotein(a) elevation. J Clin Lipidol. 2024; 18(5):e738-45.
80. Tsimikas S, Gordts P, Nora C, Yeang C, Witztum JL. Statin therapy increases lipoprotein(a) levels. Eur Heart J. 2020; 41(24):2275-84.
81. Agarwala A, Ballantyne C, Stone NJ. Primary Prevention Management of Elevated Lipoprotein(a). JAMA Cardiol. 2023;8(1): 96-7.
82. O'Donoghue ML, Fazio S, Giugliano RP, Stroes ESG, Kanevsky E, Gouni-Berthold I, et al. Lipoprotein(a), PCSK9 Inhibition, and Cardiovascular Risk. Circulation. 2019; 139(12):1483-92.
83. Warden BA, Minnier J, Watts GF, Fazio S, Shapiro MD. Impact of PCSK9 inhibitors on plasma lipoprotein(a) concentrations with or without a background of niacin therapy. J Clin Lipidol. 2019;13(4):580-5.
84. Bittner VA, Szarek M, Aylward PE, Bhatt DL, Diaz R, Edelberg JM, et al. Effect of Alirocumab on Lipoprotein(a) and Cardiovascular Risk After Acute Coronary Syndrome. J Am Coll Cardiol. 2020;75(2): 133-44.
85. Chasman DI, Shiffman D, Zee RY, Louie JZ, Luke MM, Rowland CM, et al. Polymorphism in the apolipoprotein(a) gene, plasma lipoprotein(a), cardiovascular disease, and low-dose aspirin therapy. Atherosclerosis. 2009;203(2):371-6.
86. Lacaze P, Bakshi A, Riaz M, Polekhina G, Owen A, Bhatia HS, et al. Aspirin for Primary Prevention of Cardiovascular Events in Relation to Lipoprotein(a) Genotypes. J Am Coll Cardiol. 2022;80(14):1287-98.
87. Bhatia HS, Trainor P, Carlisle S, Tsai MY, Criqui MH, DeFilippis A, et al. Aspirin and

Cardiovascular Risk in Individuals with Elevated Lipoprotein(a): The Multi-Ethnic Study of Atherosclerosis. J Am Heart Assoc. 2024;13(3):e033562.
88. Langsted A, Nordestgaard BG. Antisense Oligonucleotides Targeting Lipoprotein(a). Curr Atheroscler Rep. 2019;21(8):30.
89. Schreml J, Gouni-Berthold I. Apolipoprotein(a) antisense oligonucleotides: a new treatment option for lowering elevated lipoprotein(a)? Curr Pharm Des. 2017;23(10):1562-70.
90. O'Donoghue ML, Rosenson RS, Gencer B, López JAG, Lepor NE, Baum SJ, et al. Small Interfering RNA to Reduce Lipoprotein(a) in cardiovascular disease. N Engl J Med. 2022;387(20):1855-64.
91. Nicholls SJ, Nissen SE, Fleming C, Urva S, Suico J, Berg PH, et al. Muvalaplin, an Oral Small Molecule Inhibitor of Lipoprotein(a) Formation: A Randomized Clinical Trial. JAMA. 2023;330(11):1042-53.
92. Nissen SE, Wang Q, Nicholls SJ, Navar AM, Ray KK, Schwartz GG, et al. Lipoprotein(a) A Phase 2 Randomized Clinical Trial. JAMA. 2024;332(23):1992-2002.
93. Tokgozoglu L, Orringer C, Ginsberg HN, Catapano AL. The year in cardiovascular medicine 2021: Dyslipidaemia. Eur Heart J. 2022;43(8):807-17.

CHAPTER 9

Heart Disease in Women

■ INTRODUCTION

Picture a person having a heart attack—the image in most people's mind would be of a man clutching his chest in severe pain. This association of men and heart attacks is so embedded that the risk in women often goes underappreciated and therefore underdiagnosed and undertreated.[1-3] The notion that women at all ages have natural protection against heart disease and heart attacks is false and needs to be dispelled and be replaced by the fact that heart disease is the leading cause of death in women.[3-7] Without recognition of this fact and action driven by it women may not get optimal preventive care and may not get timely and appropriate treatment of heart disease and heart attacks (acute myocardial infarctions or AMIs).[2,5,7-9]

■ VARIED EPIDEMIOLOGY REPORTS

US Statistics on Heart Disease and Stroke

One report noted that women had a higher 30-day mortality rate after a new cardiovascular event than men.[3] Another one noted that heart attack rate increased with age in both men and women but for one difference—in men it peaked at 65–74 years of age and then declined while in women it continued to steadily increased and surpassed men's rate at age 85 years and up.[10] At every age group, except ≥85 years, women had fewer heart attacks.[10]

London Life Sciences Prospective Population (LOLIPOP) Study

This 20-year study on the cumulative incidence of coronary artery disease (CAD) among South Asians and Europeans, on further gender-stratified analysis, found that the incidence of CAD in South Asian females was substantially higher than White females and comparable to that of White European males.[11]

Institute of Health Metrics and Evaluation (IHME)

IHME calculated that over 40% of deaths from heart disease in young women (<50 years of age) were from two countries, India and China, and showed markedly divergent trends—increasing in India and decreasing in China.[12]

The VIRGO (Variation in Recovery: Role of Gender on Outcomes of Young AMI Patients)

The VIRGO case-control study evaluated the prevalence, odds ratio, and population attributable fraction (PAF). Women who had an AMI had higher PAF for several factors including diabetes, hypertension, and depression.[13]

The conclusions of the studies synopsized above do not fully reconcile with the findings of the recent landmark Prospective Urban Rural Epidemiology (PURE) study that encompassed participants from urban and rural areas of high-income countries (HICs), middle-income countries (MICs), and low-income countries (LICs). The data generated in this study allow gender comparisons and well-buttressed conclusions.[14,15]

THE PROSPECTIVE URBAN RURAL EPIDEMIOLOGY STUDY

In this large international prospective cohort study of 202,072 participants (119,799 women and 82,273 men) aged 35–70 years from 1,030 communities living in 27 HICs, MICs, and LICs from Asia, Africa, Europe, South America, North America, and the Middle East were followed and their health data recorded for a median of 9.5 years.[14,15]

The mean age of women was 50.8 years compared with 51.7 years for men. Less than half of the participants lived in a rural community (43.2% women and 44.2% men) and around 20% of both women and men included in the study were from a low-income country). Fewer women were current smokers, or consumed alcohol or engaged in high levels of physical activity than men. They had lower education and more "probable" depression than men.[14,15]

Women had higher mean total cholesterol (TC), LDL cholesterol (LDL-C), HDL cholesterol (HDL-C), non-HDL cholesterol (NHDL-C), and apolipoprotein A1(Apo A1) than men but had lower mean concentrations of triglycerides (TG), apolipoprotein B (ApoB), ratio of ApoB to ApoA1, and ratio of TC/HDL-C. Waist circumference (WC) and waist–hip ratio were lower but mean body mass index (BMI) was higher in women than in men. Systolic and diastolic blood pressures and fasting blood glucose were also lower in women than in men.[15]

Major Findings and Conclusions[14,15]

- The burden of cardiovascular risk factors (CVRF) is lower in women than men across countries at all economic levels and geographical regions.
- Primary prevention measures are used more frequently in women than in men and are accompanied by lower incidence of cardiovascular disease (CVD) and mortality.
- Secondary prevention measures after a cardiac event—cardiac investigations, and coronary interventions (stents, CABG)—are less frequent in women than in men, but women did not experience a higher rate of recurrent CVD events or death (over a median follow up of 9.5 years).
- Women had lower 30-day mortality after a new CVD event compared with men (22% in women versus 28% in men; $p < 0.0001$) **(Fig. 1)**.
- Outcomes are better in women than in men, both in those with and without previous CVD.
- The differences in treatments and in outcomes in both women and men from LICs and MICs compared with HICs are much larger than the differences between sexes globally or within groups of countries.
- Understanding and narrowing these gaps on CVD prevention and treatment between LICs and MICs versus HICs deserve greater attention.

Overall, the 30-day case fatality rates after a major adverse cardiovascular event (MACE)—myocardial infarction, stroke, or heart failure—were lower in women (22%) than in men (28%) **(Fig. 1)**. Other bars in the figure show the marked difference in

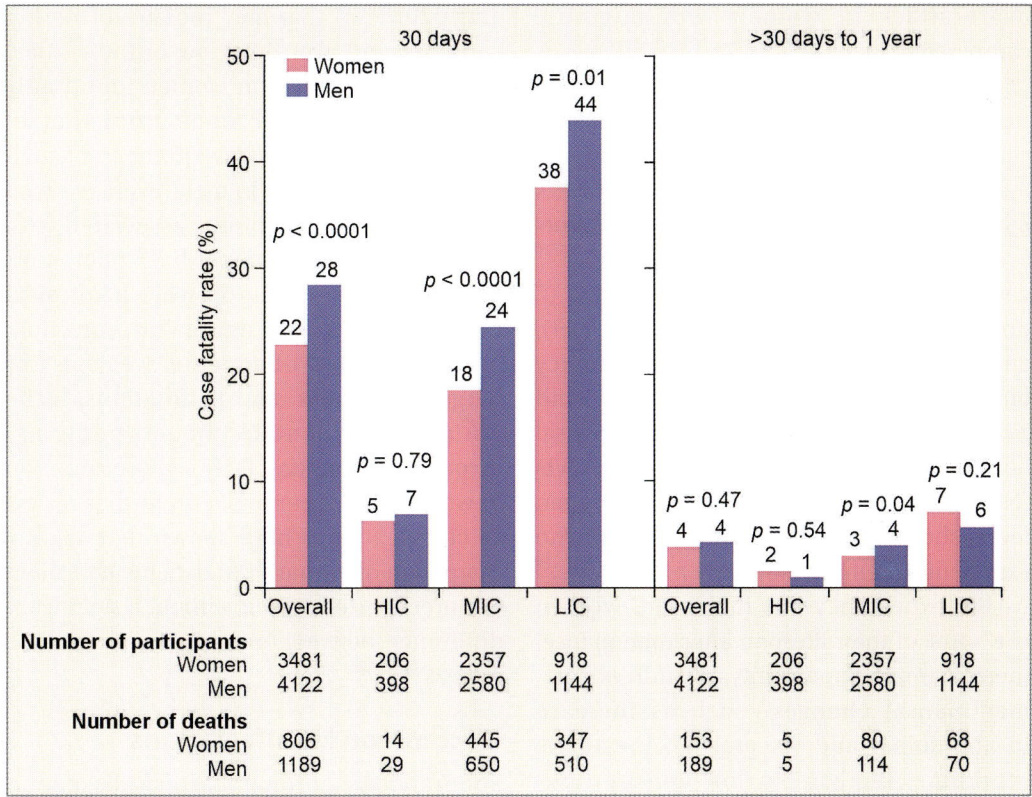

Fig. 1: Case fatality rates after an incident myocardial infarction, stroke, or heart failure event in women and men by country economic status. (Case fatality rates adjusted for age. Participants with a history of cardiovascular diseases were excluded.)
Source: Reproduced with permission from Walli-Attaei M, Joseph P, Rosengren A, Chow CK, Rangarajan S, Lear SA, et al. Variations between women and men in risk factors, treatments, cardiovascular disease incidence, and death in 27 high-income, middle-income, and low-income countries (PURE): a prospective cohort study. Lancet. 2020;396(10244):97-109.[14]

30-day case fatality rates between HICs (5% in women and 7% in men; $p = 0.79$) and MICs (18% in women and 24% in men) and LICs (38% in women and 44% in men).[14]

GENDER-SPECIFIC DIFFERENCES IN RISKS, CLINICAL ASPECTS, AND TREATMENT

Risks

The PURE study showed that the established major CVRFs pose less of a risk burden in women than in men. However, there are several gender-specific vulnerabilities in women that should not be ignored.[16] Autoimmune diseases, a recognized risk-enhancing factor for atherosclerotic cardiovascular disease (ASCVD),[17,18] are more common in women than in men.[17] Migraine, much more common in women than men, is associated with the risk of stroke; less known is that it increases (by about 20%) the hazard for heart attack.[19] A Danish population-based cohort study found a significantly higher risk of premature heart attack in women with migraine compared to men (22% vs. 7%).[20,21]

Most pertinent among the vulnerabilities to CVD in women are those associated with their life events: Early and late menarche,[18] polycystic ovary syndrome,[22,23] bilateral oophorectomy,[24] fertility treatments (especially unsuccessful ones),[25,26] gestational diabetes,[27,28] hypertension,[13,29] pre-eclampsia,[13,30] menopausal (early, peri, and postmenopausal),[31] adverse pregnancy outcome (recurrent miscarriages),[31-33] and frequent and long hot flashes.[24] Menopausal hormone therapy (MHT), to mitigate the CVD risk associated with the decline in estrogen levels should be considered in women who experience premature or early menopause.[24] As life expectancy has increased, women live ~40% of their lifespan after menopause, there is ample opportunity, to address postmenopausal changes—such as increase in abdominal and visceral fat, metabolic syndrome, increase in low-density lipoprotein cholesterol (LDL-C) and triglycerides, changes in carbohydrate metabolism and to implement preventative measures and medication(s) to reduce their CVD risk.[24]

The generally used 10-year ASCVD risk assessment tool, to initiate and guide statin therapy, has limitations. US-based National Health and Nutrition surveys (NHANES) showed that over 60% of American women have a low short-term (10-year) CVD risk, yet a high lifetime risk.[34] Better alternatives to the 10-year assessment tool are discussed and tabulated in a later chapter (Chapter 13, Table 4) and these are applicable to women.

Clinical Aspects

The most common presenting manifestation of acute coronary syndrome (ACS) for both men and women is chest pain or severe discomfort (squeezing, burning, and tightness) that may radiate to the left shoulder and arm.[35] Review of the clinical presentation of ACS in women found only small differences or none from that of men.[36,37] Women may have more associated symptoms compared to men (average of 2.6 vs. 1.8).[35] These symptoms associated with ACS were middle or upper back pain, neck pain, jaw pain, shortness of breath, paroxysmal nocturnal dyspnea, nausea or vomiting, indigestion, loss of appetite, weakness or fatigue, dizziness, and palpitations.[36] The notion that silent (without symptoms) myocardial infarction (MI) is more common in women is not borne out on further review as cohort studies have shown that slightly more than one-quarter of patients had silent or unrecognized MI but without a significant difference between genders (women 26%, men 27%).[36,38]

Uncommon Manifestations

Spontaneous coronary artery dissection (SCAD) is a tear in one of the epicardial coronary arteries and may range from intimal rupture to intramural hematoma and false lumen formation. It is a significant risk for young women including postpartum women as it leads to AMI, tachyarrhythmias, and heart failure.[39] Takotsubo syndrome ("broken heart syndrome")—a sudden weakening or ballooning of a part of heart muscle (cardiomyopathy), usually presents after a significant emotional or physical stressor that may be related to a surge of catecholamines occurs more in women (more in post-menopausal women) than in men.[40,41] Myocardial infarction in the absence of obstructive coronary artery disease (MINOCA) is defined as MI with mild or no obstructive CAD on angiogram.[42,43] Heterogeneous causes of MINOCA include coronary vasospasm, coronary embolism, coronary microvascular dysfunction, and SCAD.[44] MINOCA affects 5–15% of patients undergoing cardiac catheterization for MI. MINOCA patients are more likely to be women and are less likely to have dyslipidemia.

Treatment

Deficiencies in the treatment of heart disease in women are many and strikingly so in ACS. The early and basic ones are the failure to recognize symptoms of a heart attack, delays in transportation to the hospital in an ambulance with lights and sirens and failure to use aspirin and resuscitation measures.[45,46] The importance of prompt diagnosis and initial treatment cannot be overstressed as it reduces heart damage, complications, and death.[47,48] Gender disparities in ST-segment elevation myocardial infarction (STEMI) outcomes are reported worldwide. A meta-analysis of 56 studies of 705,098 patients (31% women) with STEMI showed that the women were older, had more comorbidities and received less antiplatelet therapy and primary percutaneous coronary intervention (PPCI) than the men in the study. Women experienced significantly longer delays to first medical contact (mean difference 42.5 minutes) and door-to-balloon time (mean difference 4.9 minutes). Women had increased rates of in-hospital mortality [odds ratio (OR) 1.91, 95% confidence interval (CI) 1.84–1.99, $p < 0.00001$], repeat MI (OR 1.25, 95% CI 1.00–1.56, $p = 0.05$), stroke (OR 1.67, 95% CI 1.27–2.20, $p < 0.001$), and major bleeding (OR 1.82, 95% CI 1.56–2.12, $p < 0.00001$) compared with males. Though the older age of women was the major driver of excess mortality, the disparities in the care given (antiplatelet therapy, PPCI, longer time to medical contact and longer time from presentation to PCI time) are contributors to the gender gap. The excess rates of repeat MI and stroke in women are likely from less use of PCI and less use of antiplatelet therapy.[49] Women are less likely to undergo coronary artery revascularization procedures (CARPs)[50-52] and receive fewer guideline recommended therapies than men during and after a myocardial infarction.[2,48]

PREMATURE HEART DISEASE IN WOMEN

There is a paucity of population wide or community-based studies that focus solely on premature heart disease in women. Most of the information available now is gleaned from clinics, hospital registries and databases and these are mostly from the US and Europe. An important one, cited earlier in this chapter, is from the IHME that over 40% of deaths from heart disease in young women (<50 years of age) were from two countries, India and China with markedly divergent trends—increasing in India and decreasing in China.[12]

Another noteworthy US study sought to answer the question whether young women (defined as <55 years of age) with ACS were a high risk group based on age and gender.[53] They analyzed data from 3,237 men and women (admitted with an ACS event from 1999 to 2006). Women <55 years of age represented 8% (259) of the entire cohort, and features of these 259 young women were compared to older women. Young women were more likely to be smokers (51 vs. 14%, $p < 0.001$) and obese (44 vs. 34%, $p = 0.006$). Young women had more diabetes and hypertension than young men. Mortality was lowest among young women and did not change over time. Young women received less treatment with aspirin, beta blockers, lipid-lowering agents, and angiotensin-converting enzyme (ACE) inhibitors, and underwent fewer coronary angiography and stenting than young men (44% vs. 59%, p < 0.001). Rehospitalization was higher among young women than young men (37% vs. 27%, p < 0.001), with no change over time.[53]

A Study from India

Research Institute and Rajasthan University of Health Sciences reported on consecutive patients who underwent percutaneous intervention (PCI) during a 3½-year-period. Of the 936 women, 299 (31.9%) were between the ages of 45 and 60 years, and 61 (6.5%) were under the age of 45 years.[54] Thus, more than one in three women (38.4%) were under 60 years of age and had premature (45–60 years) or very premature (<45 years) CAD. (Note that the age cut-off of 45 years for very premature disease used is at variance with that of IHME). In interpreting the results of this study, it should be kept in mind, as the authors point out, that these results are of a highly select group who required PCI and therefore they are not to be considered representative of the general population or of all young women in the state. Nonetheless the results as shown on **Table 1** are stunning as nearly 60% of women under 45 years of

TABLE 1: Clinical and angiographic profile of very premature (<45 years), premature (45–60 years) and non-premature (>60 years) coronary artery disease (CAD) Indian women in Jaipur, India.

Variables	Total women #936 (100%)	Age >60 years #576 (62%)	Age 45–60 years #299 (31.9%)	Age <45 years #61 (6.5%)	p-value
1A. Risk factors					
Hypertension	64%	69%	60%	38%	<0.001
Diabetes	40%	41%	43%	26%	0.233
Tobacco smoking	8%	7%	9%	13%	0.044
Chronic kidney disease	1%	2%	1%	0%	0.108
Uninsured status	42%	39%	44%	59%	0.003
1B. Lipids					
TC (mean mg/dL)	154	152	164	177	0.009
TC >200 mg/dL	14%	12%	17%	18%	0.031
TC >170 mg/dL	28%	25%	34%	30%	0.027
NHDL-C mg/dL (mean)	93	87	106	107	0.001
NHDL-C >130 mg/dL	25%	21%	33%	26%	0.003
NHDL-C >100 mg/dL	47%	42%	54%	62%	<0.001
LDL-C (mean) mg/dL	104	105	103	104	0.901
LDL-C >100 mg/dL	43%	44%	41%	49%	0.959
LDL-C >70 mg/dL	68%	67%	71%	64%	0.673
Triglycerides (TG) (median) mg/dL	135	138	133	139	0.763

Contd...

Contd...

Variables	Total women #936 (100%)	Age >60 years #576(62%)	Age 45–60 years #299 (31.9%)	Age <45 years #61 (6.5%)	p-value
TG >150 mg/dL	38%	38%	38%	38%	0.935
Statin therapy	46%	49%	42%	38%	0.013
1C. Severity of CAD					
STEMI	36%	37%	40%	42%	0.245
NSTEMI	58%	60	60%	58%	0.414
Ejection fraction <45%	54%	56%	48%	51%	0.293
Single-vessel disease	1%	3%	44%	41%	0.885
Double-vessel disease	42%	35%	37%	41%	0.818
Triple-vessel disease	36%	23%	18%	18%	0.425
Left main disease	5%	4%	4%	5%	0.885

(LDL-C: low-density lipoprotein cholesterol; NHDL-C: non-high-density lipoprotein cholesterol; NSTEMI: non-ST elevation myocardial infarction; STEMI: ST elevation myocardial infarction; TC: total cholesterol)
Source: Reproduced with permission from Sharma SK, Makkar JS, Bana A, Sharma K, Kasliwal A, Sidana SK, et al. Premature coronary artery disease, risk factors, clinical presentation, angiography and interventions: Hospital based registry. Indian Heart J. 2022;74(5):391-7.[54]

age had multivessel disease and one-half of women under 45 years of age exhibited left ventricular dysfunction indicating the severity of heart disease.

The degree of severity of CAD in young women is not easily explicable based on just the major risk factors for CAD. In the <45 age group only 13% had a history of tobacco smoking, hypertension and diabetes were present at 38% and 26% respectively and total cholesterol of >200 mg/dL was recorded in 18%. However, NHDL-C was over 100 mg/dL in 62% (38% were on statin therapy). This leads to the question—are there factors that are unaccounted?

One of the factors high on the list of unaccounted suspects is genetically determined increased lipoprotein(a) [Lp(a)], a potent atherogenic lipoprotein (fully discussed in the previous chapter).[55,56] Orth-Gomer and associates[57] showed that Lp(a) levels were linked to the age-adjusted odds ratio for CAD in the highest versus the lowest quartile of Lp(a). After adjustment for age, smoking, education, BMI, systolic blood pressure, TC, TG, and HDL-C, the odds ratio was 2.9 (95% CI, 1.6–5.0). The odds ratios for symptomatic CAD (angina and MI) were 5.1 (95% CI, 1.4–18.4) and 2.4 (95% CI, 1.3–4.5) in premenopausal and postmenopausal women, respectively. The five-fold increase in risk in premenopausal women by Lp(a) makes it a more powerful risk factor for CAD than diabetes when PAFs are taken into account.[58] The CV risk caused by Lp(a) is further magnified with elevated NHDL-C.[59,60] However, despite its value Lp(a) level is seldom measured in India.

HEART HEALTH ISSUES FACED BY WOMEN IN INDIA

Following up on the earlier discussion on gender-specific deficiencies globally (mostly from the US and Europe), this concluding segment focuses on issues of heart health care of women in India. Indian women who experience a heart attack, reportedly, are at a higher risk of death compared to women in developed countries attributable mainly to underrecognition, undertreatment, and to social and environmental hurdles.[61-65]

Underrecognition

The high lifetime risk of heart disease in women is not fully appreciated by neither physicians nor by the public. As mentioned earlier, Lp(a) levels are not checked. Although Indian women have lower rates of tobacco use than men, they share the other risk factors—diabetes, hypertension, high cholesterol, and obesity. Women are more exposed to indoor air pollution and have less opportunity for regular physical exercise. The responsibility of caring for dependents often falls on women, leading to stress, and limited personal time. Besides, women experience weight gain, metabolic syndrome, diabetes, and increase in LDL-C after menopause. Cardiovascular consequences of adverse pregnancy outcomes are not often recognized and therefore are not monitored.

Delayed Treatment and Under Treatment

Diagnosis of ACS is often delayed because of a low index of suspicion in physicians and by transportation delays and consequently critical treatments are delayed. Most cardiac care hospitals and facilities require payment in advance before a time-critical treatment such as PCI or thrombolytic therapy is initiated. This factor alone is a formidable hurdle for many in the low socio-economic level.[14] A study from Kerala showed only one-third of patients with STEMI received the indicated thrombolytic therapy. This study also revealed deficiency in guideline-based treatment of ACS as one-third of non-ST elevation myocardial infarction (NSTEMI) patients received thrombolytic therapy that is contraindicated.[62]

Social and Environmental Hurdles

Cultural barriers and potential bias can delay women from seeking timely medical care, especially in receiving life-saving PCI or clot-busting medications (thrombolytics) compared to men. Poverty, unemployment, and limited social support restrict access to healthcare. (Societal pressures can also limit women's ability to prioritize their health. Lack of education may hinder managing risk factors and navigating healthcare, leading to unhealthy choices, and delayed diagnoses.[65]

The number and scope of issues that women face are huge but are reducible with concerted action, resources, and resolve. A good start would include the following elements:[66-68]

- Educating women with knowledge about healthy diet, importance of regular physical exercise, avoidance or reduction in indoor air pollution, smoking cessation, and major risk factors (hypertension, diabetes, high cholesterol, and tobacco smoking).
- Dismantling gender bias in healthcare, improving healthcare access and ensuring culturally sensitive care of women in all venues.
- Health risk screening programs in young women (as early as in their teen years): Lp(a), total cholesterol, blood pressure, fasting blood sugar, etc.

- Follow-up plan for those with screening results outside of normal.
- Lowering the threshold for statin therapy and individualizing medication regimens based on each woman's risk profile.

This multi-pronged approach, to overcome gender disparity in cardiac care of women, needs active participation, support and advocacy from individuals, groups, physicians, other healthcare providers and action from benefactors, policy leaders and from governments at all levels.

■ KEY TAKEAWAYS

- Heart disease is the leading cause of death in women worldwide. Awareness of this fact—by the general public and by physicians and health care givers—is the first necessary step for early diagnosis and timely and appropriate treatment.
- Some important conclusions of the landmark PURE study are (1) the overall burden of cardiovascular risk factors is lower in women than men across countries at all economic levels and geographical regions; (2) primary prevention was better in women than men but the reverse was true for secondary prevention; (3) overall, the 30 day case-fatality ratio after a MACE was lower in women than men; and (4) differences in treatments and outcomes related to the income of the countries.
- Importantly, there are several gender-specific factors that increase CVD risk. Menopause causes hormonal changes (cessation of estradiol and continued testosterone production), changes body composition (more visceral fat, decrease in muscle mass) and metabolism (increase in LDL-C and TG) and increases the pace of atherosclerosis. Both early menarche and early menopause increase CVD risk.
- Gender-specific vulnerabilities in women—especially those related to pregnancy (diabetes, hypertension, and preeclampsia) and menopause (early menopause, perimenopausal symptoms, post-menopausal metabolic changes)—need to be appropriately managed.
- The common presentations (symptoms) of ACS are similar in women and men, though women may have more associated symptoms.
- Critical deficiencies are noted in the care of ACS in women. These include delays in recognition, transport and treatment in medications (aspirin, antiplatelet therapy, and thrombolytics) to primary percutaneous coronary interventions (PPCI). Coronary artery bypass (CABG) surgery is done less in women than men. Guideline-directed medical therapy is also less used in women.
- Some clinical cardiac syndromes (SCAD, Takotsubo syndrome, and MINOCA), though uncommon, disproportionately affect women more than men.
- Premature onset of CAD is suspected in women from India. Severe disease was seen in consecutive patients, including younger women, who underwent PCI in a tertiary center in Rajasthan. The degree of severity in young women, especially those <45 years of age, raises the existence of undetected risk factor(s) such as increased lipoprotein(a).
- In addition to the gender-specific deficiencies noted in high-income countries, women in India face many other social, cultural, and environmental hurdles that call for remediation.

■ REFERENCES

1. Enas EA, Senthilkumar A, Juturu V, Gupta R. Coronary artery disease in women. Indian Heart J. 2001;53(3):282-92.
2. Madan M, Qiu F, Sud M, Graham MM, Saw J, Wijeysundera H, et al. Clinical Outcomes in Younger Women Hospitalized with an Acute Myocardial Infarction: A Contemporary Population-Level Analysis. Can J Cardiol. 2022;38(11):1651-60.
3. Martin SS, Aday AW, Almarzooq ZI, Anderson CAM, Arora P, Avery CL, et al. 2024 Heart Disease and Stroke Statistics: A Report of US and Global Data from the American Heart Association. Circulation. 2024;149(8):e347-e913.
4. Choi J, Daskalopoulou SS, Thanassoulis G, Karp I, Pelletier R, Behlouli H, et al. Sex- and gender-related risk factor burden in patients with premature acute coronary syndrome. Can J Cardiol. 2014;30(1):109-17.

5. Bairey Merz CN, Andersen H, Sprague E, Burns A, Keida M, Walsh MN, et al. Knowledge, Attitudes, and Beliefs Regarding Cardiovascular Disease in Women: The Women's Heart Alliance. J Am Coll Cardiol. 2017;70(2):123-32.
6. Gaur K, Mohan I, Kaur M, Ahuja S, Gupta S, Gupta R. Escalating ischemic heart disease burden among women in India: Insights from GBD, NCDRisC and NFHS reports. Am J Prev Cardiol. 2020;2:100035.
7. Cushman M, Shay CM, Howard VJ, Jiménez MC, Lewey J, McSweeney JC, et al. Ten-Year Differences in Women's Awareness Related to Coronary Heart Disease: Results of the 2019 American Heart Association National Survey: A Special Report from the American Heart Association. Circulation. 2021;143(7):e239-48.
8. Garcia M, Mulvagh SL, Merz CN, Buring JE, Manson JE. Cardiovascular Disease in Women: Clinical Perspectives. Circ Res. 2016; 118(8):1273-93.
9. Liu J, Elbadawi A, Elgendy IY, Megaly M, Ogunbayo GO, Krittanawong C, et al. Age-Stratified Sex Disparities in Care and Outcomes in Patients With ST-Elevation Myocardial Infarction. Am J Med. 2020; 133(11):1293-1301 e1.
10. Tsao CW, Aday AW, Almarzooq ZI, Anderson CAM, Arora P, Avery CL, et al. Heart Disease and Stroke Statistics-2023 Update: A Report from the American Heart Association. Circulation. 2023;147(8):e622.
11. Kooner A. Preliminary results from LOLIPOP study. Heart. 2024.
12. Healthdata.org. (2024). GBD compare. [online] Available from www.healthdata.org IHME/GHDx/GBD compare. [Last accessed May, 2025].
13. Lu Y, Li SX, Liu Y, Rodriguez F, Watson KE, Dreyer RP, et al. Sex-Specific Risk Factors Associated with First Acute Myocardial Infarction in Young Adults. JAMA Netw Open. 2022;5(5):e229953.
14. Walli-Attaei M, Joseph P, Rosengren A, Chow CK, Rangarajan S, Lear SA, et al. Variations between women and men in risk factors, treatments, cardiovascular disease incidence, and death in 27 high-income, middle-income, and low-income countries (PURE): a prospective cohort study. Lancet. 2020;396(10244):97-109.
15. Walli-Attaei M, Rosengren A, Rangarajan S, Chow CK, Rangarajan S, Lear SA, et al. Metabolic, behavioural, and psychosocial risk factors and cardiovascular disease in women compared with men in 21 high-income, middle-income, and low-income countries: an analysis of the PURE study. Lancet. 2022; 400(10355):811-21.
16. Wong ND, Budoff MJ, Ferdinand K, Graham IM, Michos ED, Reddy T, et al. Atherosclerotic cardiovascular disease risk assessment: An American Society for Preventive Cardiology clinical practice statement. Am J Prev Cardiol. 2022;10:100335.
17. Conrad N, Verbeke G, Molenberghs G, Goetschalckx L, Callender T, Cambridge G, et al. Autoimmune diseases and cardiovascular risk: a population-based study on 19 autoimmune diseases and 12 cardiovascular diseases in 22 million individuals in the UK. Lancet. 2022;400(10354):733-43.
18. Grundy SM, Stone NJ, Bailey AL, Beam C, Birtcher KK, Blumenthal RS, et al. 2018 AHA/ACC/AACVPR/AAPA/ABC/ACPM/ADA/AGS/APhA/ASPC/NLA/PCNA Guideline on the Management of Blood Cholesterol: Executive Summary: A Report of the American College of Cardiology/American Heart Association Task Force on Clinical Practice Guidelines. J Am Coll Cardiol. 2019; 73(24):3168-209.
19. Mahmoud AN, Mentias A, Elgendy AY, Qazi A, Barakat AF, Saad M, et al. Migraine and the risk of cardiovascular and cerebrovascular events: a meta-analysis of 16 cohort studies including 1 152 407 subjects. BMJ Open. 2018; 8(3):e020498.
20. Fuglsang CH, Pedersen L, Schmidt M, Vandenbroucke JP, Botker HE, Sorensen HT. Migraine and risk of premature myocardial infarction and stroke among men and women: A Danish population-based cohort study. PLoS Med. 2023;20(6):e1004238.
21. Fuglsang CH, Pedersen L, Schmidt M, Vandenbroucke JP, Botker HE, Sorensen HT.

The combined impact of migraine and gestational diabetes on long-term risk of premature myocardial infarction and stroke: A population-based cohort study. Headache. 2024;64(9):1124-34.
22. Sangaraju SL, Yepez D, Grandes XA, Talanki Manjunatha R, Habib S. Cardio-Metabolic Disease and Polycystic Ovarian Syndrome (PCOS): A Narrative Review. Cureus. 2022;14(5):e25076.
23. Osibogun O, Ogunmoroti O, Michos ED. Polycystic ovary syndrome and cardiometabolic risk: Opportunities for cardiovascular disease prevention. Trends Cardiovasc Med. 2020;30(7):399-404.
24. El Khoudary SR, Aggarwal B, Beckie TM, Hodis HN, Johnson AE, Langer RD, et al. Menopause Transition and Cardiovascular Disease Risk: Implications for Timing of Early Prevention: A Scientific Statement from the American Heart Association. Circulation. 2020;142(25):e506-32.
25. Westerlund E, Brandt L, Hovatta O, Wallen H, Ekbom A, Henriksson P. Incidence of hypertension, stroke, coronary heart disease, and diabetes in women who have delivered after in vitro fertilization: a population-based cohort study from Sweden. Fertil Steril. 2014;102(4):1096-102.
26. Dayan N, Filion KB, Okano M, Kilmartin C, Reinblatt S, Landry T, et al. Cardiovascular Risk Following Fertility Therapy: Systematic Review and Meta-Analysis. J Am Coll Cardiol. 2017;70(10):1203-13.
27. Daly B, Toulis KA, Thomas N, Gokhale K, Martin J, Webber J, et al. Increased risk of ischemic heart disease, hypertension, and type 2 diabetes in women with previous gestational diabetes mellitus, a target group in general practice for preventive interventions: A population-based cohort study. PLoS Med. 2018;15(1):e1002488.
28. Goueslard K, Cottenet J, Mariet AS, Giroud M, Cottin Y, Petit JM, et al. Early cardiovascular events in women with a history of gestational diabetes mellitus. Cardiovasc Diabetol. 2016;15:15.
29. Gupta S, Dhamija JP, Mohan I, Gupta R. Qualitative Study of Barriers to Adherence to Antihypertensive Medication among Rural Women in India. Int J Hypertens. 2019;2019:5749648.
30. Hürter H, Vontelin van Breda S, Vokalova L, Brandl M, Baumann M, Hösli I, et al. Prevention of pre-eclampsia after infertility treatment: Preconceptional minimalisation of risk factors. Best Pract Res Clin Endocrinol Metab. 2019;33(1):127-32.
31. Crump C, Sundquist J, McLaughlin MA, Dolan SM, Govindarajulu U, Sieh W, et al. Adverse pregnancy outcomes and long term risk of ischemic heart disease in mothers: national cohort and co-sibling study. BMJ. 2023;380:e072112.
32. Wang YX, Minguez-Alarcon L, Gaskins AJ, Wang L, Ding M, Missmer SA, et al. Pregnancy loss and risk of cardiovascular disease: the Nurses' Health Study II. Eur Heart J. 2022;43(3):190-9.
33. O'Kelly AC, Michos ED, Shufelt CL, Vermunt JV, Minissian MB, Quesada O, et al. Pregnancy and Reproductive Risk Factors for Cardiovascular Disease in Women. Circ Res. 2022;130(4):652-72.
34. Marma AK, Berry JD, Ning H, Persell SD, Lloyd-Jones DM. Distribution of 10-year and lifetime predicted risks for cardiovascular disease in US adults: findings from the National Health and Nutrition Examination Survey 2003 to 2006. Circ Cardiovasc Qual Outcomes. 2010;3(1):8-14.
35. Mehta LS, Beckie TM, DeVon HA, Grines CL, Krumholz HM, Johnson MN, et al. Acute Myocardial Infarction in Women: A Scientific Statement from the American Heart Association. Circulation. 2016;133(9):916-47.
36. Canto JG, Goldberg RJ, Hand MM, Bonow RO, Sopko G, Pepine CJ, et al. Symptom presentation of women with acute coronary syndromes: myth vs reality. Arch Intern Med. 2007;167(22):2405-13.
37. Canto JG, Shlipak MG, Rogers WJ, Malmgren JA, Frederick PD, Lambrew CT, et al. Prevalence, clinical characteristics, and mortality among patients with myocardial infarction presenting without chest pain. Jama. 2000;283(24):3223-9.

38. Boland LL, Folsom AR, Sorlie PD, Taylor HA, Rosamond WD, Chambless LE, et al. Occurrence of unrecognized myocardial infarction in subjects aged 45 to 65 years (the ARIC study). Am J Cardiol. 2002;90(9):927-31.
39. Tweet MS, Kok SN, Hayes SN. Spontaneous coronary artery dissection in women: What is known and what is yet to be understood. Clin Cardiol. 2018;41(2):203-10.
40. Akashi YK. Epidemiology and pathophysiology of Takotsubo syndrome. Nat Rev Cardiol. 2015;12:387-97.
41. Singh T, Khan H, Gamble DT, Scally C, Newby DE, Dawson D. Takotsubo Syndrome: Pathophysiology, Emerging concepts, and Clinical implications. Circulation. 2022; 145:1002-19.
42. Alpert JS, Serpytis R, Serpytis P, Chen QM. Myocardial Infarction with Nonobstructive Coronary Arteries (MINOCA). Am J Med. 2019;132(3):267-8.
43. Safdar B, Spatz ES, Dreyer RP, Beltrame JF, Lichtman JH, Spertus JA, et al. Presentation, Clinical Profile, and Prognosis of Young Patients with Myocardial Infarction with Nonobstructive Coronary Arteries (MINOCA): Results from the VIRGO Study. J Am Heart Assoc. 2018;7(13):e009174.
44. Bakhshi H, Gibson CM. MINOCA: Myocardial infarction no obstructive coronary artery disease. Am Heart J Plus. 2023;33: 100312.
45. Cho L, Davis M, Elgendy I, Epps K, Lindley KJ, Mehta PK, et al. Summary of Updated Recommendations for Primary Prevention of Cardiovascular Disease in Women: JACC State-of-the-Art Review. J Am Coll Cardiol. 2020;75(20):2602-18.
46. The Lancet. Cardiology's problem women. Lancet. 2019;393(10175):959.
47. Knuuti J, Wijns W, Saraste A, Capodanno D, Barbato E, Funck-Brentano C, et al. 2019 ESC Guidelines for the diagnosis and management of chronic coronary syndromes. Eur Heart J. 2020;41(3):407-77.
48. Roeters van Lennep JE, Tokgozoglu LS, Badimon L, Dumanski SM, Gulati M, Hess CN, et al. Women, lipids, and atherosclerotic cardiovascular disease: a call to action from the European Atherosclerosis Society. Eur Heart J. 2023;44(39):4157-73.
49. Shah T, Haimi I, Yang Y, Gaston S, Taoutel R, Mehta S, et al. Meta-Analysis of Gender Disparities in In-hospital Care and Outcomes in Patients with ST-Segment Elevation Myocardial Infarction. Am J Cardiol. 2021; 147:23-32.
50. Zaman MJ, Junghans C, Sekhri N, Chen R, Feder GS, Timmis AD, et al. Presentation of stable angina pectoris among women and South Asian people. CMAJ. 2008;179(7): 659-67.
51. Zaman MJ, Crook AM, Junghans C, Fitzpatrick NK, Feder G, Timmis AD, et al. Ethnic differences in long-term improvement of angina following revascularization or medical management: a comparison between south Asians and white Europeans. J Public Health (Oxf). 2009;31(1):168-74.
52. Bucholz EM, Strait KM, Dreyer RP, Lindau ST, D'Onofrio G, Geda M, et al. Editor's Choice-Sex differences in young patients with acute myocardial infarction: A VIRGO study analysis. Eur Heart J Acute Cardiovasc Care. 2017;6(7):610-22.
53. Davis M, Diamond J, Montgomery D, Krishnan S, Eagle K, Jackson E. Acute coronary syndrome in young women under 55 years of age: clinical characteristics, treatment, and outcomes. Clin Res Cardiol. 2015;104(8):648-55.
54. Sharma SK, Makkar JS, Bana A, Sharma K, Kasliwal A, Sidana SK, et al. Premature coronary artery disease, risk factors, clinical presentation, angiography and interventions: Hospital based registry. Indian Heart J. 2022;74(5):391-7.
55. Ridker PM, Moorthy MV, Cook NR, Rifai N, Lee IM, Buring JE. Inflammation, Cholesterol, Lipoprotein(a), and 30-Year Cardiovascular Outcomes in Women. N Engl J Med. 2024;391(22):2087-97.
56. Sawhney JPS, Kumar A, Tyagi K, Madan K. Prevalence of lipoprotein(a) in acute coronary syndrome and its association with severity of heart disease among patients admitted to a tertiary care hospital. Atherosclerosis. 2023;379:117162.

57. Orth-Gomer K, Mittleman MA, Schenck-Gustafsson K, Wamala SP, Eriksson M, Belkic K, et al. Lipoprotein(a) as a determinant of coronary heart disease in young women. Circulation. 1997;95(2):329-34.
58. Enas EA. Lipoprotein(a) as a determinant of coronary heart disease in young women: a stronger risk factor than diabetes? Circulation. 1998;97(3):293-5.
59. Rifai N, Ma J, Sacks FM, Ridker PM, Hernandez WJ, Stampfer MJ, et al. Apolipoprotein(a) size and lipoprotein(a) concentration and future risk of angina pectoris with evidence of severe coronary atherosclerosis in men: The Physicians' Health Study. Clin Chem. 2004;50(8):1364-71.
60. Kronenberg F, Mora S, Stroes ESG, Ference BA, Arsenault BJ, Berglund L, et al. Lipoprotein(a) in atherosclerotic cardiovascular disease and aortic stenosis: a European Atherosclerosis Society consensus statement. Eur Heart J. 2022;43(39):3925-46.
61. Xavier D, Pais P, Devereaux PJ, Xie C, Prabhakaran D, Reddy KS, et al. Treatment and outcomes of acute coronary syndromes in India (CREATE): a prospective analysis of registry data. Lancet. 2008;371(9622):1435-42.
62. Mohanan PP, Mathew R, Harikrishnan S, Krishnan MN, Zachariah G, Joseph J, et al. Presentation, management, and outcomes of 25 748 acute coronary syndrome admissions in Kerala, India: results from the Kerala ACS Registry. Eur Heart J. 2013;34(2):121-9.
63. Gupta R, Yusuf S. Challenges in management and prevention of ischemic heart disease in low socioeconomic status people in LLMICs. BMC Med. 2019;17(1):209.
64. O'Neil A, Scovelle AJ, Milner AJ, Kavanagh A. Gender/Sex as a Social Determinant of Cardiovascular Risk. Circulation. 2018;137(8):854-64.
65. Mathew A, Hong Y, Yogasundaram H, Nagendran J, Punnoose E, Ashraf SM, et al. Sex and Medium-term Outcomes of ST-Segment Elevation Myocardial Infarction in Kerala, India: A Propensity Score-Matched Analysis. CJC Open. 2021;3(12 Suppl):S71-S80.
66. Akintoye E, Afonso L, Bengaluru Jayanna M, Bao W, Briasoulis A, Robinson J. Prognostic Utility of Risk Enhancers and Coronary Artery Calcium Score Recommended in the 2018 ACC/AHA Multisociety Cholesterol Treatment Guidelines Over the Pooled Cohort Equation: Insights From 3 Large Prospective Cohorts. J Am Heart Assoc. 2021;10(12):e019589.
67. Agarwala A, Patel J, Blaha M, Cainzos-Achirica M, Nasir K, Budoff M. Leveling the playing field: The utility of coronary artery calcium scoring in cardiovascular risk stratification in South Asians. Am J Prev Cardiol. 2023;13:100455.
68. Joseph P, Kutty VR, Mohan V, Kumar R, Mony P, Vijayakumar K, et al. Cardiovascular disease, mortality, and their associations with modifiable risk factors in a multi-national South Asia cohort: a PURE substudy. Eur Heart J. 2022;43(30):2831-40.

CHAPTER 10

Angina Pectoris: Shift from Invasive Treatment to Medical Management

■ INTRODUCTION

Angina, the classic symptom of coronary artery disease (CAD), is caused by restriction of oxygen-carrying blood to the heart muscle from plaque buildup in the coronary arteries. The pattern of chest discomfort can be crushing pain, pressure, tightness, or squeezing (Chapter 2). Stable angina, the most common type, features predictable episodes triggered by exertion or stress that typically resolve with rest or medication. The main focus of treatment for several decades was a mechanistic one, to open up the blocks with percutaneous coronary intervention (PCI) with stents or with coronary artery bypass graft (CABG) surgery. There has been a sharp and marked shift in the management of angina away from the mechanistic approach to guideline-directed medical therapy (GDMT) that tackles the underlying causes of CAD through lifestyle changes and medications. Invasive treatments are reserved now for select cases such as uncontrolled angina that significantly hinders the quality of life.[1-4] The magnitude of the shift in the management of angina since the 1990s in the US is illustrated in **Figure 1 and Table 1**.[5,6]

Cardiac catheterization and CABG surgery, once dominant,[7-11] have seen a marked decrease since 2000 **(Table 1)**. CABG surgery continues to have a role in select complex cases and PCI procedures have come down from its peak especially in those with stable CAD. Besides, the improved armamentarium of effective drugs, the increased recognition and control of major risk factors tobacco smoking, hypertension, diabetes, and cholesterol have resulted in a decline in CAD complications and in the use of invasive procedures.

In the sections that follow we explain the key studies that led to a rethinking of the management of angina and stable CAD from invasive procedures to GDMT that combines lifestyle changes and medications and go on to tabulate the key components of GDMT and the pharmacologic management of angina.

■ INSIGHTS FROM THE LANDMARK ISCHEMIA STUDY

This large National Institute of Health (NIH)-funded study (5,179 participants at a cost of $100 million) investigated the effectiveness of adding coronary artery revascularization procedures (CARP) to GDMT for stable CAD patients with moderate or severe ischemia. One half of the participants received GDMT only, the other half received GDMT plus CARP (PCI or CABG). The results confirmed and solidified conclusions of several smaller prior cardiovascular outcome trials (CVOTs).[13-16] The International Study of Comparative Health Effectiveness with Medical and Invasive Approaches (ISCHEMIA) study excluded patients with left main CAD and acute coronary syndrome (ACS), where the

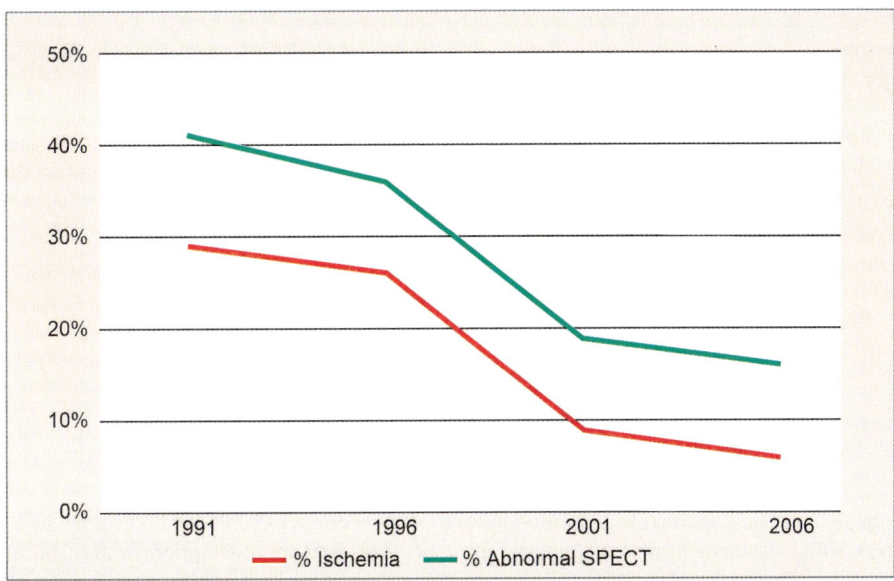

Fig. 1: Progressive decline frequency of abnormal and ischemic single photon computed tomography (SPECT) myocardial perfusion imaging (MPI) over the years.
Source: Adapted from Rozanski A, Gransar H, Hayes SW, Min J, Friedman JD, Thomson LE, et al. Temporal trends in the frequency of inducible myocardial ischemia during cardiac stress testing: 1991 to 2009. J Am Coll Cardiol. 2013;61(10):1054-65.[6]

TABLE 1: Trends of coronary interventions in the US from 1994 to 2014.[12]			
Procedure/Intervention	*1994*	*2004*	*2014*
Coronary catheterization	1,160,000	1,500,000	1,000,000
Coronary artery bypass graft (CABG)	570,000	570,000	375,000
Percutaneous transluminal coronary angioplasty (PTCA)	400,000	800,000	475,000

Note: Decrease of coronary interventions in the United States from 2004 to 2014. By 2014 annual cardiac catheterizations decreased to one million, coronary artery bypass surgery to 375,000 and percutaneous transluminal coronary intervention to 475,000.[12]

benefits of CARP are well-established. Additionally, people with a high degree of left main stenosis identified through blinded computed tomography were not included. Death rates were similar in both groups. An important observation was that approximately 20% of patients initially randomized to the conservative approach eventually received CARP. This crossover did not demonstrate any harm associated with delaying intervention. The key findings of the ISCHEMIA trial and their implications are shown on **Table 2**.[15,17-20]

LIMITATIONS OF CORONARY ARTERY REVASCULARIZATION PROCEDURES

The commonly held notion that the risk of heart attack is determined solely by the severity of stenosis (blockage) of coronary

TABLE 2: Rethinking coronary artery revascularization procedures (CARP) for stable coronary artery disease (CAD)—insights from ISCHEMIA trial.[15,17-20]

	Key findings	Implications for treatment
Manage angina with Guideline-directed Medical Therapy (GDMT)	Patients with minimal or no chest pain can be managed with GDMT even in the presence of moderate or severe ischemia	GDMT should be the mainstay of treatment for most patients, with CARP reserved for those with uncontrolled angina
No survival benefit	Extended follow-up for 7 years showed no significant difference in overall survival between the two strategies. This is particularly true in those with severe ischemia	Routine CARP does not improve survival in stable CAD patients
Relieving ischemia with CARP	No difference in outcome between patients with moderate and severe ischemia	ISCHEMIA trial questions the routine use of stress testing followed by CARP for silent ischemia
Delaying/avoiding CARP	No harm was found among those switched from conservative to invasive arm because of intractable angina	Unnecessary CARPs can be avoided by a measured approach prioritizing GDMT and intervening in only those with intractable angina
Cost savings	Up to 80% of patients with occasional chest pain managed by medication can avoid CARP	A more conservative approach can lead to significant cost savings for healthcare systems
Repeat procedures	Atherosclerosis progression may necessitate repeating CARP every 7–10 years, even with LDL levels <70 mg/dL	Aggressive low-density lipoprotein cholesterol (LDL-C) lowering (to 40–50 mg/dL) may be necessary to maximize the long-term benefits of CARP
The CARP paradox	The US performs more CARPs per 100,000 persons than Canada, yet Canada has lower CAD mortality	A less intervention-heavy approach may yield better outcomes. Besides, a 50% reduction in CARP in the US was associated with continuing decline CAD in the US
Low rates of major adverse cardiovascular event (MACE)	Annual MACE rates were low at 2% in both groups possibly due to better control of risk factors	Reduce MACE rates to 2% per year with GDMT

arteries is open to question as severe stenosis may not always lead to a heart attack, and mild blockage may cause a heart attack as plaque rupture may happen in an area without severe stenosis.[21-24] Research studies and clinical trials have further informed us: (1) The severity of a single blockage does not necessarily correlate with total plaque burden and total plaque burden correlates well with ACS. Computed coronary angiography (CTCA), in post-hoc analysis of the previously discussed ISCHEMIA cohort data showed that the total plaque volume correlated with myocardial infarction and death.[25] Coronary artery calcium (CAC) score reliably assesses the total plaque burden; (2) *Paradox of remodeling:* Arteries widening (remodeling) to accommodate plaque buildup, while appearing helpful, might be linked to increased heart attack risk, potentially

TABLE 3: Key components of guideline-directed medical treatment (GDMT).[13,14,17,26,28,29]

A heart-healthy diet	Rich in whole grains, nuts, fruits, legumes, and vegetables and markedly restricting saturated fat and instead use of monounsaturated and polyunsaturated fats (Chapter 16)
Aim for 150–300 minutes of physical activity per week	Aim for <4 hours of sitting daily and walk more as this simple change can improve your heart health, reduce chronic disease risk, and boost your overall well-being. Younger adults should strive for 10,000 steps a day and seniors >65 years should strive for 4,000 or more steps
Smoking cessation and nicotine exposure	This is crucial as it markedly reduces the risk of major adverse cardiovascular event (MACE) after an ACS by 70–80%
Maintaining healthy weight and waist circumference	For Indians a healthy BMI is <23; healthy waist circumference is 80 cm for women and 90 cm for men (Chapter 3)
Maintaining healthy blood pressure	Maintaining blood pressure <120/80 mm Hg (Chapter 5)
Maintaining fasting blood sugar <100 mg/dL	Hemoglobin A1C <7% if diabetes is present (Chapter 6)
Maintaining lower lipid goals	• *Individuals with ASCVD:* Goal of LDL-C <70 mg/dL and NHDL-C; <100 mg/dL • *Indians at very high-risk for primary prevention:* Goal of LDL-C <50 and NHDL-C <80 mg/dL (Chapter 15)
Adequate sleep	Getting 7–8 hours of sleep plus others in Life's essential 8 (Chapter 17)
Cardiac rehabilitation	Reduces recurrent heart attack, stroke, and death by 25–30% after ACS
Full adherence to anti-anginal and secondary prevention medications	Aspirin, or clopidogrel, angiotensin converting enzyme (ACE) inhibitor or angiotensin receptor blocker (ARB) statins and beta-blockers can reduce recurrent MACE by 75–80%

harboring more dangerous plaque; and (3) to pay attention to plaque characteristics not just severity of blockage as CTCA scans show that heart attack-causing lesions may only have mild narrowing.[22,23,26]

The ISCHEMIA study highlighted the benefits of GDMT as a first-line treatment for stable CAD. While CARP offers faster angina relief, it does not necessarily translate to improved survival rates. The study delineated the importance of careful patient selection and a measured approach that prioritizes GDMT and reserves CARP for those who continue to have angina on GDMT. Other than in ACS, an invasive approach with CARP is not to be considered as a life-saving modality.[18,27]

Coronary artery disease is a systemic disease (atherosclerosis) requiring systemic treatment rather than a focal disease requiring focal treatment. Thus, rather than favoring a mechanistic approach that focuses solely on blockages and how to open them, a more comprehensive approach to management of CAD, a manifestation is required. GDMT combines lifestyle changes and medications **(Table 3)**, targets inflammation and lipid buildup in the coronary arteries and throughout the systemic arteries and improves patient outcomes.[30-32]

■ STABLE ANGINA: MEDICATIONS

Medications used in the management of stable angina comprise ones that relieve symptoms and ones that aim to prevent heart attacks and strokes. Preventive medications are indicated in both primary prevention (before a heart attack) and in secondary [after a heart attack or other major adverse cardiovascular event (MACE)] prevention.

- *First line:*
  - Nitrates—sublingual; oral forms both short acting and long acting.
  - Calcium channel blockers—non-dihydropyridines (e.g., diltiazem, felodipine, and amlodipine).
  - Be aware that short acting nifedipine is not recommended as it may cause reflex tachycardia.
  - Beta-blockers, especially in those with previous heart attacks and poor heart function (left ventricular ejection fraction <40%).
- *Second and third line:*
  - Ranolazine
  - Ivabradine
- *Secondary prevention:*
  - Aspirin
  - *Clopidogrel:* Though aspirin and clopidogrel may be considered in select patients exercise caution because of the high risk of bleeding.
  - Angiotensin converting enzyme (ACE) inhibitor or angiotensin receptor blocker (ARB)
  - Statins (Chapter 13) are important in secondary and primary prevention.
  - Beta-blockers for 1 year following ACS
- *New drugs:* Glucagon-like peptide-1 receptor agonists (GLP-1 RAs) and sodium glucose co-transporter 2 (SGLT2) inhibitors are two classes of drugs that show great promise in reducing CAD progression and in reducing MACEs in patients (especially in those with type 2 diabetes). However, their role in the management of stable angina is not yet clear. A relatively small recent controlled trial (EMPT-ANGINA) of a SGLT2 drug showed beneficial antianginal effects in patients with diabetes.[33]

CURRENT AMERICAN CLINICAL PRACTICE GUIDELINES

The ISCHEMIA trial has significantly reshaped the 2021 American College of Cardiology and American Heart Association (ACC/AHA) guidelines (main points are given below) for coronary revascularization in stable CAD.[34]

- Guideline-directed medical therapy is the preferred initial approach, even for high-risk patients with extensive disease.
- The role of both PCI and CABG surgery is defined and the indications clarified.
  - For patients with significant left main disease, surgical revascularization is indicated to improve survival relative to that likely to be achieved with medical therapy.
  - Surgical revascularization may be reasonable to improve survival in triple-vessel CAD.
- In patients undergoing CARP adequate information about benefits, risks, therapeutic consequences, and potential alternatives in the performance of CARP should be given, with sufficient time for informed decision-making to improve clinical outcomes.
- Overall, the guidelines suggest that GDMT alone may be sufficient for as many as 80% of the patients with CARP reserved for those with uncontrolled angina.[34]

DIVERGENT MANAGEMENT OF CORONARY ARTERY DISEASE IN THE US AND INDIA

While CARP (both PCI and CABG) have declined in the US, there has been a rise in

CARP in India. Between 2013 and 2018, PCI procedures in India more than doubled. Of note, 12% of PCIs were in young adults (<40 years of age) consistent with increased premature CAD in India.[35] However, premature onset alone would not be sufficient to explain the degree of divergence in usage of PCIs between the two countries. The overemphasis of PCI in India leads to two considerations: Overestimation of the advantages of PCI and/or the underestimation of what GDMT can do.

This imbalance between PCI and GDMT needs to be addressed as GDMT can improve patient outcomes, is cost effective and avoids procedure-related risks, reduce healthcare costs and financial strain for patients and bring cardiac care in alignment to proven practices. We suggest the following steps:

- Comprehensive educational initiatives targeting both physicians and patients on the long-term preventive power of GDMT and its efficacy in managing CAD.
- Evidence-based guidelines that prioritize GDMT as the first-line of treatment, and reserve invasive procedures to specific, high-risk scenarios (e.g., ACS) where invasive procedures such as PCI can offer the most benefit.
- Conducting robust studies in India comparing benefits, risks, and outcomes of and cost-effectiveness of PCI and GDMT within the Indian context.

TESTS WITH IMPROVED DIAGNOSTIC PRECISION TO GUIDE TREATMENT

The diagnosis of angina is gaining remarkable precision with advancements such as computed tomographic coronary angiography (CTCA) and fractional flow reserve computed tomography (FFRCT). Traditionally, diagnosing angina relied on subjective symptoms and stress tests, which have limitations. Symptoms can vary, and stress tests may not be definitive for all patients, especially those with atypical presentations. The 2021 ACC/AHA guidelines recommend CTCA as a Class I recommendation for suitable patients with stable chest pain.[4]

Computed tomographic coronary angiography offers a noninvasive way to visualize coronary arteries, providing a detailed anatomical picture of the extent of plaque buildup and narrowing. This allows for improved detection of CAD and identification of specific blockages contributing to angina. This procedure also helps differentiate critical blockages causing significant ischemia (oxygen deficiency) that contribute to angina from less critical blockages that may not require immediate intervention.

Fractional flow reserve computed tomography builds on CTCA by functionally assessing the impact of blockages on blood flow within the coronary arteries and can differentiate between patients who would best benefit from CARP from those who are unlikely to benefit. The Assessing Diagnostic Value of Non-invasive FFRCT in Coronary Care (ADVANCE) Registry found that a positive FFRCT result, indicating a significant blockage, led to treatment changes in two-thirds of patients compared to using CTCA alone, highlighting its use to avoid invasive coronary angiograms in patients with blockages that do not significantly impact blood flow. This combined approach with FFRCT offers a more precise approach to diagnosing angina, optimizing treatment decisions, and potentially reducing unnecessary interventions.[36]

CHRONIC CORONARY DISEASE: A PATIENT-CENTERED APPROACH TO MANAGEMENT

Chronic coronary disease (CCD) encompasses a spectrum of heart conditions, including those with prior heart attack, weakened heart muscle (cardiomyopathy), chest pain (angina), blocked arteries, and high coronary plaque burden (high CAC score). The updated 2023 ACC/AHA guidelines prioritize both extending lifespan and improving quality of life for CCD patients. The main recommendations of the guidelines are:

- The use of GDMT in all patients with CCD.[37]
- Coronary artery calcium score to assess risk and for prompt therapeutic intervention (mostly GDMT) in patients with high CAC score to prevent a MACE. A CAC score >300 is associated with a 3–7-fold high risk of a MACE.[38]
- Coronary artery revascularization procedure is appropriate in two specific scenarios:[37,39]
  1. Relief of severe angina that limits daily activities despite optimal medical therapy,
  2. Improve survival in high-risk patients with severe left main artery disease or multivessel disease with severely weakened heart function [left ventricular ejection fraction (LVEF) ≤35%]. In these patients, coronary artery bypass (CABG) surgery combined with medication(s) is recommended.
- Caution against unnecessary cardiac tests: Routine periodic anatomic or ischemic testing in the absence of a change in clinical or functional status is not recommended for risk stratification or to guide therapeutic decision-making for patients with CCD.[37]

■ KEY TAKEAWAYS

- Guideline-directed medical treatment (GDMT) utilizes a powerful combination of heart-healthy lifestyle modifications (diet, exercise, and sleep smoking cessation) and effective medications that control cardiac risk factors, relieve angina, are cardioprotective and prevent MACE. Key elements of GDMT and antianginal and preventive medications are tabulated and detailed in the text.
- Coronary artery bypass graft (CABG) surgery and percutaneous coronary intervention (PCI) procedures are no longer the primary treatment modalities for angina and stable CAD. This shift away from invasive procedures reflects a better understanding that CAD is a systemic disease and therefore addressing the underlying causes with GDMT is more apt and effective.
- Coronary revascularization procedures (CARP) that include CABG and PCI are limited to select patients in two scenarios: (1) Severe angina (that limits daily activities) despite optimal medication management; (2) Severe left main artery disease or multivessel disease with severely diminished left ventricular ejection fraction (LVEF).
- Guideline-directed medical treatment is the right choice for all patients with stable angina and many with chronic coronary disease (CCD).
- Several medications—first line and second line—are available for angina management. Secondary prevention to prevent major adverse cardiovascular events (MACE) is to be emphasized in all patients with angina.
- *Newer imaging tests:* Computed tomographic coronary arteriography (CCTA) and fractional flow reserve computed tomography (FFRCT) are more precise in diagnosing angina than currently used tests and are better guides to management.
- There is a remarkable divergence in the management of CAD between the US and India. While cardiovascular revascularization procedures (both CABG and PCI) have markedly decreased in the US, in India PCIs have very markedly increased. This is due to an overestimation of the benefits of PCI and an underestimation of the benefits of GDMT.

- Research generated and evidence-based guidelines and educational efforts that target both doctors and the public are needed to increase the use of proven GDMT in India.

REFERENCES

1. Favaloro RG. 50th anniversary historical article. Surgical treatment of acute myocardial infarction. J Am Coll Cardiol. 1999;33(6):1435-41.
2. Knuuti J, Wijns W, Saraste A, Capodanno D, Barbato E, Funck-Brentano C, et al. 2019 ESC Guidelines for the diagnosis and management of chronic coronary syndromes. Eur Heart J. 2020;41(3):407-77.
3. Gruntzig AR, Senning A, Siegenthaler W. Nonoperative dilatation of coronary-artery stenosis: Percutaneous transluminal coronary angioplasty. N Engl J Med. 1979; 301:61-8.
4. Gulati M, Levy PD, Mukherjee D, Amsterdam E, Bhatt DL, Birtcher KK, et al. 2021 AHA/ACC/ASE/CHEST/SAEM/SCCT/SCMR Guideline for the Evaluation and Diagnosis of Chest Pain: Executive Summary: A Report of the American College of Cardiology/American Heart Association Joint Committee on Clinical Practice Guidelines. Circulation. 2021;144(22):e368-e454.
5. Rozanski A, Berman D. Optimizing the Assessment of Patient Clinical Risk at the Time of Cardiac Stress Testing. JACC Cardiovasc Imaging. 2020;13(2 Pt 2):616-23.
6. Rozanski A, Gransar H, Hayes SW, Min J, Friedman JD, Thomson LE, et al. Temporal trends in the frequency of inducible myocardial ischemia during cardiac stress testing: 1991 to 2009. J Am Coll Cardiol. 2013; 61(10):1054-65.
7. Favaloro RG. Saphenous vein autograft replacement of severe segmental coronary artery occlusion: Operative technique. Ann Thorac Surg. 1998;5:334-9.
8. Favaloro RG. Critical analysis of coronary artery bypass graft surgery: a 30-year journey. J Am Coll Cardiol. 1998;31(4 Suppl B):1B-63B.
9. Favaloro RG. Saphenous vein graft in the surgical treatment of coronary artery disease. Operative technique. J Thorac Cardiovasc Surg. 1969;58(2):178-85.
10. Goldman S, Zadina K, Moritz T, Ovitt T, Sethi G, Copeland JG, et al. Long-term patency of saphenous vein and left internal mammary artery grafts after coronary artery bypass surgery: results from a Department of Veterans Affairs Cooperative Study. J Am Coll Cardiol. 2004;44(11):2149-56.
11. Tsao CW, Aday AW, Almarzooq ZI, Anderson CAM, Arora P, Avery CL, et al. Heart Disease and Stroke Statistics-2023 Update: A Report from the American Heart Association. Circulation. 2023;147(8):e93-e621.
12. Virani SS, Alonso A, Aparicio HJ, Benjamin EJ, Bittencourt MS, Callaway CW, et al. Heart Disease and Stroke Statistics-2021 Update: A Report from the American Heart Association. Circulation. 2021;143(8):e254-e743.
13. Bittner V, Bertolet M, Barraza Felix R, Farkouh ME, Goldberg S, Ramanathan KB, et al. Comprehensive Cardiovascular Risk Factor Control Improves Survival: The BARI 2D Trial. J Am Coll Cardiol. 2015;66(7):765-73.
14. Boden WE, O'Rourke RA, Teo KK, Hartigan PM, Maron DJ, Kostuk WJ, et al. Optimal Medical Therapy with or without PCI for Stable Coronary Disease. N Engl J Med. 2007;356(15):1503-16.
15. Al-Lamee R, Thompson D, Dehbi HM, Sen S, Tang K, Davies J, et al. Percutaneous coronary intervention in stable angina (ORBITA): a double-blind, randomised controlled trial. Lancet. 2018;391(10115):31-40.
16. Weintraub WS, Spertus JA, Kolm P, Maron DJ, Zhang Z, Jurkovitz C, et al. Effect of PCI on quality of life in patients with stable coronary disease. N Engl J Med. 2008;359(7):677-87.
17. Maron DJ, Hochman JS, Reynolds HR, Bangalore S, O'Brien SM, Boden WE, et al. Initial Invasive or Conservative Strategy for Stable Coronary Disease. N Engl J Med. 2020;382(15):1395-1407.
18. Chaitman BR, Alexander KP, Cyr DD, Berger JS, Reynolds HR, Bangalore S, et al.

Myocardial infarction in the ISCHEMIA Trial: impact of different definitions on incidence, prognosis, and treatment comparisons. Circulation. 2021;143(8):790-804.
19. Boden WE, Stone PH. To stent or not to stent? Treating angina after ISCHEMIA: why a conservative approach with optimal medical therapy is the preferred initial management strategy for chronic coronary syndromes: insights from the ISCHEMIA trial. Eur Heart J. 2021;42(14):1394-400.
20. Bradley SM, Gluckman TJ. If the Fates Allow: The Zero-Sum Game of ISCHEMIA-EXTEND. Circulation. 2023;147(1):20-22.
21. Arbab-Zadeh A, Fuster V. The myth of the "vulnerable plaque": transitioning from a focus on individual lesions to atherosclerotic disease burden for coronary artery disease risk assessment. J Am Coll Cardiol. 2015; 65(8):846-55.
22. Arbab-Zadeh A, Fuster V. The Risk Continuum of atherosclerosis and its implications for defining CHD by coronary angiography. J Am Coll Cardiol. 2016;68(22): 2467-78.
23. Mortensen MB, Dzaye O, Steffensen FH, Bøtker HE, Jensen JM, Rønnow Sand NP, et al. Impact of plaque burden versus stenosis on ischemic events in patients with coronary atherosclerosis. J Am Coll Cardiol. 2020; 76(24):2803-13.
24. Motoyama S, Ito H, Sarai M, Kondo T, Kawai H, Nagahara Y, et al. Plaque characterization by coronary computed tomography angiography and the likelihood of acute coronary events in mid-term follow-up. J Am Coll Cardiol. 2015;66(4):337-46.
25. Nurmohamed NS, Min JK, Anthopolos R, Reynolds HR, Earls JP, et al. Atherosclerosis quantification and cardiovascular risk: the ISCHEMIA trial. Eur Heart J. 2024;45(36): 3735-47.
26. Ferraro R, Latina JM, Alfaddagh A, Michos ED, Blaha MJ, Jones SR, et al. Evaluation and management of patients with stable angina: beyond the ischemia paradigm: JACC state-of-the-art review. J Am Coll Cardiol. 2020;76(19):2252-66.
27. Ambrosch A, Muhlen I, Kopf D, Augustin W, Dierkes J, König W, et al. LDL size distribution in relation to insulin sensitivity and lipoprotein pattern in young and healthy subjects. Diabetes Care. 1998;21(12):2077-84.
28. Nabel EG, Braunwald E. A tale of coronary artery disease and myocardial infarction. N Engl J Med. 2012;366(1):54-63.
29. Stone PH, Libby P, Boden WE. Fundamental pathobiology of coronary atherosclerosis and clinical implications for chronic ischemic heart disease management—the plaque hypothesis: a narrative review. JAMA Cardiol. 2023; 8(2):192-201.
30. Nissen SE, Bakaeen FG. Coronary revascularization strategies: making sense of sparse, limited-quality data. JAMA. 2020; 324(2):154-6.
31. Chacko L, J PH, Rajkumar C, Nowbar AN, Kane C, Mahdi D, et al. Effects of percutaneous coronary intervention on death and myocardial infarction stratified by stable and unstable coronary artery disease: a meta-analysis of randomized controlled trials. Circ Cardiovasc Qual Outcomes. 2020;13(2):e006363.
32. Antman EM, Braunwald E. Managing stable ischemic heart disease. N Engl J Med. 2020;382(15):1468-70.
33. Mansouri MH, Mansouri P, Sadeghi M, Hashemi SM, Khosravi A, Behjati M, et al. Antianginal effects of empagliflozin in patients with type 2 diabetes and refractory angina; a randomized, double-blind placebo-controlled trial (EMPT-ANGINA Trial). Clin Cardiol. 2024;47(1):e24158.
34. Lawton JS, Tamis-Holland JE, Bangalore S, Bates ER, Beckie TM, Bischoff JM, et al. 2021 ACC/AHA/SCAI Guideline for Coronary Artery Revascularization: A Report of the American College of Cardiology/American Heart Association Joint Committee on Clinical Practice Guidelines. J Am Coll Cardiol. 2022;79(2):e21-e129.
35. Arramraju SK, Janapati RK, Sanjeeva Kumar E, Mandala GR. National interventional council data for the year 2018-India. Indian Heart J. 2020;72(5):351-5.

36. Fairbairn TA, Nieman K, Akasaka T, Nørgaard BL, Berman DS, Raff G, et al. Real-world clinical utility and impact on clinical decision-making of coronary computed tomography angiography-derived fractional flow reserve: lessons from the ADVANCE Registry. Eur Heart J. 2018;39(41):3701-11.
37. Virani SS, Newby LK, Arnold SV, Bittner V, Brewer LC, Demeter SH, et al. 2023 AHA/ACC/ACCP/ASPC/NLA/PCNA Guideline for the Management of Patients with Chronic Coronary Disease: A Report of the American Heart Association/American College of Cardiology Joint Committee on Clinical Practice Guidelines. Circulation. 2023;148(9):e9-e119.
38. Grandhi GR, Mirbolouk M, Dardari ZA, Al-Mallah MH, Rumberger JA, Shaw LJ, et al. Interplay of Coronary Artery Calcium and Risk Factors for Predicting CVD/CHD Mortality: The CAC Consortium. JACC Cardiovasc Imaging. 2020;13(5):1175-86.
39. Rao SV, Reynolds HR, Hochman JS. Chronic Coronary Disease Guidelines. Circulation. 2023;148(9):729-31.

CHAPTER 11

Acute Coronary Syndrome: Management and Secondary Prevention

▪ INTRODUCTION

Earlier in this book, the process of atherosclerosis, plaque formation within coronary arteries, and consequent clinical manifestations were described (Chapter 2, Table 2). While angina pectoris is the characteristic symptom associated with coronary artery disease (CAD), the most important manifestation is acute coronary syndrome (ACS). Among the three types of ACS, ST-segment elevation myocardial infarction (STEMI) from complete occlusion of an artery is the most serious and consequential one. The others are non-ST segment elevation myocardial infarction (NSTEMI) from a non-occlusive clot and unstable angina similar to NSTEMI but without troponin elevation.

Here in this chapter, a few historical highlights are shared as we traverse the past decades and document the marked decline in acute myocardial infarctions (AMIs) in the US, unmistakably linked to a much better understanding of plaques and clots that cause over 70% of heart attacks (AMIs) and sudden cardiac deaths.[1-4] The knowledge accrued from much basic and clinical research then translated to improved diagnostic accuracy and prompt effective interventions, secondary prevention, and vastly improved prognosis of heart attacks.

▪ A TRIP THROUGH THE DECADES

Between 1950 and 1970, about two-thirds of deaths from AMI occurred before the patients reached a hospital. Those who reached the hospital alive were placed throughout the hospital, far away from nurses' stations, so that the patient's total bed rest would not be disturbed. Confined to strict bed rest for weeks, often isolated from family and heavily sedated, nearly a third succumbed to the ordeal. Physicians at the time believed this rigorous bed rest was essential for survival—a stark testament to the limited understanding of heart attack management in that era. The following case history of a patient, none other than the President of the US, reflects the standard of care then and the events in later years illustrate the progression of atherosclerosis with stroke and recurrent heart attacks. President Dwight Eisenhower had a heart attack in 1955.[5] He was treated with total bed rest for 48 days in the hospital; upon discharge, he was advised to continue bed rest for another 6 months at the White House and to cut down his smoking from four packs (80 cigarettes) to one pack per day. Subsequently he had a stroke in 1957 and a second heart attack in 1965. Altogether, he had seven heart attacks and 14 cardiac arrests until death from heart failure in 1969.

A simple change from strict bed rest to "armchair treatment", pioneered in the 1950s by Drs Lown and Levine, alone, decreased mortality rates.[6-9] The development of coronary care units in 1961, capable of monitoring electrocardiogram (ECG/EKG), and to perform closed-chest cardiac resuscitation and direct current defibrillation reduced in-hospital mortality of AMI by half.[10,11]

By the 1970s, in-hospital mortality from heart attack had plummeted to around 15%, with another 10% succumbing within a year (often from heart failure due to larger infarctions).[2] The 1970s and 1980s saw a surge in coronary artery revascularization procedures (CARP)—coronary artery bypass surgery (CABG)[12] and percutaneous coronary intervention (PCI).[13] Since the 1980s, increased use of guideline-directed medical treatment (GDMT) (details in previous chapter), driven by advances in cardiovascular treatments led to a dramatic decline in both the number and severity of AMI. This decrease is reflected in a substantial drop in AMI deaths, with only about 110,000 deaths attributed to AMI in the US in 2020.[3,4,14] The decrease is not just in the number of AMIs, but also in their severity. Notably, STEMI, the most severe type of heart attack, now accounts for only 25–30% of all heart attacks in the US.[15] Mortality rates have continued to drop and today only 5% of patients admitted for ACS in the US die in the hospital.[15] Unfortunately many, especially those in the rural areas die before they get to the hospital.[16]

THE PLAQUE HYPOTHESIS: IMPETUS FOR CURRENT TREATMENTS

Groundbreaking cardiovascular outcome trials (CVOTs) have fundamentally challenged the traditional focus on narrowed arteries (stenosis) as the sole culprit behind heart attacks. These studies demonstrated that CARPs—CABG and PCI—provided minimal additional benefit beyond relieving angina and paved the way to the "plaque hypothesis," proposed by Stone et al.[17] The plaque hypothesis is that the total amount of plaque burden throughout the arteries, as shown on **Figure 1**, is better in predicting the risk of a heart attack rather that the blocks themselves.[17-19]

Figure 2 is a representation of what happens when the fibrous cap of vulnerable plaque breaks to trigger thrombus formation. The interaction of the fluid phase in the blood (coagulation proteins and factors) with the solid state in the plaque's core (macrophages and many factors) determines the clinical consequences—a partial or transient coronary artery occlusion that may be silent or cause unstable angina or a persistent and occlusive thrombus that cause an acute myocardial infarction. Intrinsic factors in

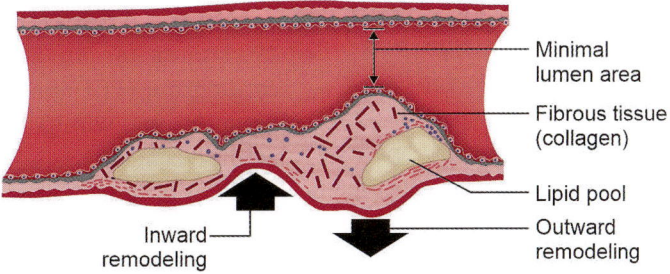

Fig. 1: Most of the coronary artery segment shows atherosclerotic plaque with both inward and outward remodeling and contained lipid pools and narrowing of the luminal area.
Source: Adapted from Stone PH, Libby P, Boden WE. Fundamental Pathobiology of Coronary Atherosclerosis and Clinical Implications for Chronic Ischemic Heart Disease Management-The Plaque Hypothesis: A Narrative Review. JAMA Cardiol. 2023;8(2):192-201.[17]

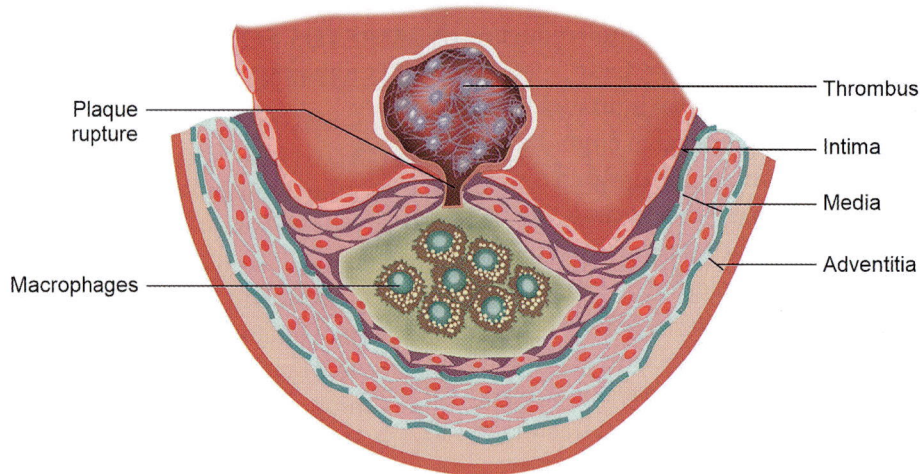

Fig. 2: The layers of the coronary artery (adventitia, media, and intima) are shown and an intraluminal thrombus resulting from the rupture of a vulnerable plaque is schematically shown.
Source: Adapted from Stone PH, Libby P, Boden WE. Fundamental Pathobiology of Coronary Atherosclerosis and Clinical Implications for Chronic Ischemic Heart Disease Management-The Plaque Hypothesis: A Narrative Review. JAMA Cardiol. 2023;8(2):192-201.[17]

the blood, such as high lipoprotein(a) [Lp(a)] favor thrombus formation. Intrinsic high-risk plaque characteristics can now be identified by CT coronary angiogram.

This shift in thinking from detection and grading of the degree of coronary artery occlusion/stenosis to the pathogenesis of plaque formation, factors that increase the risk of rupture and thrombus formation and the many blood, cellular and tissue factors that are operative aligns perfectly with the growing success of medications such as statins, beta-blockers, sodium-glucose cotransporter 2 (SGLT2) inhibitors, and glucagon-like peptide-1 (GLP-1) agonists. This new era of proactive cardiovascular care prioritizes early and comprehensive use of these medications to potentially stabilize vulnerable plaques and prevent future cardiovascular events. Thus, the focus has shifted from solely addressing existing blockages to preventing plaque-related complications altogether.[20-24]

DIAGNOSIS AND MANAGEMENT OF ACUTE CORONARY SYNDROME

Each year, an estimated 1.2 million individuals in the US are hospitalized with ACS.[4,15] STEMI accounts for about 30% of these hospitalizations, while NSTEMI and unstable angina account for the remaining 70%.[15] The European Cardiology Society guideline offers an easy-to-remember "ACS." Acronym for initial triage and assessment:

- "A" stands for an abnormal electrocardiogram (ECG/EKG), which should be performed within 10 minutes of first medical contact.
- "C" for clinical context, considering symptom presentation and any patient history available
- "S" for clinical stability, which is crucial for immediate care decisions.

The first priority, in a patient with chest pain suspected to be cardiac in origin, is to determine the type of ACS without any delay. This is an emergency where the time factor makes the difference between life and death. EKG and high-sensitivity troponin blood test are to be performed within 10 minutes of emergency department (ED) arrival.[4,14]

ST-SEGMENT ELEVATION MYOCARDIAL INFARCTION

ST-segment elevation on EKG and elevated troponin confirm the diagnosis of STEMI. The next immediate step is coronary angiography to pinpoint the blockage within the coronary artery. Following Andreas Gruntzig's pioneering balloon angioplasty in 1979,[13] stents were introduced to address the issue of re-narrowing arteries. Drug-eluting stents used now are successful in reducing restenosis rates.

Primary Percutaneous Coronary Intervention

Primary percutaneous coronary intervention (PPCI) within 90 minutes of STEMI diagnosis to an equipped and staffed facility is the goal (total of 120 minutes if a transfer to such a facility is needed). PPCI has revolutionized heart attack treatment by reopening blocked arteries in patients experiencing STEMI.[25-27] While the priority and focus of PPCI in STEMI patients is the blocked culprit artery to restore blood flow, there are benefits to open all other major blockages to reduce complications and mortality. However, this decision to address the nonculprit arteries should be based on multiple factors that include coronary anatomy, hemodynamic stability, and kidney function of the patient.[4] Compared to thrombolytic therapy, PCI offers several advantages:

- *Faster clot removal:* Percutaneous coronary intervention directly removes clots leading to quicker reperfusion while thrombolytics attempt to dissolve them.
- *Improved outcomes:* Studies show PCI reduces cardiovascular death risk by 31% and heart attack risk by 26% compared to 18% for thrombolytics.[4,28]
- *Reduced restenosis:* Drug-eluting stents used in PCI significantly decrease the chance of re-narrowing arteries compared to older methods.

However, disparities in access to PCI exist, with uninsured patients receiving this life-saving treatment less frequently, even in developed countries like the US and Canada. PCI is a very widely used procedure in the US: in 96% of patients with STEMI, in over 60% of NSTEMI and in 20% of stable angina.[28]

Other indications for PCI: Besides its primary role in the acute management of STEMI, PCI may benefit patients in the following situations:[29]

- *Rescue angioplasty:* Reopening a blocked artery after failed angioplasty
- *Treating recurrent ischemia:* Addressing post-heart attack chest pain
- *Preventing ischemia:* Preventing future angina episodes in high-risk patients
- PCI is an option for AMI patients not undergoing CABG surgery.

Thrombolytic (fibrinolytic) therapy is the next best alternative to PCI, if PCI is not available or not possible within 120 minutes (either at the initial hospital or after transfer). Thrombolytic medication is advised at a full dose for those under 75 years and a half dose for those 75 years and over if they have no contraindications such as bleeding or a recent stroke. Following thrombolytic therapy, transfer to a facility with PCI capabilities within 24 hours is advised.[4]

Thrombolytic Therapy

Thrombolytic therapy has a long history. Building on cardiac catheterization advancements, intracoronary thrombolysis emerged

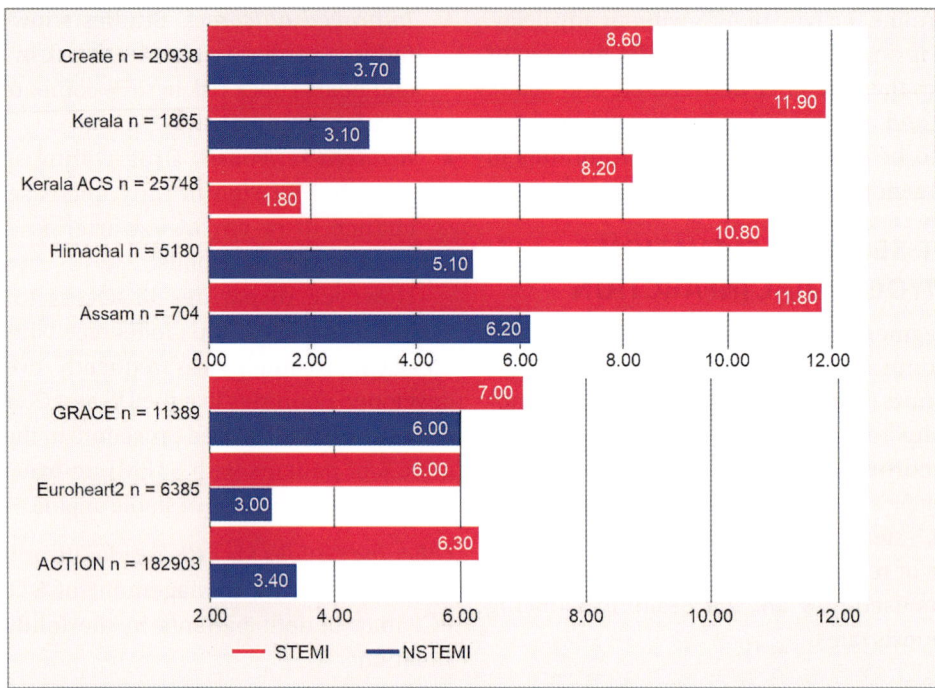

Fig. 3: Short-term mortality in acute coronary syndrome (ACS) patients with ST-segment elevation myocardial infarction (STEMI) and non-ST segment elevation myocardial infarction (NSTEMI) in India [Create and states in India (Kerala and others) compared to Canada (GRACE), Europe (Euroheart2), and the US (ACTION) registries].
Source: Adapted from Gupta R, Khedar RS, Gaur K, Xavier D. Low quality cardiovascular care is an important coronary risk factor in India. Indian Heart J. 2018;70(Suppl 3):S419-S430.[31]

in 1958. Streptokinase, the first drug used in 1976, improved outcomes significantly as large trials showed an 18% mortality reduction at 21 days. By the 1980s, this therapy became the standard therapy for STEMI. Faster-acting agents such as tissue plasminogen activator (t-PA) followed, offering better survival rates but with a slightly increased risk of stroke. Importantly, these benefits were most pronounced in high-risk heart attack patients.[4,15,30]

As shown in **Figure 3**, short-term mortality is much higher after STEMI as contrasted to NSTEMI. Important to note that the overall short-term mortality following STEMI and NSTEMI in India is twice that of Europe and the US.[31]

NON-ST-SEGMENT ELEVATION MYOCARDIAL INFARCTION

Non-STEMI is three times more common than STEMI in the US while STEMI is the most common form of ACS in India **(Fig. 3)**. NSTEMI involves blockages in multiple coronary arteries and requires diligence in diagnosis using troponin tests and echocardiograms, even with a normal or an apparently normal EKG. Treatment varies based on risk level and individual circumstance. In patients at high-risk or at very high-risk such as those experiencing ongoing chest pain, dynamic or persistent EKG changes, hemodynamic instability and life-threatening arrhythmias, an early invasive approach of coronary angiography followed by CARP involving PCI or CABG, to restore blood flow is appropriate. The choice between PCI and CABG is based on multiple considerations—patient preference, clinical status, underlying diseases and assessment of operative risk. CABG surgery offers potentially longer-lasting results, PCI offers a faster recovery[3] and both improve the quality of life.[28,32] Others at a lower risk can be managed conservatively with medications—aspirin, a P2Y12 platelet inhibitor, and an anticoagulant to prevent further clotting.[4,14] In the US about 60% of NSTEMI patients undergoing angiography receive PCI, 10% receive CABG, and 30% are treated with medications.[15]

Unstable Angina

The distinction between unstable angina and NSTEMI hinges on troponin levels. Two consecutive normal high-sensitivity troponin measurements within a few hours can nearly rule out a heart attack with 99% accuracy. For low-risk patients with normal troponin levels, shared decision-making between physician and patient preferences is important when choosing between medications (conservative) or CARP (invasive) to address angina. GDMT, as explained in the previous chapter, targets the basic pathogenetic processes in the coronary arteries and systemically while CARP aims locally to open and or bypass block(s) in the coronary arteries.[14,33]

■ OTHER VARIANTS

Myocardial Infarction in the Absence of Obstructive Coronary Artery Disease

Myocardial infarction in the absence of obstructive coronary artery (MINOCA) is a rare presentation (5–6% of AMI cases) and requires fulfillment of the following diagnostic criteria.[34]

- Acute myocardial infarction (criteria discussed earlier) and corroborative evidence of at least one among the following—symptoms (e.g., angina), new ischemic ST-segment ECG changes, new Q wave on ECG, abnormal imaging (new wall motion abnormality or loss of viable myocardium), coronary thrombus on angiography. Vasospastic angina is a form of MINOCA associated with dramatic changes in ECG during chest pain.[35]
- Nonobstructive coronary arteries on angiography inclusive of normal coronary arteries, mild luminal irregularities, and moderate stenosis (<50%).
- No other specific alternate diagnosis to explain the clinical presentation.

Younger age and women and those of black, Maori, or Pacific race and Hispanic ethnicity are represented disproportionately among MINOCA patients than those with obstructive AMI. It is also noted in some studies that traditional risk factors for CAD are less frequent in MINOCA patients than in their counterparts.[35]

Vasospastic Angina

Vasospastic angina (VSA) was first described in 1959 by Myron Prinzmetal as "the variant form of angina pectoris" on the basis of medical history and ECG.[36] This condition is currently categorized as an endotype of MINOCA. However, VSA may lead to life-threatening arrhythmia, AMI, and sudden death. The clinical presentation may be neglected, and the diagnosis missed. VSA classically present at rest, unlike most cases of angina, though in some patients, vasospasm may be triggered by physical exertion and or, emotional/mental stress and is associated with transient ECG changes (ST-segment elevation, depression and/or T-wave changes). Provocative testing during coronary angiography is suggested as the gold standard test but is rarely used.

Angina with nonobstructive coronary arteries is not benign as the reduced coronary blood flow puts the patient at increased risk of AMI and sudden death.[35] Calcium channel blockers (CCBs) are the first-line treatment for coronary artery spasm.[37]

PROGNOSIS OF ACUTE MYOCARDIAL INFARCTION: AGE A MAJOR FACTOR

Mortality rates from AMI have markedly improved over the past several decades. As a reference point, the case fatality rate (CFR) of AMI was over 35% in 1970 for those ≥65 years of age (~15% for those <65) and dropped to under 10 for those over 65 in 2010. While the improvement in CFR is very impressive the marked difference in CFR between those under age of 65 and those over 65 continues.[38] Compared to AMI patients younger than 65 years, the 10-year mortality rate doubles for those over 65 and triples for those over 75 years old.[23,39] The plausible explanation relates to multiple factors:
- Cumulative exposure to risk factors—lipid score (Chapter 7), pack years of smoking, years of diabetes, hypertension, etc.
- Lack of/or suboptimal primary prevention
- Comorbid diseases
- Frailty—a geriatric syndrome characterized by decreased resilience to stressors, can increase vulnerability to complications after a heart attack.
- Reduced functional capacity hinder recovery and limit participation in cardiac rehabilitation programs

Importance of prompt and appropriate treatment of ACS and care in an appropriate setting (coronary care unit, continuous monitoring, and skilled nursing care) cannot be overstressed. PPCI, thrombolytics and medications such as beta-blockers, aspirin and other antiplatelet drugs are credited with the dramatic reduction in in-hospital mortality of AMI to <5% in the US.[4] The aforementioned drugs started in the hospital during an AMI, as tertiary prevention, not only reduces in-hospital mortality but also prevents major adverse cardiovascular event (MACE) and overall cardiovascular mortality.

SECONDARY PREVENTION: EFFECTIVE BUT UNDERUTILIZED

The term "secondary prevention" refers to measures to prevent a future MACE after the first heart attack. A quarter or more of the many millions who survive a heart attack face a heightened risk of a MACE (heart attack, stroke, and heart failure) in the subsequent 5-10 years. This risk can be reduced very markedly (75-80%) with medications coupled with life-style modifications. However, the reality is that this level of reduction is not achieved as exemplified by reports from Sweden and Finland. The Swedish study that followed elderly patients after ACS for up to 8 years found that adherence to secondary prevention medications was low and yearly blood pressure and cholesterol measurements were done respectively on only 62% and 28% of them.[40] A large Finnish follow-up study of patients after an MACE for 5 years reported that 42% had recurrent MACE or had died and that their risk was highest in the first 6 months (13.4 per 100 patient-years). Important to note that 70% of the patients had an LDL-C of over 70 mg/dL that begs the question—how they would have fared if they had their LDL-C lowered and maintained at 40 mg or less the level linked to lowest MACE.[41] The deficiencies in secondary prevention measures are much more in countries that have less financial resources.

Aspirin, an inexpensive drug of proven benefit over a long time in secondary prevention, presents a striking example of the disparity in use between countries based on financial resources (as noted below).[42]
- Low-income countries (LICs): 17%
- Lower-middle-income countries (LMICs): 25%
- Upper-middle-income countries (UMICs): 51%
- High-income countries (HICs): 65%

Antithrombotic and anticoagulants: P2Y12 receptor blockers (clopidogrel, ticlopidine, ticagrelor, prasugrel, and cangrelor) are antiplatelet drugs. To avoid bleeding complications the P2Y12 drug should be withheld before the initial coronary angiogram and initiated only after a decision not to do an immediate CABG surgery.[43]

Dual antiplatelet therapy (DAPT) with both aspirin and a P2Y12 receptor blocker after a heart attack reduces the risk of a recurrent heart attack, but the benefit wanes over time. Following an STEMI, DAPT is given typically for 12 months. In patients with a high risk of bleeding the course of DAPT can be shorter, based on assessment of the risk versus benefit.[4,22] Patients with more severe CAD may require a longer course of DAPT but at the cost of a higher risk of bleeding. Newer-generation drug-eluting stents (DES) typically require a longer duration of DAPT compared to bare-metal stents (BMS).

Angiotensin converting enzyme inhibitor (ACE-I) reduces the incidence of re-infarction in patients after a heart attack (AMI). About 10% of patients on ACE-I may develop a dry cough within 1–2 weeks of starting the drug. In such patients an effective substitute is an *angiotensin receptor blocker* (ARB).

Beta-blockers used early after a heart attack reduce the risk of a repeat heart attack by 27% and decrease mortality rate by 8%. Specific beta-blockers such as bisoprolol, carvedilol, metoprolol succinate, and nebivolol not only help to prevent re-infarctions but also to manage heart failure. However, the 2023 ACC/AHA guidelines do not recommend routine long-term use of a beta blocker in CAD but recommends its use selectively in patients after a recent heart attack, when heart function is reduced, or when other reason(s) for its use exists.[4,44]

High-intensity statins are the bedrock of treatment for ACS patients. These medications (rosuvastatin 20–40 mg/day and atorvastatin 40–80 mg/day) can lower LDL-C levels by >50%. The LDL-C target is <70 mg/dL for all cardiovascular disease (CVD) patients, and <55 mg/dL) for very high-risk atherosclerotic cardiovascular disease (ASCVD) patients. Considering the heightened risk of heart disease and heart attacks at lower LDL-C in Indians, it is our personal opinion that Indians who have ASCVD should aim for a lower LDL-C of <50–55 mg/dL. Newer studies suggest that very low LDL-C (as low as 20 mg/dL) is well tolerated and may improve long-term outcomes in patients who are at high risk.[45-47]

Polypill: The SECURE clinical trial evaluated the benefits of a single tablet containing aspirin, ACE inhibitor (ramipril) and a statin (atorvastatin 20–40 mg) in 2,499 older patients with at least one major cardiovascular risk factor (CVRF) and a history of heart attack within the previous 6 months. The patients were followed for a median of 36 months.[48] Medication adherence was higher in those in the polypill group. This study showed a significantly lower risk of MACE (30%) than in the control group that received usual care. This recently reported study opens the door to a simplified and effective secondary prevention approach across the world that somewhat evens the field for countries with less financial resources.

DISPARITY BETWEEN HIGH-INCOME COUNTRIES AND LOWER-MIDDLE-INCOME COUNTRIES IN THE CARE OF PATIENTS WITH ACUTE CORONARY SYNDROME

Today, a patient with ACS in an emergency room in a HIC, such as the US, would get expedited diagnostic testing and if STEMI is diagnosed, receive PCI with stenting and the indicated medications within hours (and not days). In the hospital the patient would be mobilized early and discharged within days with instructions on continued medications, cardiac rehabilitation and lifestyle modifications. However, the reality in low- and middle-income countries (LMICs) like India is often different.

- Diagnosis may be missed or delayed especially in younger patients and vegetarians without many of the traditional risk factors because of less awareness of premature disease in Indians and on the risk factors and many risk-enhancing factors (RENFs) (Chapter 3).
- Studies from western countries have reported that the diagnosis of ACS was delayed in South Asian patients and they were less likely than white patients to receive timely PCI. However, this could not be attributed to atypical presentation, as was conventionally believed, as classic (typical) moderate-to-severe intensity midsternal chest pain or discomfort was the most common presenting ACS symptom across all ethnic groups.[49,50]
- Percutaneous coronary intervention is not available as the primary option on a 24-hour basis in most emergency departments and hospitals. In addition, the cost may be prohibitive for some of the patients.
- When PCI is not available, thrombolysis is the right option. Besides availability, the cost for the patient may be prohibitive. The policy that requires the patient/family to pay in advance of treatment is a major barrier for timely treatment.
- Overestimation of the benefits of CARP. A common misconception is that coronary bypass surgery or stent(s) offer a "one-and-done" cure. This calls for improved physician and patient education to dispel this myth and to focus on the crucial role of lifestyle changes and on guideline-directed medical treatment (as detailed in the previous chapter).
- Most glaring and tragic is the low rate of adherence to secondary prevention medications of proven worth. Four medications, taken long term, markedly reduce mortality after a heart attack. In LIC the use of these medications is abysmally low **(Table 1)**.

Several factors contribute to this sorry state in the LICs that include poverty, medication affordability, low literacy rate, access to health care and early medication abandonment by both doctors and patients.

TABLE 1: Differences in the use of secondary prevention drugs in high-income country (HIC) and lower-middle-income country (LMIC).[51,52]

Drug category	HIC	LIC
Antiplatelets	62%	9%
ACEI or ARBs	50%	5%
Beta-blockers	40%	10%
High-intensity statin therapy	67%	3%
Availability of all four drugs in urban communities	95%	25%
Availability of all four drugs in rural communities	90%	3%

(ACEI: angiotensin-converting enzyme; ARBs: angiotensin receptor blockers; HIC: high-income country; LIC: low-income country; Of note, most of the patients in LIC were represented by India and other countries in South Asia)

These cry out for attention and remedial initiatives.[44,53,54] A 2025 follow-up of the PURE study participants showed that the current secondary prevention strategies continue to leave out the majority of people with cardiovascular disease untreated or undertreated in most parts of the world, with little improvement over the past 15 years.[55]

■ KEY TAKEAWAYS

- Prior to 1970 a heart attack (myocardial infarction) was like a death knell; mortality was high and those who survived often succumbed to another attack or a stroke as the pathogenetic mechanisms were obscure and there were no effective treatments. Since then, our understanding of the importance of plaque burden, rupture and thrombosis and application of acute interventional treatments (PCI) and use of secondary prevention measures (lifestyle factors and medications) have drastically improved the prognosis of heart attacks.
- The diagnostic steps for chest pain have been streamlined and made time efficient by ACS (acronym for abnormal EKG, clinical context, and clinical stability). Those with elevated ST-segment and high troponin—STEMI—promptly undergo PPCI to open up the blocked artery and reperfuse the myocardium. In others with NSTEMI, the most common form of ACS in the US, treatment varies based on risk level and individual circumstance. In patients at high-risk (e.g., ongoing chest pain, dynamic or persistent EKG changes, hemodynamic instability, life-threatening arrhythmias, an early invasive approach) PCI or CABG is indicated to restore blood flow. Others at lower risk can be managed conservatively with medications—aspirin, a P2Y12 platelet inhibitor, and an anticoagulant to prevent further clotting.
- Primary percutaneous coronary intervention has revolutionized heart attack treatment in the US and is now the gold standard for both STEMI (used in 96% of cases) and NSTEMI (over 60% of cases). PCI has a low incidence of adverse events (e.g., cerebral hemorrhage) and has dramatically reduced mortality. In-hospital deaths from STEMI have fallen to around 3%, and from NSTEMI to around 2%. This remarkable triumph is not only from the timely and targeted treatment of ACS in the acute critical phase but also from the reduction in heart attacks by improved recognition and management of risk factors for heart disease.
- Besides the advances in acute management (often called tertiary management) there are major advances in secondary prevention (after an initial heart attack) to prevent another heart attack or stroke. Lifestyle changes and GDMT are vital steps. Specifically, use of and long-term adherence to four medications—antiplatelet, ACEI or ARB, beta blocker, statin—together reduce the risk of another heart attack (reinfarction) by 80%.
- Polypill, a single tablet containing aspirin, angiotensin-converting-enzyme (ACE) inhibitor (ramipril) and statin (atorvastatin) have been shown to be effective in reducing MACEs after an initial heart attack. Patient's adherence to taking a polypill is higher than in taking multiple tablets.
- However, sadly, the impressive improvements in heart attack care are not achieved in low- and middle-income countries (LMICs) because of deficiencies in both acute care as well as in secondary prevention.
- Primary percutaneous coronary intervention, the gold standard of treatment for ACS, is not often used as the primary mode in India due to limitations on access (PCI-capable hospitals and interventional cardiologists) and affordability. Thrombolytic therapy remains the standard. Secondary prevention measures are largely lacking as exemplified by the dismally low use of medications of proven benefit.

■ REFERENCES

1. Arbustini E, Dal Bello B, Morbini P, Burke AP, Bocciarelli M, Specchia G, et al. Plaque erosion is a major substrate for coronary thrombosis in acute myocardial infarction. Heart. 1999;82(3):269-72.
2. Sugane H, Kataoka Y, Otsuka F, Nakaoku Y, Nishimura K, Nakano H, et al. Cardiac outcomes in patients with acute coronary syndrome attributable to calcified nodule. Atherosclerosis. 2021;318:70-5.

3. Collet JP, Thiele H, Barbato E, Barthélémy O, Bauersachs J, Bhatt DL, et al. 2020 ESC Guidelines for the management of acute coronary syndromes in patients presenting without persistent ST-segment elevation. Eur Heart J. 2021;42(14):1289-367.
4. Gulati M, Levy PD, Mukherjee D, Amsterdam E, Bhatt DL, Birtcher KK, et al. 2021 AHA/ACC/ASE/CHEST/SAEM/SCCT/SCMR Guideline for the Evaluation and Diagnosis of Chest Pain: Executive Summary: A Report of the American College of Cardiology/American Heart Association Joint Committee on Clinical Practice Guidelines. Circulation. 2021;144(22):e368-e454.
5. Gilbert RE. Eisenhower's 1955 heart attack: medical treatment, political effects, and the "behind the scenes" leadership style. Politics Life Sci. 2008;27(1):2-21.
6. Levine SA, Lown B. The "chair" treatment of acute thrombosis. Trans Assoc Am Physicians. 1951;64:316-27.
7. Levine SA, Lown B. "Armchair" treatment of acute coronary thrombosis. J Am Med Assoc. 1952;148(16):1365-9.
8. Mitchell AM, Lown B, Levine SA. The armchair treatment of acute myocardial infarction. Am J Nurs. 1953;53(6):674-6.
9. Reed GW, Rossi JE, Cannon CP. Acute myocardial infarction. Lancet. 2017;389(10065): 197-210.
10. Julian DG. Treatment of cardiac arrest in acute myocardial ischaemia and infarction. Lancet. 1961;2(7207):840-4.
11. Nabel EG, Braunwald E. A tale of coronary artery disease and myocardial infarction. N Engl J Med. 2012;366(1):54-63.
12. Favaloro R. A revival of Paul Dudley White: An overview of present medical practice and of our society. Circulation. 1999;99(12): 1525-37.
13. Gruntzig AR, Senning A, Siegenthaler W. Nonoperative dilatation of coronary-artery stenosis: Percutaneous transluminal coronary angioplasty. N Engl J Med. 1979;301: 61-8.
14. Bhatt DL, Lopes RD, Harrington RA. Diagnosis and Treatment of Acute Coronary Syndromes: A Review. JAMA. 2022;327(7): 662-75.
15. Martin SS, Aday AW, Almarzooq ZI, Anderson CAM, Arora P, Avery CL, et al. 2024 Heart Disease and Stroke Statistics: A Report of US and Global Data from the American Heart Association. Circulation. 2024;149(8):e347-e913.
16. Grey C, Jackson R, Schmidt M, Ezzati M, Asaria P, Exeter DJ, et al. One in four major ischaemic heart disease events are fatal and 60% are pre-hospital deaths: a national data-linkage study (ANZACS-QI 8). Eur Heart J. 2017;38(3):172-80.
17. Stone PH, Libby P, Boden WE. Fundamental Pathobiology of Coronary Atherosclerosis and Clinical Implications for Chronic Ischemic Heart Disease Management-The Plaque Hypothesis: A Narrative Review. JAMA Cardiol. 2023;8(2):192-201.
18. Perel P, Avezum A, Huffman M, Pais P, Rodgers A, Vedanthan R, et al. Reducing Premature Cardiovascular Morbidity and Mortality in People with Atherosclerotic Vascular Disease: The World Heart Federation Roadmap for Secondary Prevention of Cardiovascular Disease. Glob Heart. 2015;10(2):99-110.
19. Boden WE, O'Rourke RA, Teo KK, Hartigan PM, Maron DJ, Kostuk WJ, et al. Optimal Medical Therapy with or without PCI for Stable Coronary Disease. N Engl J Med. 2007;356(15):1503-16.
20. Randomised trial of intravenous streptokinase, oral aspirin, both, or neither among 17,187 cases of suspected acute myocardial infarction: ISIS-2. ISIS-2 (Second International Study of Infarct Survival) Collaborative Group. Lancet. 1988;2(8607):349-60.
21. Bhatt DL, Hulot JS, Moliterno DJ, Harrington RA. Antiplatelet and anticoagulation therapy for acute coronary syndromes. Circ Res. 2014;114(12):1929-43.
22. Udelson JE, Kelsey MD, Nanna MG, Fordyce CB, Yow E, Clare RM, et al. Deferred Testing in Stable Outpatients with Suspected Coronary Artery Disease: A Prespecified Secondary Analysis of the PRECISE Randomized Clinical Trial. JAMA Cardiol. 2023; 8(10):915-24.
23. Krumholz HM, Normand ST, Wang Y. Twenty-Year Trends in Outcomes for Older

24. Adults with Acute Myocardial Infarction in the United States. JAMA Netw Open. 2019;2(3):e191938.
24. Kochar A, Chen AY, Sharma PP, Pagidipati NJ, Fonarow GC, Cowper PA, et al. Long-Term Mortality of Older Patients with Acute Myocardial Infarction Treated in US Clinical Practice. J Am Heart Assoc. 2018; 7(13):e007230.
25. DeWood MA, Spores J, Notske R, Mouser LT, Burroughs R, Golden MS, et al. Prevalence of total coronary occlusion during the early hours of transmural myocardial infarction. N Engl J Med. 1980;303(16):897-902.
26. DeWood MA, Stifter WF, Simpson CS, Spores J, Eugster GS, Judge TP, et al. Coronary arteriographic findings soon after non-Q-wave myocardial infarction. N Engl J Med. 1986;315(7):417-23.
27. Chacko L, J PH, Rajkumar C, Nowbar AN, Kane C, Mahdi D, et al. Effects of Percutaneous Coronary Intervention on Death and Myocardial Infarction Stratified by Stable and Unstable Coronary Artery Disease: A Meta-Analysis of Randomized Controlled Trials. Circ Cardiovasc Qual Outcomes. 2020;13(2):e006363.
28. Bhatt DL. Percutaneous Coronary Intervention in 2018. JAMA. 2018;319(20):2127-8.
29. O'Gara PT, Kushner FG, Ascheim DD, Casey DE Jr, Chung MK, de Lemos JA, et al. 2013 ACCF/AHA guideline for the management of ST-elevation myocardial infarction: executive summary: a report of the American College of Cardiology Foundation/American Heart Association Task Force on Practice Guidelines. Circulation. 2013;127(4):529-55.
30. DeWood MA, Notske RN, Berg R, Jr, Ganji JH, Simpson CS, Hinnen ML, et al. Medical and surgical management of early Q wave myocardial infarction. I. Effects of surgical reperfusion on survival, recurrent myocardial infarction, sudden death and functional class at 10 or more years of follow-up. J Am Coll Cardiol. 1989;14(1):65-77.
31. Gupta R, Khedar RS, Gaur K, Xavier D. Low quality cardiovascular care is an important coronary risk factor in India. Indian Heart J. 2018;70(Suppl 3):S419-30.
32. Bavry AA, Kumbhani DJ, Rassi AN, Bhatt DL, Askari AT. Benefit of early invasive therapy in acute coronary syndromes: a meta-analysis of contemporary randomized clinical trials. J Am Coll Cardiol. 2006;48(7):1319-25.
33. Chiang CH, Chiang CH, Pickering JW, Stoyanov KM, Chew DP, Neumann JT, et al. Performance of the European Society of Cardiology 0/1-Hour, 0/2-Hour, and 0/3-Hour Algorithms for Rapid Triage of Acute Myocardial Infarction: An International Collaborative Meta-analysis. Ann Intern Med. 2022;175(1):101-13.
34. Tamis-Holland JE, Jneid H, Reynolds HR, Agewall S, Brilakis ES, Brown TM, et al. Contemporary Diagnosis and Management of Patients with Myocardial Infarction in the Absence of Obstructive Coronary Artery Disease: A Scientific Statement from the American Heart Association. Circulation. 2019;139(18):e891-e908.
35. Jenkins K, Pompei G, Ganzorig N, Brown S, Beltrame J, Kunadian V. Vasospastic angina: a review on diagnostic approach and management. Ther Adv Cardiovasc Dis. 2024; 18:17539447241230400.
36. Sternbach G. William Heberden and Myron Prinzmetal: angina pectoris. J Emerg Med. 1991;9(1-2):81-3.
37. Baroz A, Musayeb Y, De Grauwe S, Roffi M, Iglesias JF. [Vasospastic angina: an underdiagnosed pathology]. Rev Med Suisse. 2024;20(885):1560-66.
38. Dalen JE, Alpert JS, Goldberg RJ, Weinstein RS. The epidemic of the 20(th) century: coronary heart disease. Am J Med. 2014;127(9):807-12.
39. Wang Y, Leifheit EC, Krumholz HM. Trends in 10-Year Outcomes Among Medicare Beneficiaries Who Survived an Acute Myocardial Infarction. JAMA Cardiol. 2022;7(6):613-22.
40. Bentzel S, Ljungman C, Hjerpe P, Schiöler L, Manhem K, Bengtsson Boström K, et al. Long-term secondary prevention and outcome following acute coronary syndrome: real-world results from the Swedish Primary Care Cardiovascular Database. Eur J Prev Cardiol. 2024;31(7):812-21.

41. Cholesterol Treatment Trialists' (CTT) Collaboration; Baigent C, Blackwell L, Emberson J, Holland LE, Reith C, et al. Efficacy and safety of more intensive lowering of LDL cholesterol: a meta-analysis of data from 170,000 participants in 26 randomised trials. Lancet. 2010;376(9753):1670-81.
42. Yoo SGK, Chung GS, Bahendeka SK, Sibai AM, Damasceno A, Farzadfar F, et al. Aspirin for Secondary Prevention of Cardiovascular Disease in 51 Low-, Middle-, and High-Income Countries. JAMA. 2023; 330(8):715-24.
43. Dawson LP, Chen D, Dagan M, Bloom J, Taylor A, Duffy SJ, et al. Assessment of Pretreatment with Oral P2Y12 Inhibitors and Cardiovascular and Bleeding Outcomes in Patients with Non-ST Elevation Acute Coronary Syndromes: A Systematic Review and Meta-analysis. JAMA Netw Open. 2021; 4(11):e2134322.
44. Virani SS, Newby LK, Arnold SV, Bittner V, Brewer LC, Demeter SH, et al. 2023 AHA/ACC/ACCP/ASPC/NLA/PCNA Guideline for the Management of Patients with Chronic Coronary Disease: A Report of the American Heart Association/American College of Cardiology Joint Committee on Clinical Practice Guidelines. Circulation. 2023;148(9):e9-e119.
45. Lloyd-Jones DM, Allen NB, Anderson CAM, Black T, Brewer LC, Foraker RE, et al. Life's Essential 8: Updating and Enhancing the American Heart Association's Construct of Cardiovascular Health: A Presidential Advisory from the American Heart Association. Circulation. 2022;146(5): e18-e43.
46. Mach F, Baigent C, Catapano AL, Koskinas KC, Casula M, Badimon L, et al. 2019 ESC/EAS Guidelines for the management of dyslipidaemias: lipid modification to reduce cardiovascular risk. Eur Heart J. 2020;41(1):111-88.
47. Grundy SM, Stone NJ, Bailey AL, Beam C, Birtcher KK, Blumenthal RS, et al. 2018 AHA/ACC/AACVPR/AAPA/ABC/ACPM/ADA/AGS/APhA/ASPC/NLA/PCNA Guideline on the Management of Blood Cholesterol: Executive Summary: A Report of the American College of Cardiology/American Heart Association Task Force on Clinical Practice Guidelines. J Am Coll Cardiol. 2019;73(24):3168-209.
48. Castellano JM, Pocock SJ, Bhatt DL, Quesada AJ, Owen R, Fernandez-Ortiz A, et al. Polypill Strategy in Secondary Cardiovascular Prevention. N Engl J Med. 2022; 387(11):967-77.
49. Zaman MJ, Junghans C, Sekhri N, Chen R, Feder GS, Timmis AD, et al. Presentation of stable angina pectoris among women and South Asian people. CMAJ. 2008;179(7): 659-67.
50. King-Shier K, Quan H, Kapral MK, Tsuyuki R, An L, Banerjee S, et al. Acute coronary syndromes presentations and care outcomes in white, South Asian and Chinese patients: a cohort study. BMJ Open. 2019;9(3):e022479.
51. Yusuf S, Islam S, Chow CK, Rangarajan S, Dagenais G, Diaz R, et al. Use of secondary prevention drugs for cardiovascular disease in the community in high-income, middle-income, and low-income countries (the PURE Study): a prospective epidemiological survey. Lancet. 2011;378(9798):1231-43.
52. Gupta R, Gaur K. Epidemiology of Ischemic Heart Disease and Diabetes in South Asia: An Overview of the Twin Epidemic. Curr Diabetes Rev. 2021;17(9):e100620186664.
53. Sigamani A, Gupta R. Revisiting secondary prevention in coronary heart disease. Indian Heart J. 2022;74(6):431-40.
54. Mathews R, Wang W, Kaltenbach LA, Thomas L, Shah RU, Ali M, et al. Hospital Variation in Adherence Rates to Secondary Prevention Medications and the Implications on Quality. Circulation. 2018;137(20): 2128-38.
55. Joseph P, Avezum Á, Ramasundarahettige C, Mony PK, Yusuf R, Kazmi K, et al. Secondary prevention medications in 17 countries grouped by income level (PURE): A prospective cohort study. J Am Coll Cardiol. 2025; 85(5):436-7.

Interrelated Disorders and Diseases: Cardiovascular Kidney Metabolic Syndrome, Atrial Fibrillation, Stroke, and Heart Failure

INTRODUCTION

Cardiovascular disease (CVD) encompasses a broad spectrum of conditions beyond coronary artery disease (CAD). Among them atrial fibrillation (AF), stroke, and heart failure (HF) have interrelationships with CAD (used synonymously as heart disease in this book) that not only increase the morbidity but also present challenges to optimal management. To know the metabolic underpinnings of CVD, the interconnected pathophysiologic relationships and to implement a comprehensive approach to prevention and treatment, it is fundamental to understand the basics of the "cardiovascular kidney metabolic (CKM) syndrome".[1]

CARDIOVASCULAR KIDNEY METABOLIC SYNDROME

Previously (Chapter 3) we defined metabolic syndrome and named it as a cardiovascular risk-enhancing factor.[2] To recap, metabolic syndrome requires three out of the following five criteria—fasting glucose (>100 mg/dL), triglycerides (>150 mg/dL), HDL (<40 mg/dL men, <50 mg/dL women), blood pressure (>130/85 mm Hg), abdominal obesity (by waist circumference) (in men ≥102 cm and women ≥88 cm and amended to ≥90 cm and ≥80 cm for Indian men and women) for diagnosis.[3] CKM syndrome adds kidney disease (proteinuria and or glomerular filtration rate <60 mL/min) to metabolic syndrome. The components of CKM syndrome and pathways and interrelationships are depicted in **Figure 1**.[4]

Increase in body mass index (BMI) and obesity are associated with the risk of progression of kidney disease likely related to glomerular hyperfiltration.[4] Further, adiposity, diabetes, and hypertension have combined effects on the glomeruli. Additionally, visceral fat increases leptin and adipokines that stimulate aldosterone production and importantly may cause an increase in kidney and systemic inflammation and oxidative stress. The likely pathways—through oxidative stress, endothelial dysfunction, activation of the sympathetic system, activation of the renin-angiotensin-aldosterone system and others—that adversely affect cardiac function are schematically represented in **Figure 1**.

Cardiovascular kidney metabolic syndrome, if untreated, advances in stages to worsening CVD and kidney failure. Early identification of CKM syndrome and early intervention are necessary to halt or reduce disease progression and end organ damage. Lifestyle modifications, including weight management, diet, and exercise, form the foundation of prevention and treatment. The integration of these into a broader healthcare management plan is essential to improve patient outcomes. The development of effective therapies that target multiple components of CKM syndrome is a promising

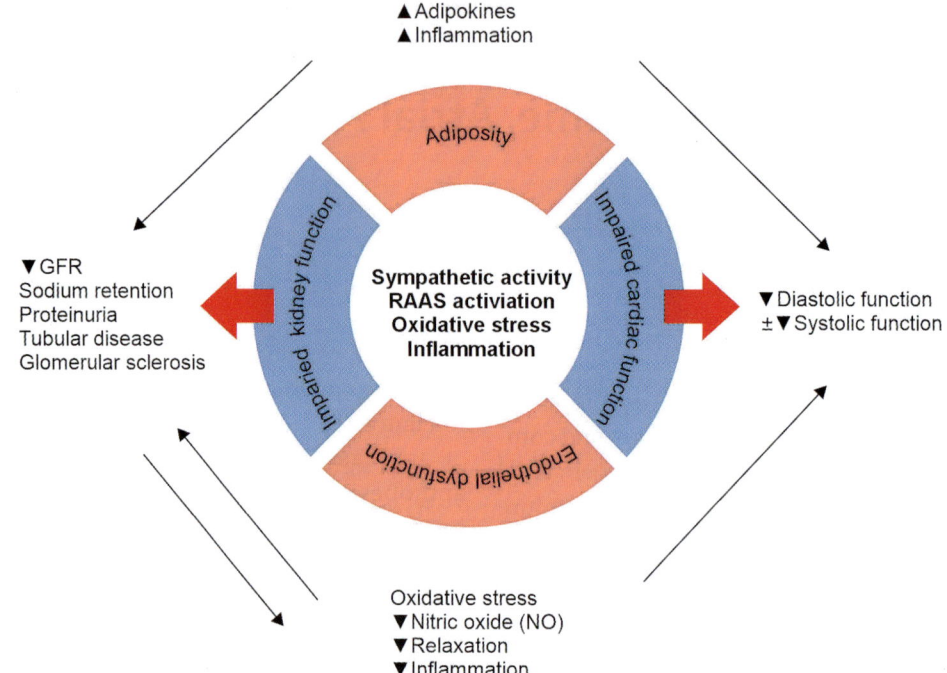

Fig. 1: Central adiposity (adipokines and inflammation), causative and contributing factors (with interrelationships) that decrease cardiac and renal function and result in the cardiovascular kidney metabolic syndrome. (GFR: glomerular filtration rate; RAAS: renin-angiotensin-aldosterone system)
Source: Adapted from Sowers JR, Whaley-Connell A, Hayden MR. The Role of Overweight and Obesity in the Cardiorenal Syndrome. Cardiorenal Med. 2011;1(1):5-12.[4]

area of research. The 0–4 stages of CKM, their manifestations, implications, and treatments are listed in **Table 1**.[1]

■ ATRIAL FIBRILLATION

Atrial fibrillation (AFib or AF) is an irregular heart rhythm (arrhythmia) with rapid beats that originates in the upper heart chambers (atria) that affects many people (estimated 50 million globally)[5] and can lead to serious medical conditions like a stroke or HF.[6] Symptoms associated with AF are mainly heart palpitations, dizziness, and shortness of breath. It may precipitate angina (Chapter 10) and may cause syncope (fainting). However, it can occur without any of these symptoms or with just fatigue as the only symptom. Based on the duration of episodes, AF can be classified as paroxysmal, persistent, persistent-longstanding, and permanent. Paroxysmal AF lasts <7 days and terminates spontaneously or with treatment. Persistent AF lasts >7 days and may require medication or electrical cardioversion to terminate. Persistent long standing AF lasts >1 year or is one that cannot be converted to sinus rhythm, or for which a decision was made not to attempt conversion.[5] While there are many conditions that predispose to AF such as hyperthyroidism, chronic obstructive pulmonary disease (COPD), and sleep apnea, the components of CKM syndrome (topic of this chapter) are common and important predisposing factors for AF.[5]

TABLE 1: Definitions, implications, and management of five stages of cardiovascular kidney metabolic (CKM) syndrome.[1]

Stages	Criteria and management implications
Stage 0: A foundation for prevention	Individuals without established CVD, kidney, or metabolic disease. Primordial prevention—adopting healthy habits early in life. Lifestyle modifications, such as regular physical activity, a balanced diet, and weight management, during childhood and adolescence, markedly reduce the risk of developing CKM syndrome (Chapters 15–17)
Stage 1: Excess or dysfunctional adiposity	• Individuals with overweight/obesity or abdominal adiposity without the presence of metabolic factors other than prediabetes. BMI over 23 kg/m^2 (>25 for Whites) • Waist circumference (WC) >80/90 cm for Indian women/men (88/102 cm for US women/men) and fasting blood glucose >100–124 or HbA1C between 5.7 and 6.4 • By identifying these factors early, preventive measures can be taken to avoid future metabolic syndrome. An estimated 80 million Americans have stage 1 CKM
Stage 2: Metabolic risk factors	• Individuals with metabolic risk factors such as hypertriglyceridemia, hypertension, diabetes, metabolic syndrome, or CKD • SGLT2 inhibitors can be prioritized for those with CKD given their protective impact on kidney function decline, HF hospitalizations and MACE • GLP-1RAs can be prioritized for those with obesity or HbA1c ≥9% • Metformin use with SGLT2 inhibitor or GLP-1RA is advised for those with HbA1c ≥7.5% to help achieve glycemic targets with minimal side effects and better affordability

Stage 3: Subclinical CVD	• Stage 2 plus subclinical CVD (CAC score is >1 or by CTCA or by angiography)
	• Subclinical heart failure is diagnosed when NT-proBNP ≥125 pg/mL, hs-troponin T ≥14 ng/L for women and ≥22 ng/L for men, or by echocardiographic parameters. Combination of the two parameters indicates the highest risk for HF
	• *Risk equivalents of subclinical CVD include:*
	  – Very high-risk CKD (stage G4 or G5 CKD) or very high risk per KDIGO classification
	  – High predicted 10-year CVD risk equivalents (very high-risk CKD or high predicted CVD risk (>20%). The goal of management in stage 3 CKM is to prevent progression to clinical CVD and kidney failure

Stage 4: Clinical CVD *Stage 4A:* No kidney failure *Stage 4B:* With kidney failure	Clinical CVD (CAD, stroke, PAD, HF, and AF) among individuals with excess adiposity. The goal of management in stage 4 CKM is to optimize care and secondary prevention for patients with CVD and concurrent metabolic factors, CKD, or both. In all patients with ASCVD, use of aspirin or P2Y12 inhibitors in addition to high-intensity statin therapy is indicated. Many individuals with diabetes and ASCVD will fall into this subpopulation. For those with very high-risk ASCVD intensified LDL lowering therapy with statin, with ezetimibe and a PCSK9 inhibitors could be considered for with an LDL-C goal <55 mg/dL (Chapters 12 and 13)

(AF: atrial fibrillation; ASCVD: atherosclerotic cardiovascular disease; BMI: body mass index; CAC: coronary artery calcium; CKD: chronic kidney disease; CTCA: computerized tomographic angiography; CKD: chronic kidney disease; GLP-1RA: glucagon-like polypeptide 1 receptor antagonist; HbA1C: hemoglobin A1c; HF: heart failure; KDIGO: Kidney Disease Improving Global Outcomes; MACE: major adverse cardiovascular events; NT-proBNP: N-terminal pro-B-type natriuretic peptide; PCSK9: proprotein convertase subtilisin/kexin type 9; P2Y12: purinergic receptor P2Y, G-protein coupled 12; SGLT2: sodium-glucose cotransporter-2)

Flowchart 1: Mechanisms and pathways leading to atrial fibrillation (AF); the pathways that contribute to the development of AF create a substrate for reentry and provide triggers that can initiate arrhythmic activity.

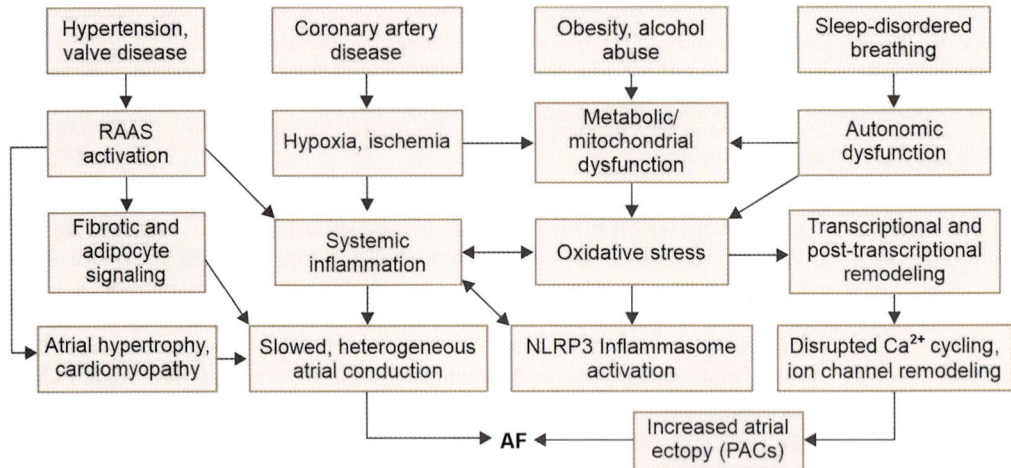

(NLRP3: NOD-like receptor protein 3; PAC: premature atrial contraction; RAAS: renin-angiotensin-aldosterone system)
Source: With permission from Joglar JA, Chung MK, Armbruster AL, Benjamin EJ, Chyou JY, Cronin EM, et al. 2023 ACC/AHA/ACCP/HRS Guideline for the Diagnosis and Management of Atrial Fibrillation: A Report of the American College of Cardiology/American Heart Association Joint Committee on Clinical Practice Guidelines. J Am Coll Cardiol. 2024;83(1):109-279.[5]

Coronary Artery Disease and Atrial Fibrillation

Coronary artery disease and atrial fibrillation share a complex **(Flowchart 1)** and bidirectional **(Fig. 2)** relationship. Both conditions often share common risk factors (e.g., hypertension, obesity, metabolic syndrome) underscoring the importance of a comprehensive approach to cardiovascular health.[5] **Flowchart 1** illustrates the pathogenetic mechanisms of and pathways to atrial fibrillation.

Management

Management of AF has evolved with a strong emphasis on preventing stroke and improving patient outcomes. The American College of Cardiology/American Heart Association (ACC/AHA) AF guidelines of 2023 provide a framework for prevention, risk assessment, and treatment strategies.

- *Risk factors:* It is of fundamental importance to treat and manage risk factors—such as obesity, hypertension, diabetes, dyslipidemia, and sleep apnea. By adopting a heart-healthy lifestyle, through diet, exercise, and smoking cessation, individuals can reduce their risk of developing AF.[5]
- *Risk stratification:* The CHA2DS2-VASc score is commonly used to assess the annual risk of ischemic stroke, guiding anticoagulation decisions. For patients with AF and an annual risk of ischemic stroke of 2%, oral anticoagulation is strongly recommended.
- *Anticoagulation:* Direct oral anticoagulants (e.g., apixaban, argatroban, and dabigatran) are preferred over Vitamin K

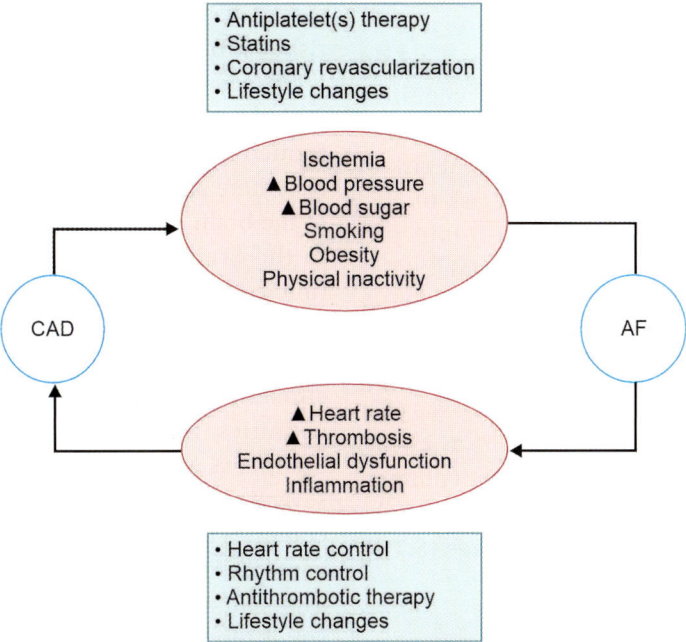

Fig. 2: The bidirectional mechanisms that are at work between coronary artery disease (CAD) and atrial fibrillation (AF). The main drivers (within the pink ovals) and the directionality by arrows are shown. Treatments/Interventions that can stop or modify the cycle are shown within the green rectangles.
Source: Adapted from Batta A, Hatwal J, Batta A, Verma S, Sharma YP. Atrial fibrillation and coronary artery disease: An integrative review focusing on therapeutic implications of this relationship. World J Cardiol. 2023;15(5):229-43.[7]

antagonists (e.g., warfarin) due to their safety and efficacy profile.
- *Rate control versus rhythm control:* The choice between these strategies depends on individual patient factors, including symptom burden, comorbidities, and patient preference. Examples of rate control drugs are digoxin, metoprolol, carvedilol, verapamil, diltiazem, and examples of rhythm control drugs are procainamide, disopyramide, flecainide, sotalol, propafenone, dofetilide, and amiodarone, etc.[5]

Procedural Interventions

- *Electrical cardioversion:* A commonly used procedure to convert AF to sinus rhythm.
- *Catheter ablation:* This invasive procedure is an option for patients with persistent or recurrent AF who are refractory to medical therapy or have significant symptoms.
- *Left atrial appendage closure (LACC):* LAAC is an invasive procedure performed by an electrophysiologist. By closing off the left atrial appendage (LAA), a common source of blood clots, LAAC prevents blood from pooling and forming clots.[8,9]

The Food and Drug Administration (FDA) of the US recently qualified the "Apple Watch AFib History feature" as a medical device development tool. This marks a notable advancement in cardiac monitoring that has great potential to improve patient care and aid further research on AF.

Adverse Outcomes of AF

Meta-analyses have shown a 2.4-fold risk of stroke,[10] 1.5-fold risk of cognitive impairment or dementia,[6] 1.5-fold risk of myocardial infarction (MI),[11] 2-fold risk of sudden cardiac death,[11] 5-fold risk of HF,[5] 1.6-fold risk of CKD,[10] and 1.3-fold risk of peripheral artery disease (PAD).[10] AF is associated with a 1.5- to 2-fold increased risk of death, with higher mortality in women than in men.[5] In Medicare beneficiaries (elderly), the most frequent outcome in the 5 years after diagnosis of AF was death (19.5% at 1 year; 48.8% at 5 years);[12] the next most common was HF (13.7%), followed by new-onset stroke (7.1%), gastrointestinal hemorrhage (5.7%), and MI (3.9%).[12]

■ STROKE

Stroke, a "brain attack", is a life-threatening condition that occurs when blood flow to the brain is interrupted, leading to brain cell damage from lack of oxygen. Stroke is a leading cause of death and disability worldwide. Over 12 million people worldwide will have their first stroke each year and 6.5 million will die as a result. One in four adults over the age of 25 years will have a stroke in their lifetime.[13] In the US every year, >795,000 people have a stroke. About 185,000 strokes—nearly one in four—are in people who have had a previous stroke.[14] The death rate for stroke has decreased from 41.1 per 100,000 in 2021 to 39.5 per 100,000 in 2022.[14] Stroke reduces mobility in more than one half of stroke survivors aged 65 years and older.[14,15] The South-East Asia Region bears a significant portion of the world's stroke burden, accounting for over 40% of global stroke mortality. The countries in this region include India, Indonesia, Bangladesh, Sri Lanka, Korea etc. Among stroke survivors in this region, up to one-third experience severe disabilities, while the rest face a high risk of stroke recurrence.[16]

There are two main types of stroke:[17] (1) Ischemic stroke caused by a blood clot that formed in the brain (thrombosis) or formed elsewhere and traveled through blood vessels to the brain (embolism) blocking blood flow to the brain, and (2) Hemorrhagic stroke (intracerebral or into the subarachnoid space) caused by tears or rupture of a blood vessel. About 80–85% of all strokes are ischemic strokes.[17] Compared to people of European countries, hemorrhagic stroke is higher in Southeast Asians.[16] However, over the past several decades hemorrhagic strokes in Asian countries have decreased, likely due to better control of hypertension. Lacunar strokes are a specific type of ischemic stroke caused by small blood vessel blockages. While often asymptomatic, repeated lacunar strokes can lead to cognitive impairment and other neurological issues.[18] A transient ischemic attack (TIA), or "mini-stroke", is a temporary blockage of blood flow to the brain, causing stroke-like symptoms without lasting damage. However, it serves as a critical warning sign for potential future stroke. Understanding the different types of stroke, their risk factors, and symptoms is essential for early detection and intervention.[15,19,20]

Early Detection

Early detection of a stroke is critical as loss of time leads to loss of brain function.[21] Stroke happens suddenly and most often without any warning. Unlike a heart attack, pain is not a symptom of a brain attack (stroke). An exception is severe headache as the main symptom in subarachnoid hemorrhage.

FAST: It is a useful acronym to remember for early detection.
- Face drooping
- Arm weakness

- Speech difficulty
- Time to call 911 in the US or emergency service system number

Acute Management

In patients with ischemic strokes, the priority is to restore circulation to affected brain areas. If this is done promptly it may prevent permanent damage or at least limit the damage. In patients with hemorrhagic strokes, treatment depends on the location and severity of the bleeding. Aims are to reduce the amount of bleeding by reducing blood pressure and to prevent further bleeding by improving clotting **(Table 2)**.

Stroke Rehabilitation

Stroke rehabilitation aims to help patients recover to adapt to the changes in their brain and to regain abilities they had before their stroke. This can be done on multiple fronts through speech therapy, physical therapy, occupational therapy, and cognitive therapy. Trained professionals with support facilities in each of these areas are key factors in reducing disability and in returning patients to productive lives.[22]

Risk Factors

As was stated in the preceding section on atrial fibrillation, AFib is a significant and independent risk factor for stroke. Stroke and heart disease share numerous common risk factors. The INTERSTROKE study—a global analysis involving over 26,000 participants, identified 10 modifiable risk factors contributing significantly to stroke occurrence worldwide.[19,20] These factors include:

- *Hypertension:* The most potent risk factor, contributing to 54% of stroke burden.
- *Physical inactivity:* Linked to 36% of stroke cases
- *High cholesterol:* Contributing to 27% stroke burden
- *Unhealthy diet:* Responsible for 23% of stroke cases
- *Psychosocial factors (depression, stress):* Contributing to 17% of stroke burden
- *Smoking:* Linked to 12% of stroke cases
- *Abdominal obesity:* Contributing to 10% of stroke burden
- *Alcohol consumption:* Responsible for 6% of stroke cases

While stroke and heart disease share many of the risk factors listed above, their prevalence and mortality rates vary markedly across different populations **(Table 3)**. Historically, Asian populations, especially China, have had higher stroke mortality rates compared to heart disease. This is in contrast to the US and global patterns where heart disease mortality rate is higher than stroke mortality. India follows the global pattern. Stroke mortality in Indians as shown on the table is less than one half of heart disease

TABLE 2: Management of ischemic stroke and hemorrhagic stroke.

Ischemic stroke	Hemorrhagic stroke
Thrombolytic drugs (within 3–4.5 hours)	Blood pressure management
Thrombectomy (if there is no significant brain damage), by catheter through a major vessel	Reversal of any medication that might increase bleeding (vitamin K, clotting factor infusions)
Blood pressure management	Use of medications. Surgery, in some cases, may be needed to reduce pressure on the brain

TABLE 3: Differences in mortality rates per 100,000 for stroke and heart disease in selected countries (2019).[23]

Countries	Stroke death rate per 100,000		Heart disease death rate per 100,000	
	All ages	15–49 years	All ages	15–49 years
India	50	7	115	24
China	154	12	138	12
US	58	3	148	10
Global	85	9	114	16

Source: Healthdata.org. (2024). The Institute of Health Metrics and Evaluation. [online] Available from www.healthdata.org IHME/GHDx/GBD [Last accessed May, 2024].[23]

mortality for all ages and less than one third for those under 50 years.[23,24]

Prevention

Prevention is of paramount importance in reducing the global burden of stroke. The decline in stroke rates in the US and many countries attributed to control of high blood pressure control and other risk factors, underscores the importance of effective public health interventions.[25] However, the rising prevalence of obesity, diabetes, and sedentary lifestyles poses a challenge to sustaining this progress, particularly in lower- and middle-income countries. Understanding regional and demographic differences is crucial to develop targeted prevention and treatment strategies.[25,26] A healthy diet,[27] regular physical activity, maintaining a healthy weight and other "Life's Essential 8" (Chapter 17) can reduce the incidence of stroke and its impact after a stroke.[28]

■ HEART FAILURE

Heart failure is a major public health issue globally with an estimated prevalence of 64 million people and with high mortality and morbidity.[29] The incidence of HF seems to be declining in developed countries, but its prevalence is increasing due to aging of the population, increased survival after heart attacks and HF on improved treatment. The common understanding of HF is one of the inadequate pumping of the ventricle (systolic) or inadequate filling of the ventricle (diastolic). A universal definition of HF proposed is: A clinical syndrome caused by different diseases with symptoms and/or signs caused by a structural and/or functional cardiac abnormality and corroborated by elevated natriuretic peptide levels and/or objective evidence of pulmonary or systemic congestion.[30,31] Common symptoms of HF are shortness of breath at exertion or rest (especially at night lying in bed) coughing or wheezing, fatigue, swelling (especially in the feet and ankles), weight changes, and lack of appetite.

Prevalence and Epidemiology

A meta-analysis based on echocardiographic screening studies from 1997 to 2014 in the general population from developed countries reported a prevalence of HF in 11.8% of those ≥60 years and about 1% among those <60 years.[32,33] Epidemiological studies have limitations related to differences in definitions of HF, population selection and lack of data from some areas. There is a concerning lack of epidemiological data from countries outside Europe and North America, especially from lower and middle-income countries, even though they carry a heavy cardiovascular disease burden.[31] The 2021 AHA Heart Disease and Stroke Statistics reported a prevalence of HF of about 2.5% based on self-reported data.[14] It is projected that the prevalence of HF will increase due to the aging of the population. Most recent projections for the US suggest an increase in the prevalence of HF by about 46% from 2012 to 2030, with a corresponding increase in healthcare costs of about 127%.[34] The incidence of HF in India is estimated to be at least between 0.5 and 1.7 cases per 1,000 person-years, for a total of 492,000 to 1.8 million new cases per year.[35]

Early Detection and Staging

Advancements in diagnostic tools and biomarkers, such as natriuretic peptides (BNP and NT-proBNP) and high-sensitivity troponin have enhanced our ability to identify individuals at risk for HF and monitor disease progression. Staging of HF has also improved, facilitating tailored treatments based on disease severity.

The incorporation of biomarkers such as natriuretic peptides in early stages of HF has enabled earlier identification of high-risk individuals (Stage B) as shown in **Table 4**.

Natriuretic peptides, produced by the heart in response to increased myocardial inflammation and stress, provide diagnostic and prognostic information for patients with HF. The risk of adverse outcomes is also predicted by elevated natriuretic peptides in patients without HF.[37,38] Optimal blood pressure control and medications such as sodium-glucose cotransporter-2 (SGLT2) inhibitors, at this preclinical stage can avert disease progression and improve patient outcomes.[30]

Classification

Left ventricular ejection fraction (LVEF or EF) continues its role as the key measure for diagnosis, classification, prognosis, and treatment selection in HF. The 2022 ACC/AHA guidelines classify HF into four categories based on ejection fraction (EF) and disease history as below:[30]

- *Heart failure with reduced ejection fraction (HFrEF):* EF is below 40%.
- *Heart failure with mildly reduced ejection fraction (HFmrEF):* EF between 41 and 49%.
- *Heart failure with preserved ejection fraction (HFpEF):* EF is 50% or above.
- *Heart failure with improved EF:* EF has increased by at least 10 points from a previous low of 40% or less.

TABLE 4: Stages of heart failure.[30]

Stages	Description	Characteristics
Stage A	At high risk of HF	Without structural heart disease or symptoms of HF
Stage B	Pre-HF	With structural heart disease without signs or symptoms of HF; persistently elevated biomarkers—high-sensitivity troponin; BNP ≥35 pg/mL or NT-proBNP of ≥125 pg/mL
Stage C	Symptomatic HF	With structural heart disease, with prior or current symptoms of HF
Stage D	Advanced HF	Refractory HF requiring specialized interventions[36]

(BNP: B-type natriuretic peptide; HF: heart failure; NT-proBNP: N-terminal pro-B–type natriuretic peptide)

Heart Failure with Reduced Ejection Fraction

Heart failure with reduced ejection fraction is a serious condition resulting from the heart's inability to pump blood effectively. Hospitalized HFrEF patients face a mortality rate comparable to, or even exceeding, that of many metastatic cancers, underscoring the need for prompt and effective treatment to improve outcome.[36,39] The 2022 HF guidelines recommend a standardized approach using "quadruple therapy" with angiotensin receptor-neprilysin inhibitor, beta-blocker, SGLT2 inhibitor, and mineralocorticoid receptor antagonist as the foundation for managing HFrEF **(Table 5)**.

Guideline-directed medical therapy (GDMT), as on **Table 5**, has revolutionized the management of HFrEF and has markedly improved patient outcomes, reduced hospitalizations and mortality. However, there are disparities in GDMT utilization due to cost, patient adherence, and healthcare system barriers that need to be overcome to fully realize the benefits of GDMT.[44-46]

Device-based therapies are useful in select groups of patients. Implantable cardioverter-defibrillators (ICDs) are recommended for patients with an EF below 35% to prevent sudden cardiac death.[49] While effective in preventing fatal arrhythmias, ICDs may not improve quality of life and can lead to complications such as device infections or to activating inappropriately. Cardiac resynchronization therapy (CRT), that involves the pacing of both ventricles, is beneficial for patients with HFrEF and wide QRS complex. CRT has been shown to reduce morbidity and mortality in this population. The choice of device therapy depends on various factors, including the HF, patient preferences, and available resources. The left ventricular assist device (LVAD),

TABLE 5: Quadruple medical therapy for heart failure with reduced ejection fraction (HFrEF).[30,40-45]

Angiotensin receptor-neprilysin inhibitors (ARNIs)	ARNIs have superior efficacy in reducing hospitalization and mortality compared to traditional therapies. However, if their high cost makes it prohibitive ACE inhibitors are the preferred alternative over angiotensin receptor blockers (ARBs)
Beta-blockers	Beta-blockers are staple medications for HFrEF that improve survival and reduce complications. The overall efficacy of different beta-blockers is comparable and should be incorporated into the treatment regimen to optimize outcomes
SGLT2 inhibitors	Initially developed for diabetes management, SGLT2 inhibitors have emerged as breakthrough drugs for heart failure that reduce hospitalizations, improve survival, and enhance quality of life of patients with HF regardless of their diabetes status[46-48]
Mineralocorticoid receptor antagonists (MRAs)	MRAs, spironolactone and eplerenone, block the effects of aldosterone, a hormone that can worsen HF symptoms. By inhibiting aldosterone, MRAs help to reduce fluid retention, lower blood pressure, and protect the heart to reduce morbidity and mortality. A newer agent, finerenone is a non-steroidal MRA with potential advantages over traditional MRAs
Loop diuretics	Loop diuretics (e.g., furosemide) are effective in managing fluid overload in HF, to improve shortness of breath, and reduce leg swelling. However, their role has evolved from primary treatment to supportive therapy
Digoxin	Digoxin, once the mainstay of treatment has now limited to no role because of its narrow therapeutic range and with the advent of safer and more effective drugs

a mechanical pump implanted to assist the ventricle to pump blood, is used in patients waiting for a heart transplant. It is also used as a long-term treatment in patients with end-stage HF who are not eligible for heart transplants.

Heart transplantation is the best option for those with end-stage HF. In 2023, there were 4,023 adult heart transplants done in the US. The 1-year survival rate has increased to 90%- and the 5-year survival rate is about 80% in the US and 85% and 69% worldwide for 1 year and 5 years, respectively. While transplantation offers the opportunity for an improved quality of life and extended survival, shortage of donor hearts, rigorous selection criteria, post-transplant care, and the high cost limit its application on a wider scale.[50,51]

Palliative care is very appropriate for patients with HF and particularly for those with advanced HF. Palliative care is a multidisciplinary approach to provide holistic care to improve quality of life through symptom relief, emotional support, communication and help patients and their caregivers in decision making on treatment goals.[52]

Heart Failure with Preserved Ejection Fraction (HFpEF)

HFpEF and impaired diastolic function ("stiff heart") affects millions of people worldwide and share some of the manifestations (e.g., exertional shortness of breath). Though the clinical diagnosis of HFpEF is challenging it is reasonable to suspect it in a patient of 60 or older with exertional shortness of breath with one or more of the following conditions: AF, CKD, diabetes, hypertension, and overweight/obesity.[53,54] These conditions are part of/or are connected to the CKM syndrome as described earlier. Obesity, part of metabolic syndrome, is a risk factor because of chronic inflammation that affects cardiomyocyte structure and function, hemodynamic derangements and impairment of diastolic filling **(Fig. 1)**. While operative cellular mechanisms are not yet fully understood the resulting changes in tissue cause structural remodeling of the left ventricle.

Besides lifestyle modifications, interventions, optimal control of hypertension and correction of metabolic abnormalities, SGLT2 inhibitors offer promise in improving outcomes in HFpEF patients.[48,54,55] A recent economic evaluation, which included a simulation model of US adults with HFpEF, suggests that an SGLT2-inhibitor added to standard therapy would add an annual cost of $4,500 for each patient.[55] With over 3 million individuals affected by HFpEF, the potential impact on health care spending would be very substantial.[55-57]

Glucagon-like peptide-1 (GLP-1) agonists (e.g., dulaglutide, exenatide, liraglutide, lixisenatide, and semaglutide) developed for treatment of type 2 diabetes has shown additional benefits to treat obesity and notably to treat HF including HFpEF.[58,59] Mainly by addressing the metabolic diseases and disorders (diabetes and obesity) and by other potential benefits that include lowering blood pressure and delaying progression of diabetic nephropathy GLP-1 agonists improve heart function, reduce hospitalizations and improve quality of life in patients with HF.[60] Judicious combinations of a GLP-1 agonist with established drugs for HF **(Table 5)** hold promise to improve outcomes.[57] If SGLT2 inhibition and GLP-1 agonism work together to benefit patients with HF regardless of the type (EF reduced or preserved) it would challenge the present focus on EF and shift it to their commonality of features and to common treatment approaches.[54]

Trends and Mortality

In the INTER-CHF prospective cohort study of 5,823 patients, overall mortality of HF was 16.5%: highest in Africa (34%) and India (23%), intermediate in South-East Asia (15%), and lowest in China (7%), South America (9%), and the Middle East (9%).[61] In another large cohort study, HF mortality was higher in patients from lower-income countries (26%) compared with middle-income (20%) and higher-income countries (17%).[62] The prevalence of HFpEF is increasing and deaths due to non-CV causes are increasing while prevalence of HFrEF is holding steady and the incidence (new cases) of HFrEF is decreasing. As to mortality based on the type of HF, according to the European Society of Cardiology Heart Failure registry, mortality at 1 year mainly due to CV deaths were more frequent in HFrEF (53.5%) versus HFpEF (47.2%). Conversely, non-CV mortality at 1 year was lower in HFrEF (20.1%) versus HFpEF (30.7%).[63]

■ KEY TAKEAWAYS

- Cardiovascular kidney metabolic (CKM) syndrome highlights the interconnectedness of metabolic, kidney, and heart disorders (**Fig. 1**). Recognition of these interconnections with early intervention including lifestyle modifications and targeted therapies reduce the risk of morbidity and mortality.
- Atrial fibrillation (AF) and coronary artery disease (CAD) share a complex bidirectional relationship (**Flowchart 1 and Fig. 2**) due to overlapping risk factors such as hypertension, obesity, diabetes, and dyslipidemia that calls for a comprehensive approach to cardiovascular health.
- Atrial fibrillation is associated with a 2.4-fold risk of stroke, 5-fold risk of HF, 1.5-fold risk of heart attacks, 1.6-fold of CKD, 2-fold risk of sudden cardiac death and increased mortality (1 year 19.5%, 5 years 48.8%). Prompt recognition and treatment (rhythm control, rate control by electric cardioversion and/or medications) are required. Newer anticoagulant drugs are easier on the patients.
- Stroke is a stoppage of blood flow to a part of the brain from a blood clot (ischemic) or bleed (hemorrhagic). Quick recognition (see FAST acronym in text) and transport to an acute care facility are of highest importance as time loss translates to brain loss. Immediate treatment of ischemic and hemorrhagic strokes varies. Rehabilitation (multiple disciplines) is important after acute management.
- Stroke prevention requires control of risk factors—high blood pressure, high cholesterol, and diabetes. Lifestyle modifications including diet, exercise, avoidance of alcohol and tobacco smoking are essential. Rehabilitation (multiple disciplines) is important after acute management.
- Heart failure is a clinical syndrome caused by different diseases with symptoms and/or signs caused by a structural and/or functional cardiac abnormality and corroborated by elevated natriuretic peptide levels and/or objective evidence of pulmonary or systemic congestion.
- Symptoms and consequences of HF are caused by the heart's inability to pump blood effectively due to inadequacy of the left ventricle's pumping function or due to inadequacy of filling of left ventricle. Accordingly, HF is primarily classified into two main types: Heart failure with reduced ejection fraction (EF) (HFrEF) and Heart failure with preserved ejection fraction (HFpEF).
- Treatment of HF is tailored to the stage of disease and the degree of reduction in EF. In HFrEF the standardized recommended treatment is with four drugs: ARNI, beta blocker, SGLT2 inhibitor, and MRA.
- *Device-based treatment:* ICD in patients with severely reduced EF (<35%); CART to pace ventricles in patients with HFrEF and wide QRS complex; LVAD, a mechanical pump, to assist the ventricle as a bridge to heart transplants and in some patients ineligible for transplant for a longer term. Heart transplant is the best option for advanced HF, but shortage of donor hearts, selection criteria and cost keep it out of the range for many patients.

- Heart failure with preserved ejection fraction results from CKM syndrome or its individual components and many other conditions that impair diastolic filling. Besides rigorous control of the underlying conditions and lifestyle modifications, SGLT2 inhibitor, and GLP-1 agonist are used in treatment.
- Heart failure affects many millions of people with an impact on their quality of life and mortality. 1-year mortality from cardiovascular (CV) deaths is more frequent in HFrEF than in HFpEF and conversely non-CV deaths are more frequent in HFpEF. Trends indicate a rise in prevalence of HFpEF.

REFERENCES

1. Ndumele CE, Neeland IJ, Tuttle KR, Chow SL, Mathew RO, Khan SS, et al. A Synopsis of the Evidence for the Science and Clinical Management of Cardiovascular-Kidney-Metabolic (CKM) Syndrome: A Scientific Statement from the American Heart Association. Circulation. 2023;148.
2. Grundy SM, Stone NJ, Bailey AL, Beam C, Birtcher KK, Blumenthal RS, et al. 2018 AHA/ACC/AACVPR/AAPA/ABC/ACPM/ADA/AGS/APhA/ASPC/NLA/PCNA Guideline on the Management of Blood Cholesterol: Executive Summary: A Report of the American College of Cardiology/American Heart Association Task Force on Clinical Practice Guidelines. J Am Coll Cardiol. 2019; 73(24):3168-209.
3. Alberti KG, Eckel RH, Grundy SM, Zimmet PZ, Cleeman JI, Donato KA, et al. Harmonizing the metabolic syndrome: a joint interim statement of the International Diabetes Federation Task Force on Epidemiology and Prevention; National Heart, Lung, and Blood Institute; American Heart Association; World Heart Federation; International Atherosclerosis Society; and international association for the Study of Obesity. Circulation. 2009;120(16):1640-5.
4. Sowers JR, Whaley-Connell A, Hayden MR. The Role of Overweight and Obesity in the Cardiorenal Syndrome. Cardiorenal Med. 2011;1(1):5-12.
5. Joglar JA, Chung MK, Armbruster AL, Benjamin EJ, Chyou JY, Cronin EM, et al. 2023 ACC/AHA/ACCP/HRS Guideline for the Diagnosis and Management of Atrial Fibrillation: A Report of the American College of Cardiology/American Heart Association Joint Committee on Clinical Practice Guidelines. J Am Coll Cardiol. 2024; 83(1):109-279.
6. GBD Disease and Injury Incidence and Prevalence Collaborators. Global, regional, and national incidence, prevalence, and years lived with disability for 354 diseases and injuries for 195 countries and territories, 1990–2017: a systematic analysis for the Global Burden of Disease Study 2017. Lancet. 2018;392(1789-858):1789-1858.
7. Batta A, Hatwal J, Batta A, Verma S, Sharma YP. Atrial fibrillation and coronary artery disease: An integrative review focusing on therapeutic implications of this relationship. World J Cardiol. 2023;15(5):229-43.
8. Madhavan MV, Howard JP, Brener MI, Der Nigoghossian C, Chen S, Makkar R, et al. Long-Term Outcomes of Randomized Controlled Trials Comparing Percutaneous Left Atrial Appendage Closure to Oral Anti-coagulation for Nonvalvular Atrial Fibrillation: A Meta-Analysis. Struct Heart. 2023; 7(1):100096.
9. Jiang H, Koh TH, Vengkat V, Fei G, Ding ZP, Ewe SH, et al. An Updated Meta-Analysis on the Clinical Outcomes of Percutaneous Left Atrial Appendage Closure Versus Direct Oral Anticoagulation in Patients with Atrial Fibrillation. Am J Cardiol. 2023;200:135-43.
10. Dai H, Zhang Q, Much AA, Maor E, Segev A, Beinart R, et al. Global, regional, and national prevalence, incidence, mortality, and risk factors for atrial fibrillation, 1990-2017: results from the Global Burden of Disease Study 2017. Eur Heart J Qual Care Clin Outcomes. 2021;7(6):574-82.
11. Rattanawong P, Upala S, Riang Wiwat T, Jaruvongvanich V, Sanguankeo A, Vutthikraivit W, et al. Atrial fibrillation is associated with sudden cardiac death: a systematic review and meta-analysis. J Interv Card Electrophysiol. 2018;51(2):91-104.

12. Piccini JP, Hammill BG, Sinner MF, Jensen PN, Hernandez AF, Heckbert SR, et al. Incidence and prevalence of atrial fibrillation and associated mortality among Medicare beneficiaries, 1993-2007. Circ Cardiovasc Qual Outcomes. 2012;5(1):85-93.
13. World Stroke Organization. (2025). Impact-of-stroke. [online] Available from https://www.world-stroke.org [Last accessed May, 2025].
14. Tsao CW, Aday AW, Almarzooq ZI, Anderson CAM, Arora P, Avery CL, et al. Heart Disease and Stroke Statistics-2023 Update: A Report from the American Heart Association. Circulation. 2023;147(8):e93-e621.
15. Boehme AK, Esenwa C, Elkind MS. Stroke Risk Factors, Genetics, and Prevention. Circ Res. 2017;120(3):472-95.
16. Venketasubramanian N, Yoon BW, Pandian J, Navarro JC. Stroke Epidemiology in South, East, and South-East Asia: A Review. J Stroke. 2017;19(3):286-94.
17. Feigin VL, Brainin M, Norrving B, Martins S, Sacco RL, Hacke W, et al. World Stroke Organization (WSO): Global Stroke Fact Sheet 2022. Int J Stroke. 2022;17(1):18-29.
18. Hou X, Cen K, Cui Y, Zhang Y, Feng X. Antiplatelet therapy for secondary prevention of lacunar stroke: a systematic review and network meta-analysis. Eur J Clin Pharmacol. 2023;79(1):63-70.
19. O'Donnell MJ, Chin SL, Rangarajan S, Xavier D, Liu L, Zhang H, et al. Global and regional effects of potentially modifiable risk factors associated with acute stroke in 32 countries (INTERSTROKE): a case-control study. Lancet. 2016;388(10046):761-75.
20. O'Donnell MJ, Xavier D, Liu L, Zhang H, Chin SL, Rao-Melacini P, et al. Risk factors for ischaemic and intracerebral haemorrhagic stroke in 22 countries (the INTERSTROKE study): a case-control study. Lancet. 2010; 376(9735):112-23.
21. Ahmed M, Ahsan A, Fatima L, Basit J, Nashwan AJ, Ali S, et al. Efficacy and safety of aspirin plus clopidogrel versus aspirin alone in ischemic stroke or high-risk transient ischemic attack: A meta-analysis of randomized controlled trials. Vasc Med. 2024:1358863X241265335.
22. Zhao H, Zhou L, Hu L, Chen R, Dong L, Zhao Q, et al. Summary of best evidence for rehabilitation management of patients with motor dysfunction after stroke. Zhong Nan Da Xue Xue Bao Yi Xue Ban. 2024;49(4):497-507.
23. Healthdata.org. (2024). The Institute of Health Metrics and Evaluation. [online] Available from www.healthdata.org IHME/GHDx/GBD [Last accessed May, 2024].
24. Ke C, Gupta R, Xavier D, Prabhakaran D, Mathur P, Kalkonde YV, et al. Divergent trends in ischaemic heart disease and stroke mortality in India from 2000 to 2015: a nationally representative mortality study. Lancet Glob Health. 2018;6(8):e914-23.
25. Aparicio HJ, Himali JJ, Satizabal CL, Pase MP, Romero JR, Kase CS, et al. Temporal Trends in Ischemic Stroke Incidence in Younger Adults in the Framingham Study. Stroke. 2019;50(6):1558-60.
26. Vaduganathan M, Mensah GA, Turco JV, Fuster V, Roth GA. The Global Burden of Cardiovascular Diseases and Risk: A Compass for Future Health. J Am Coll Cardiol. 2022;80(25):2361-71.
27. Papadaki A, Martinez-Gonzalez MA, Alonso-Gomez A, Rekondo J, Salas-Salvadó J, Corella D, et al. Mediterranean diet and risk of heart failure: results from the PREDIMED randomized controlled trial. Eur J Heart Fail. 2017;19(9):1179-85.
28. Lloyd-Jones DM, Allen NB, Anderson CAM, Black T, Brewer LC, Foraker RE, et al. Life's Essential 8: Updating and Enhancing the American Heart Association's Construct of Cardiovascular Health: A Presidential Advisory from the American Heart Association. Circulation. 2022;146(5):e18-e43.
29. Roth GA, Mensah GA, Johnson CO, Addolorato G, Ammirati E, Baddour LM, et al. Global Burden of Cardiovascular Diseases and Risk Factors, 1990-2019: Update from the GBD 2019 Study. J Am Coll Cardiol. 2020;76(25):2982-3021.
30. Heidenreich PA, Bozkurt B, Aguilar D, Allen LA, Byun JJ, Colvin MM, et al. 2022 AHA/ACC/HFSA Guideline for the Management of Heart Failure: A Report of the

American College of Cardiology/American Heart Association Joint Committee on Clinical Practice Guidelines. Circulation. 2022;145(18):e895-e1032.
31. Bozkurt B, Coats AJS, Tsutsui H, Abdelhamid CM, Adamopoulos S, Albert N, et al. Universal definition and classification of heart failure: a report of the Heart Failure Society of America, Heart Failure Association of the European Society of Cardiology, Japanese Heart Failure Society and Writing Committee of the Universal Definition of Heart Failure: Endorsed by the Canadian Heart Failure Society, Heart Failure Association of India, Cardiac Society of Australia and New Zealand, and Chinese Heart Failure Association. Eur J Heart Fail. 2021;23(3):352-80.
32. van Riet EE, Hoes AW, Wagenaar KP, Limburg A, Landman MA, Rutten FH. Epidemiology of heart failure: the prevalence of heart failure and ventricular dysfunction in older adults over time. A systematic review. Eur J Heart Fail. 2016;18(3):242-52.
33. Shahim B, Kapelios CJ, Savarese G, Lund LH. Global Public Health Burden of Heart Failure: An Updated Review. Card Fail Rev. 2023;9:e11.
34. Virani SS, Morris PB, Agarwala A, Ballantyne CM, Birtcher KK, Kris-Etherton PM, et al. 2021 ACC Expert Consensus Decision Pathway on the Management of ASCVD Risk Reduction in Patients with Persistent Hypertriglyceridemia: A Report of the American College of Cardiology Solution Set Oversight Committee. J Am Coll Cardiol. 2021;78(9):960-93.
35. Martinez-Amezcua P, Haque W, Khera R, Kanaya AM, Sattar N, Lam CSP, et al. The Upcoming Epidemic of Heart Failure in South Asia. Circ Heart Fail. 2020;13(10):e007218.
36. Conrad N, Judge A, Canoy D, Tran J, Pinho-Gomes AC, Millett ERC, et al. Temporal Trends and Patterns in Mortality After Incident Heart Failure: A Longitudinal Analysis of 86 000 Individuals. JAMA Cardiol. 2019;4(11):1102-11.
37. Welsh P, Campbell RT, Mooney L, Kimenai DM, Hayward C, Campbell A, et al. Reference Ranges for NT-proBNP (N-Terminal Pro-B-Type Natriuretic Peptide) and Risk Factors for Higher NT-proBNP Concentrations in a Large General Population Cohort. Circ Heart Fail. 2022;15(10):e009427.
38. Jia X, Al Rifai M, Hoogeveen R, Echouffo-Tcheugui JB, Shah AM, Ndumele CE, et al. Association of Long-term Change in N-Terminal Pro-B-Type Natriuretic Peptide with Incident Heart Failure and Death. JAMA Cardiol. 2023;8(3):222-30.
39. Shah KS, Xu H, Matsouaka RA, Bhatt DL, Heidenreich PA, Hernandez AF, et al. Heart Failure with Preserved, Borderline, and Reduced Ejection Fraction: 5-Year Outcomes. J Am Coll Cardiol. 2017;70(20):2476-86.
40. McMurray JJ, Packer M, Desai AS, Gong J, Lefkowitz MP, Rizkala AR, et al. Angiotensin-neprilysin inhibition versus enalapril in heart failure. N Engl J Med. 2014;371(11):993-1004.
41. Chatterjee S, Biondi-Zoccai G, Abbate A, D'Ascenzo F, Castagno D, Van Tassell B, et al. Benefits of beta blockers in patients with heart failure and reduced ejection fraction: network meta-analysis. BMJ. 2013;346:f55.
42. Xie W, Zheng F, Song X, Zhong B, Yan L. Renin-angiotensin-aldosterone system blockers for heart failure with reduced ejection fraction or left ventricular dysfunction: Network meta-analysis. Int J Cardiol. 2016;205:65-71.
43. Poole-Wilson PA, Swedberg K, Cleland JG, Di Lenarda A, Hanrath P, Komajda M, et al. Comparison of carvedilol and metoprolol on clinical outcomes in patients with chronic heart failure in the Carvedilol or Metoprolol European Trial (COMET): randomised controlled trial. Lancet. 2003;362(9377):7-13.
44. Moghaddam N, Hawkins NM, McKelvie R, Poon S, Joncas SX, MacFadyen J, et al. Patient Eligibility for Established and Novel Guideline-Directed Medical Therapies After Acute Heart Failure Hospitalization. JACC Heart Fail. 2023;11(5):596-606.
45. Vaduganathan M, Claggett BL, Jhund PS, Cunningham JW, Pedro Ferreira J, Zannad F, et al. Estimating lifetime benefits of comprehensive disease-modifying pharmacological

therapies in patients with heart failure with reduced ejection fraction: a comparative analysis of three randomised controlled trials. Lancet. 2020;396(10244):121-8.
46. Bassi NS, Ziaeian B, Yancy CW, Fonarow GC. Association of Optimal Implementation of Sodium-Glucose Cotransporter 2 Inhibitor Therapy with Outcome for Patients with Heart Failure. JAMA Cardiol. 2020;5(8):948-51.
47. Redfield MM, Borlaug BA. Heart Failure with Preserved Ejection Fraction: A Review. JAMA. 2023;329(10):827-38.
48. Wright AK, Carr MJ, Kontopantelis E, Leelarathna L, Thabit H, Emsley R, et al. Primary Prevention of Cardiovascular and Heart Failure Events with SGLT2 Inhibitors, GLP-1 Receptor Agonists, and Their Combination in Type 2 Diabetes. Diabetes Care. 2022;45(4):909-18.
49. Leong DP, Joseph PG, McKee M, Anand SS, Teo KK, Schwalm JD, et al. Reducing the Global Burden of Cardiovascular Disease, Part 2: Prevention and Treatment of Cardiovascular Disease. Circ Res. 2017;121(6):695-710.
50. Trela KC, Salerno CT, Chuba E, Dhawan R. Donation After Circulatory Death Heart Transplantation: A Narrative Review. J Cardiothorac Vasc Anesth. 2024;38(9):2047-58.
51. Jennings DL, Sultan L, Mingov J, Choe J, Latif F, Restaino S, et al. PCSK9 inhibitors safely and effectively lower LDL after heart transplantation: a systematic review and meta-analysis. Heart Fail Rev. 2023;28(1):149-56.
52. Meehan CP, White E, CVitan A, Jiang L, Wu WC, Wice M, et al. Factors Associated with Early Palliative Care Among Patients with Heart Failure. J Palliat Med. 2024;27(8):1001-8.
53. Golla MSG, Shams P. Heart failure with preserved ejection fraction (HFpEF). In StatPearls (Internet). Treasure Island (FL): StatPearls Publishing; 2025.
54. Cannata A, McDonagh TA. Heart Failure with Preserved Ejection Fraction. N Engl J Med. 2025;392(2):173-84.
55. Cohen LP, Isaza N, Hernandez I, Lewis GD, Ho JE, Fonarow GC, et al. Cost-effectiveness of Sodium-Glucose Cotransporter-2 Inhibitors for the Treatment of Heart Failure with Preserved Ejection Fraction. JAMA Cardiol. 2023;8(5):419-28.
56. Solomon SD, McMurray JJV, Claggett B, de Boer RA, DeMets D, Hernandez AF, et al. Dapagliflozin in Heart Failure with Mildly Reduced or Preserved Ejection Fraction. N Engl J Med. 2022;387(12):1089-98.
57. Anker SD, Butler J, Filippatos G, Ferreira JP, Bocchi E, Böhm M, et al. Empagliflozin in Heart Failure with a Preserved Ejection Fraction. N Engl J Med. 2021;385(16):1451-61.
58. Kosiborod MN, Abildstrom SZ, Borlaug BA, Butler J, Rasmussen S, Davies M, et al. Semaglutide in Patients with Heart Failure with Preserved Ejection Fraction and Obesity. N Engl J Med. 2023;389(12):1069-84.
59. Kosiborod MN, Petrie MC, Borlaug BA, Butler J, Davies MJ, Hovingh GK, et al. Semaglutide in Patients with Obesity-Related Heart Failure and Type 2 Diabetes. N Engl J Med. 2024;390(15):1394-1407.
60. Greene SJ, Butler J, Fonarow GC. Contextualizing Risk Among Patients with Heart Failure. JAMA. 2021;326(22):2261-2.
61. Dokainish H, Teo K, Zhu J, Roy A, AlHabib KF, ElSayed A, et al. Heart Failure in Africa, Asia, the Middle East and South America: The INTER-CHF study. Int J Cardiol. 2016;204:133-41.
62. Tromp J, Paniagua SMA, Lau ES, Allen NB, Blaha MJ, Gansevoort RT, et al. Age dependent associations of risk factors with heart failure: pooled population-based cohort study. BMJ. 2021;372:n461.
63. Crespo-Leiro MG, Anker SD, Maggioni AP, Coats AJ, Filippatos G, Ruschitzka F, et al. European Society of Cardiology Heart Failure Long-Term Registry (ESC-HF-LT): 1-year follow-up outcomes and differences across regions. Eur J Heart Fail. 2016;18(6):613-25; Erratum in: Eur J Heart Fail. 2017;19(3):438.

CHAPTER 13

Statins: Bedrock of Prevention and Treatment of Heart Disease

■ INTRODUCTION

The last quarter of the 20th century saw a revolution in heart health with the arrival of statins. These drugs transformed the practice of cardiology, as they became the bedrock of prevention and management of heart disease. In Chapter 2, we discussed atherosclerosis, the systemic disease that causes atherosclerotic cardiovascular disease (ASCVD), and we focused on coronary artery disease (CAD), the major component among ASCVDs. We followed up in the subsequent chapters on the major risk factors for CAD—tobacco smoking, hypertension, diabetes, and cholesterol. Among these cholesterol—specifically atherogenic lipoproteins [especially low-density lipoprotein cholesterol (LDL-C)]—are the major culprits for most of the cardiovascular deaths amounting to many millions a year. Statins target the root causes of clogged arteries and high-intensity statin therapy (HIST) has demonstrated the ability to reduce LDL-C by 50% or more and to markedly reduce major adverse cardiovascular events (MACE) such as heart attacks and strokes.

Mechanism of Action

Brown and Goldstein, Nobel Laureates (1985), found that LDL receptors on cell surfaces mediate the uptake of LDL-C—the principal carrier of cholesterol in the blood. The uptake of dietary cholesterol inhibits the cells own synthesis of cholesterol, reduces the number of LDL receptors on the cell surface, and increases the level of cholesterol in the blood. Statins are inhibitors of reductase 3-hydroxy-3-methyl-glutaryl-coenzyme A (HMG-CoA), the rate-limiting enzyme in the cholesterol biosynthetic pathway.[1-3] Statins lower cholesterol by increasing the uptake of LDL via the LDL receptor. Although LDL receptor upregulation is clearly the primary mechanism of action, these drugs also decrease the production of apolipoprotein B (Apo B) containing lipoproteins by the liver.[3-6]

■ STATINS DECREASE HEART ATTACKS AND PROLONG LIFE

Landmark studies such as the Scandinavian Simvastatin Survival Study (4S in 1994) and the West of Scotland Primary Prevention Study (WOSCOPS in 1995) demonstrated statins' remarkable ability to:[7-9]

- Reduce deaths in patients with prior heart attacks [acute myocardial infarctions (AMIs)].
- Prevent heart attacks, strokes, and death in high-risk individuals without prior heart attacks.
- Reduce the need for invasive and expensive coronary artery revascularization procedures (CARPs) such as coronary artery stent(s) and coronary artery bypass graft (CABG) surgery.[10]

- Offer lasting protection of heart disease even after stopping medication ("legacy effect").[9]

These and several subsequent studies[11-13] established statins as the bedrock for both primary prevention (preventing future heart disease)[8] and secondary prevention (managing existing disease),[7] saving countless lives and reducing healthcare expenditures.[7,10] Some of the important factors that enhance the scope and benefits of statin therapy are: intensity of statin therapy, achieved LDL-C reduction, baseline ASCVD risk, duration of the LDL-C reduction, and use in primary and secondary prevention of MACEs.[2]

Intensity of statin therapy depends on the ASCVD risk and the LDL-C reduction desired to reach a personalized goal. Different statins and the doses for different intensities are shown in **Table 1**. HIST for >50% reduction in LDL-C is recommended for patients with existing heart disease or multiple major risk factors regardless of their LDL-C level, while low-intensity statin therapy (LIST) for <30% reduction in LDL-C is recommended in others without prior heart disease. Of note, reduction in statin dose is needed only when LDL-C is down to <25 mg/dL and remains at that level.[5]

Low-density Lipoprotein Cholesterol Reduction from Statins

For each 40 mg/dL reduction in LDL-C, there is a relative reduction in MACE (20–25%) that is independent of the baseline LDL-C level and coexisting disease (diabetes or chronic kidney disease).[5] The benefits of LDL-C lowering therapy may extend to adults at a young age and those at a lower cardiovascular risk.[16] High-dose, high-potency statins such as rosuvastatin and atorvastatin can achieve impressive reductions exceeding 50%, while moderate-intensity statins can achieve a respectable 30–45% reduction **(Table 2)**. However, low potency, low-dose simvastatin (5 mg) and pravastatin (10 mg), commonly used for primary prevention in India, may be inadequate as they produce only a 15–20% reduction in LDL-C. To achieve LDL-C goal <70 mg/dL for most Indians would require at least a moderate dose of atorvastatin (10–20 mg) or rosuvastatin (5–10 mg). Statins also provide additional benefits by lowering

TABLE 1: Dose of various statin medications that qualify for various intensities of statin therapies.

	High intensity	*Moderate intensity*	*Low intensity*
LDL-C lowering	>50%	30–49%	<30%
Rosuvastatin	20 and 40 mg	5 and 10 mg	NA (not applicable)
Atorvastatin	40 and 80 mg	10 and 20 mg	NA
Simvastatin		20 and 40 mg	10 mg
Pravastatin		40 mg	10 and 20 mg
Lovastatin		40 mg	20 mg
Fluvastatin		80 mg	20 and 40 mg
Pitavastatin		1–4 mg	NA

(LDL-C: low-density lipoprotein cholesterol)
Source: Adapted Virani SS, et al., 2023 and LaRosa JC, et al., 2005.[14,15]

TABLE 2: Percent reduction in lipid parameters with increasing statin doses.				
	LDL-C (mg/dL)	Non-HDL-C (mg/dL)	Apo B (mg/dL)	Triglycerides (mg/dL)
Rosuvastatin				
5 mg/day	–39	–35	–30	–15
10 mg/day	–44	–40	–35	–19
20 mg/day	–50	–45	–39	–20
40 mg/day	–55	–50	–43	–22
Atorvastatin				
10 mg/day	–36	–33	–28	–16
20 mg/day	–41	–38	–33	–19
40 mg/day	–46	–43	–37	–21
80 mg/day	–50	–47	–41	–35

(Apo B: apolipoprotein B; HDL-C: high density lipoprotein cholesterol; LDL-C: low-density lipoprotein cholesterol)
Source: Adapted from Enas EA, et al., 2013.[2]

non-HDL cholesterol (NHDL-C), Apo B, and triglycerides (TG) **(Table 2)**.

Impact of Statin Therapy

Statin therapy is effective in reducing adverse cardiovascular events and deaths at different levels of ASCVD risk **(Figs. 1A and B)**.

Benefits versus Costs

The previously mentioned WOSCOPS, a randomized, placebo-controlled trial involving 6,595 men aged 45–64 years with elevated cholesterol randomized to receive pravastatin 40 mg daily or placebo for 5 years[8] initially, then followed for an additional 10 years, noted treatment benefits as well as cost benefits.[10] During the extended follow-up, continued benefit was noted in those who had received pravastatin ("legacy effect").[10] Ford et al.[9] reported that the treatment group fared much better than the control group. Men in the treatment group, compared to the placebo group had a 35% reduction in hospitalizations for heart failure, 24% reduction in hospitalizations for AMI, 27% reduction in cardiovascular deaths, 18% reduction in AMIs, 15% reduction in coronary revascularization procedures, and a 13% reduction in all-cause deaths. Economic analysis revealed that over a 15-year period, pravastatin treatment in 1,000 patients saved a net of £710,000 (after cost of medication that was high then, and monitoring) for the UK National Health Service and translated to a gain of 136 quality-adjusted life years (QALYs).[10]

Benefits of a Low-density Lipoprotein Cholesterol Over a Life Time

Multiple lines of evidence cement the importance of consistently maintaining a low LDL-C over a life time to maximize heart health benefits:
- *Genetic evidence:* Individuals with a natural, lifelong 40 mg/dL LDL-C reduction have a remarkable 54% lower risk of AMIs compared to the 25% lower risk achieved with statin therapy for 5 years.[18]

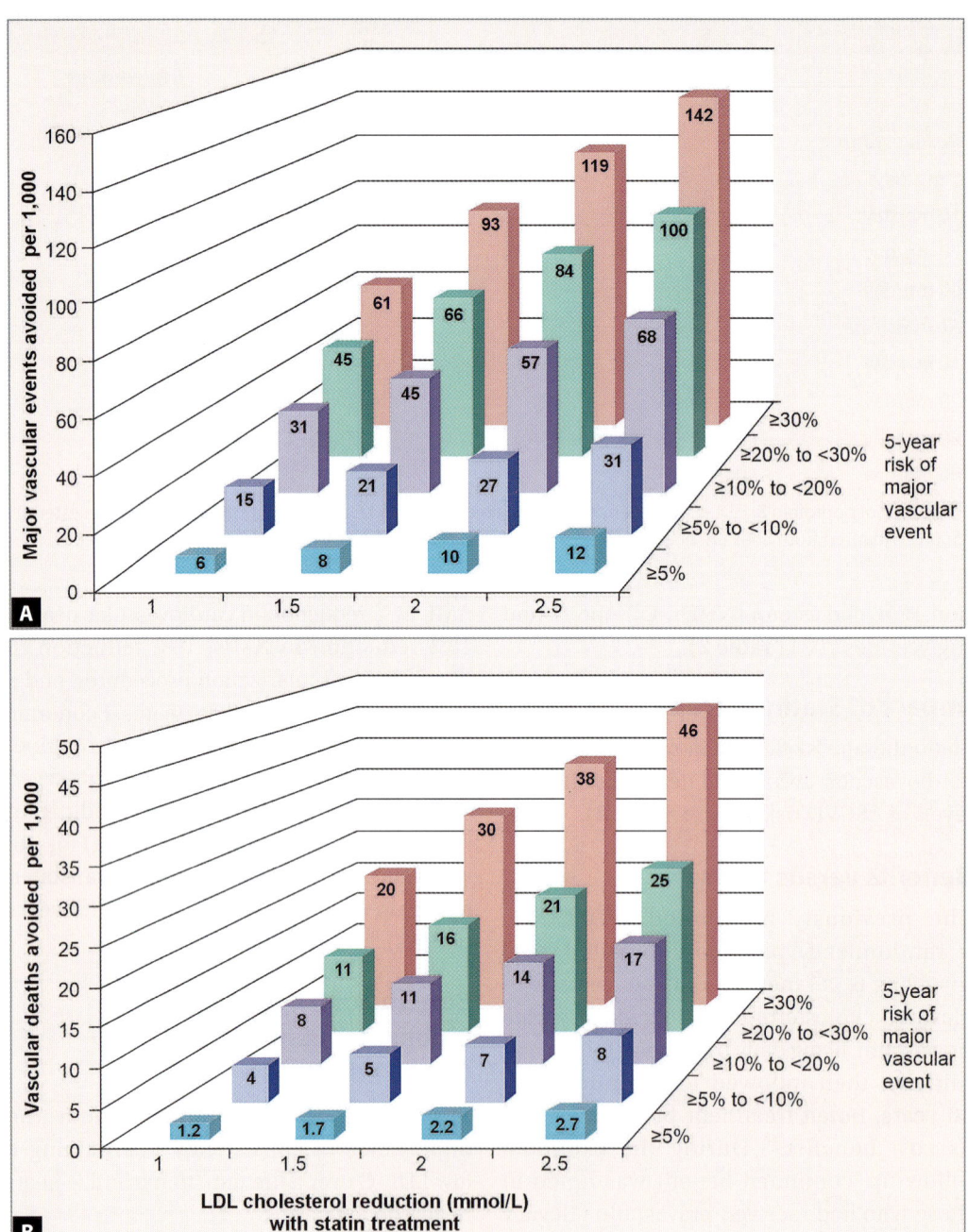

Figs. 1A and B: Predicted 5-year benefits of LDL-C reductions with statin treatment at different risk levels: (A) Major adverse cardiovascular events (MACE); (B) Cardiovascular deaths (on the vertical axis). Risk categories over a 5-year period and risk reductions achieved with a 1 mmol/L (40 mg/dL) reduction in LDL-C with statin treatment are shown. (LDL-C: low-density lipoprotein cholesterol)
Source: Reproduced with permission from Cholesterol Treatment Trialists C, et al., 2012.[17]

- *Clinical trials evidence:* A large meta-analysis showed that a 40 mg/dL LDL-C reduction results in a 17% reduction in MACE in the first year and a 29% reduction after 7 years of sustained control.[19] At any and all levels of risk factors for heart disease, Indians have a higher risk than whites for AMI and other MACE.[20] It is therefore reasonable to expect the benefits of lowering LDL-C would also be more in Indians. **Table 3** lists the rationale for the early initiation of statin therapy and sustaining it throughout life.
- *Eliminate coronary artery disease (ECAD) trial:* ECAD is a logical extension of the benefit(s) of lowering LDL-C by statin (atorvastatin 20 mg daily) in young adults (men 35–50 and women 45–59 years of age) with just one coronary risk factor to prevent MACE. Notably, healthy Indians/South Asians of this age group without any major established coronary factors qualify for enrollment in this trial as their ethnicity is counted as a risk factor. The results of the ECAD trial have the potential to be a game changer in easing the indications for statin treatment and eliminating the need for complicated risk assessment tools.[16]

Beyond Primary Prevention

Statins not only significantly reduce the initial occurrence of an MACE but is also an essential part of treatment during an MACE (e.g., AMI or a stroke). Statins have an integral and important role in secondary prevention to substantially lower the risk of recurrent MACE after a first AMI.[37-39] One study, reported that aggressive statin therapy plus a PCSK9 inhibitor that brought down and maintained LDL-C at a very low level (24 mg/dL) resulted in a "triple regression" effect on coronary plaques: decreased plaque volume, increased minimum lumen area, and improved the composition of unstable plaques to more stable ones.[40]

TABLE 3: Rationale for early initiation of primary prevention therapy in Indians.[5,21-34]

In India, heart disease, MACE, and deaths affect younger adults disproportionately	52–62% of heart disease deaths in India occur before age 70, compared to just 25% in the US. Besides, India accounts for 30% of global heart disease deaths under 50 years of age despite constituting only 18% of the world's population[21,35]
LDL-C >100 mg/dL in young adults is a serious threat	LDL-C at this range at a young age significantly increased the risk (64%) of developing heart disease within 20 years even if LDL-C is lowered later. Studies suggest a sustained and lifelong 30% reduction in LDL-C can radically slash heart disease risk by up to 90%
Early statins are key for optimal prevention	Starting statin therapy early by age 30 offers the greatest benefit in reducing the risk of heart disease. Delaying statin therapy can significantly decrease its effectiveness by 10% per decade: 54% at age 30s, 44% at 40s, 34% at 50s, and 24% at 60s[35,36]
10-year ASCVD risk calculator underestimates the CAD risk in younger adults	The US has the most liberal statin therapy threshold—10-year ASCVD risk >7.5%. Yet nearly one-half of those who had heart attack (AMI) under 50 years of age did not meet the threshold for statin therapy prior to the event. This proportion may be much higher in Indians whose risk of extremely premature (<50) deaths from heart disease is 13 times higher than in the US

(AMI: acute myocardial infarction; ASCVD: atherosclerotic cardiovascular disease; CAD: coronary artery disease; LDL-C: low-density lipoprotein cholesterol; MACE: major adverse cardiovascular events)

Adherence to Statin Therapy

After a heart attack, there is a demonstrable difference between those who adhere to statin therapy and those who do not. The latter has worse outcomes in complications and deaths while those who have good adherence experience less MACEs and less deaths.[36] A Swedish study suggested that in preventing MACEs adherence to statin therapy may be more important than the intensity of treatment.[41]

A Heart-healthy Diet and Other Prevention Modalities (Chapters 15–17)

Statin, for all its power and efficacy, is not the sole hero that protects all from heart disease and heart attacks. Statins act like magnets attracting LDL-C particles from the bloodstream. They achieve this by boosting LDL-C receptors in the liver, which act like traps. This targeted attack can be markedly enhanced by a heart-healthy diet rich in nuts, fiber, and plant sterols and by limiting saturated fat and refined carbohydrates. Such a dietary approach (Chapter 16) can significantly lower LDL-C as much as 30–40 mg/dL, potentially matching the effectiveness of low-dose statin therapy.[42,43] Dietary supplements (fish oil, cinnamon, garlic, turmeric, plant sterols, etc.) do not lower LDL-C as shown in one study that compared six dietary supplements to Rosuvastatin 5 mg daily.[44]

ALTERNATIVES TO 10-YEAR RISK ATHEROSCLEROTIC CARDIOVASCULAR DISEASE ESTIMATION IN INDIANS

Current national and international guidelines for statin therapy often rely on a 10-year ASCVD risk estimation that has limitations mainly in the underestimation of the risk (Chapter 1).

This underestimation particularly affects South Asians as the model heavily weighs the age factor and therefore young persons with multiple risk factors who would benefit from statin therapy may not meet the qualifying 10-year estimate. Studies also show nearly one-half of young Americans who had AMIs would not have qualified for statins beforehand due to this sole focus on 10-year risk.[20,45] Therefore, lifetime or 30-year risk estimations may be more suitable for young Indians considering their disproportionately high risk of heart disease under age 50. **Table 4** lists the better assessment options for the initiation of statin therapy.[26,54,55]

Coronary Artery Calcium (CAC) Scoring

CAC scoring goes beyond traditional methods to identify high-risk individuals, especially those who might be untreated or undertreated (Chapter 2). A secondary benefit of CAC score is that it may motivate individuals to adopt healthy habits and improve medication adherence.[53,56-62]

Lifetime Risk Estimation

Lifetime risk estimation can identify young adults with a high long-term risk [e.g., a 25-year-old with LDL-C of 140 mg/dL is at high risk (46%) over lifetime, but is at a low 10-year risk]. The Predicting the Risk of Cardiovascular events (PREVENT) calculator being developed (expected completion in 2025) by the American Heart Association (AHA) incorporates lifetime risk estimation and is a marked improvement over the Pooled Cohort Equation (PCE) in three domains: a wider age range of 30–79 years,

TABLE 4: Options to overcome limitations of 10-year ASCVD risk estimation for statin therapy.[20,45-53]

Using any one of the established major risk factors as a surrogate for 30-year ASCVD risk >20%[26,54,55]	A person with any one of the four established major risk factors (tobacco use, diabetes, high blood pressure, and high cholesterol) would have a 30-year ASCVD risk >20% regardless of age and would benefit from statin therapy. They also have 10-year ASCVD risk >7.5%, the threshold for statin therapy in the US
Using three or more ASCVD risk-enhancing factors (RENFs)	The 2018 ACC/AHA cholesterol guidelines introduced 13 RENFs that increase cardiovascular risk and Indian ethnicity is one among them. In addition, lipoprotein(a) >50 mg/dL and triglycerides >175 mg/dL, chronic kidney disease, and metabolic syndrome are common RENFs among Indians[45,52] (Chapter 3)
Using coronary artery calcium (CAC) scoring	A CAC score of 1–99 when associated with RENFs is an appropriate indication for statin therapy. A score above 100 equates to a 10-year ASCVD risk exceeding 7.5% warranting moderate or high intensity statin therapy. Scores exceeding 300 indicate high heart disease risk and a ≥3-fold higher risk for sudden death and therefore require high-intensity statin therapy (HIST)[53,56-62]
The PREVENT calculator	In development; incorporates a lifetime risk estimation
Simplified approach for Indians by Enas and Varkey	Indications for statin therapy by using the established and risk-enhancing factors without calculating ASCVD risk[46] **(Table 5)**

(ACC: American College of Cardiology; AHA: American Heart Association; ASCVD: atherosclerotic cardiovascular disease)

consideration of other disease states (e.g., heart failure, kidney failure, and metabolic states), and consideration of the social determinants of health, such as socioeconomic status and access to health care.[63]

Simplified Approach

In an editorial in the Indian Heart Journal,[46] we proposed a simplified approach based on risk classes tailored for Indians **(Table 5)**. Our proposal was prompted by the disappointingly low use of stains in India and our objective was to make the indications for statins easier (without risk estimations and calculations) to understand and follow. Thus, on high-risk classes (1A and 1B) as shown in **Table 5**, no extensive testing is needed. We also proposed that primary care physicians be educated and empowered to prescribe statins and to follow-up patients.

STATINS ARE SAFE BUT UNDERUSED

The World Health Organization (WHO)'s global goal is to have at least 50% of those eligible (meeting accepted indications) to take statins. However, this goal is very far from the present reality particularly in the resource-poor countries and the gap between them and in the resource-rich countries remains wide. In the US, a total of ~82 million people (~50% of eligible adults over 60 years of age and a lesser percentage of younger adults) and in other resource-rich countries one in three of eligible people receive statin therapy.[64] India is an outlier as only 5–10% who meet the indications take statins.[65] Why this disconnect between the proven and the practice? We offer our considered thoughts in the following text.

TABLE 5: Simplified approach to lipid-lowering therapy in Indians.

Conditions	Class	Statin therapy (mg/day)
Established ASCVD (AMI, stroke, coronary stent, coronary bypass surgery, carotid stenosis/stent, etc.)	1A Very strong	Atorvastatin 40–80 Rosuvastatin 20–40
Any one of the four established major factors: Diabetes: SBP >130 mg/dL; tobacco smoking; LDL-C ≥100 mg/dL, TC 170 mg/dL	1B Strong	Atorvastatin 10–20 Rosuvastatin 5–10
Any three risk-enhancing factors (RENFs) including: Indian ethnicity: Lp(a) >30 mg/dL; triglyceride ≥175 mg/dL; MetS, etc., (Chapter 3) lists all the RENFs	IIA Reasonable	Atorvastatin 10–20 Rosuvastatin 5–10
CAC score ≥100	IIB Tie breaker	Atorvastatin 10–20 Rosuvastatin 5–10
One RENF other than Indian ethnicity + CAC score >1	IIC May be considered	Atorvastatin 10–20 Rosuvastatin 5–10

(AMI: acute myocardial infarction; ASCVD: atherosclerotic cardiovascular disease; CAC: coronary artery calcium; LDL-C: low-density lipoprotein cholesterol; Lp(a): lipoprotein(a); SBP: systolic blood pressure; TC: total cholesterol)
Source: Modified from Enas and Varkey.[46]

Barriers to Statin Therapy

There are 3 types of barriers—physician, patient, system—that present singly or in various combinations. Physician barriers include insufficient knowledge—of risk factors for heart disease especially on LDL-C testing for the major risk factors, efficacy of statins, to identify patients who would benefit from them, and practice deficiencies—hesitancy in prescribing statins especially high intensity to high-risk patients, preference to mechanistic approaches (stents, CABG) over prevention and guideline directed treatment and the underestimation of benefits and overestimation of side effects of statins (a barrier that is shared by patients too). Other patient and system barriers include lack of awareness of heart disease and risk factors, poor adherence to prescribed statin and other medications, statin affordability, and concerns and misconceptions on statins.

Concerns on Statins

The 3 main areas of concerns are regarding—myopathy, stroke, and diabetes mellitus. Some people, in the early days after they start taking a statin, may experience muscle aches that most often are self-limited. Myopathy is rare (excess incidence of about 0.5 per 1,000 over 5 years), even in a high-intensity regimen with the exception of simvastatin 80 mg daily (or lower in Asian populations).[3,66] Switching from one statin to a different one is an option [The National Lipid Association (NLA) of the US defines true statin intolerance as failing at least two different statin medications]. Serious muscle breakdown (rhabdomyolysis) is extremely rare and causes extremely high creatine kinase levels (over 5–40 times the upper limit of normal) and may cause acute kidney injury. Additionally, it can be misdiagnosed and triggered by other medications.[57] A very large study of individuals receiving statin therapy for primary prevention, the incidence of rhabdomyolysis was 1 in 10,000 and the mortality <1 per 100,000.[67]

Previously referenced Cholesterol Treatment Trialists' (CTT) collaborators analyses[17,68] indicate that the annual excess risk of hemorrhagic strokes per 1.0 mmol/L LDL-C reduction might be of the order of 0.5 per 1,000 people treated over 5 years. This may be higher in populations in which hemorrhagic stroke accounts for a higher proportion of strokes (e.g., Chinese).[69] However, this risk is more than outweighed by the reduction in the overall number of strokes and notably the risk of ischemic strokes independent of predicted risk. Additionally, as shown in **Figure 1**, major occlusive vascular events and deaths are reduced.

The risk of proportional increase in diabetes on statin therapy is reported to be about 10% and the incidence of diabetes in primary prevention trials is about 5% over 5 years (the absolute excess about 0.1% per year).[70] Even if a new diagnosis of diabetes is associated with an immediate doubling of cardiovascular risk as has been suggested[71,72] in people with a 5-year risk of major vascular events of <10%, the absolute benefit expected with statin therapy is far more than their risk.[72] Additionally, long-term follow-up reports of statin trials have shown that the benefits of statin therapy in reducing major vascular events continue on treatment and persist even after cessation of treatment without adverse effects.[9,73,74]

Misconceptions

Statins do not affect growth and sexual maturation in males and females. They can be used safely, if indicated, in children. Statins do not cause or predispose to neuropathy, cataracts, or cancer.[75-78] Reduction of LDL-C with a statin does not increase the incidence of cancer [relative risk (RR) per 1.0 mmol/L, LDL-C reduction 1.00, 95% confidence interval (CI) 0.96-1.04], cancer mortality (RR 0.99, 95% CI 0.93-1.06), or other non-vascular mortality.[9,74] Statins do not cause dementia and do not worsen existing dementia. They might reduce the risk of worsening dementia even at low cholesterol levels.[76,77,79,80]

Cautions

Statins are not recommended for use during pregnancy due to potential risks to the fetus. It is important for a patient who is pregnant or planning to be pregnant to inform her physician. Statins are safe in most patients with liver disease including chronic viral hepatitis and nonalcoholic fatty liver disease (NAFLD). However, if liver enzymes get high and persist for >4 weeks (three times the upper limit of normal), statin cessation and reevaluation are advised.[75,81] Statins reduce heart disease risk in people with chronic kidney disease in stages 2-4. However, the pros and cons of the use of statins in those with end-stage renal disease (ESRD) requiring dialysis is not yet settled.

Drug-drug interactions that increase statin levels in blood can lead to muscle aches and possibly myopathy. Cyclosporine and amlodipine are drugs that can increase blood levels of statins and dosage adjustments may be needed in patients taking warfarin. Lovastatin and simvastatin are more prone to drug interactions than atorvastatin and rosuvastatin. Pravastatin appears to have the lowest potential for drug interactions.[2,75,81] Human immunodeficiency virus (HIV)-positive patients who require both statins and antiretroviral therapy may experience drug interactions and therefore require expert physician guidance. As elderly people often take multiple medications (polypharmacy), a moderate-intensity statin is preferred in the elderly to avoid potential drug interactions.[82]

■ A REMARKABLE JOURNEY

Statins have journeyed from scientific curiosity to the bedrock of cardiovascular disease (CVD) prevention and treatment. The journey continues as we explore the benefit of expanded use of statins beyond those with major risk factors and those with established ASCVD to prevention in apparently healthy individuals with genetic, ethnic, social determinants, and other known (inflammation and infection) and yet to be discovered predispositions.

■ KEY TAKEAWAYS

- Statins target the root cause—atherosclerosis—that causes plaque and obstruction to blood flow in the coronary arteries. Statin therapy has the demonstrated capability to markedly reduce LDL-C and markedly reduce MACE such as heart attacks, strokes, and deaths in those who have had an AMI (secondary prevention). Statins also reduce the need for invasive CARPs.
- Prevent AMIs, strokes, and death in individuals without prior AMIs (primary prevention). While those at high risk benefit more from primary prevention, meta-analysis of large studies shows that people at low risk (estimated 5-year risk of AMI of <10%) benefit significantly from statin therapy. Important factors in effective statin therapy are earlier initiation, longer duration, and intensity (related to risk status and desired LDL-C level).
- Currently used 10-year risk model may underestimate the true risk of heart disease in South Asians as it heavily weighs age and therefore young persons with multiple risk factors who would benefit from statin therapy would not be considered eligible. Hence, the use of any of the following three options are preferred: (1) Presence of one of the four established major risk factors: diabetes, smoking, high blood pressure, and high cholesterol as a surrogate for a 30-year ASCVD risk >20%; (2) Presence of three or more ASCVD RENFs; (3) CAC score of >100.
- We have proposed a simplified approach that eschews risk calculators and extensive tests in patients at high risk: (1) those with established ASCVD—AMI, stroke, coronary stent, coronary bypass surgery, carotid stenosis/stent, etc. and (2) those with any of the of the four established major factors: tobacco smoking, hypertension, diabetes, and hypercholesterolemia.
- In the US, the accepted normal level for total cholesterol (TC) is 170 mg/dL, LDL-C is 100 mg/dL, and NHDL-C is 130 mg/dL. In our reasoned opinion (Chapter 7), the appropriate levels of these measurements are 140 mg/dL, 70 mg/dL, and 100 mg/dL in Indians.
- Statins are used by millions of people and have an excellent safety profile and can be used even in children as young as 8 years old who are at a high risk. However, they are markedly underused in India due to several factors—physician, patient, and system—often in combination as barriers.
- Concerns that statins cause myopathy, increased stroke, and diabetes are not without basis. But the extent of risks is overblown and the benefits far outweigh the risks as detailed in the text. The misconceptions, cautions, and drug-drug interactions of statins are also explained.

■ REFERENCES

1. Goldstein JL, Brown MS. A century of cholesterol and coronaries: From plaques to genes to statins. Cell. 2015;161(1):161-72.
2. Enas EA, Kuruvila A, Khanna P, Pitchumoni CS, Mohan V. Benefits & risks of statin therapy for primary prevention of cardiovascular disease in Asian Indians—a population with the highest risk of premature coronary artery disease & diabetes. Indian J Med Res. 2013;138(4):461-91.
3. Collins R, Reith C, Emberson J, Armitage J, Baigent C, Blackwell L, et al. Interpretation of the evidence for the efficacy and safety of statin therapy. Lancet. 2016;388(10059):2532-61.
4. Enas EA, Kuruvilla A. Retracing the heroic steps from lipid hypothesis to aggressive treatment of blood cholesterol: a revolution

in preventive cardiology. In: Chopra HK, (Ed). Textbook of Cardiology. New Delhi: Jaypee Brothers Medical Publishers; 2012. pp. 180-194.
5. Grundy SM, Stone NJ, Bailey AL, Beam C, Birtcher KK, Blumenthal RS, et al. 2018 AHA/ACC/AACVPR/AAPA/ABC/ACPM/ADA/AGS/APhA/ASPC/NLA/PCNA Guideline on the Management of Blood Cholesterol: Executive Summary: A Report of the American College of Cardiology/American Heart Association Task Force on Clinical Practice Guidelines. J Am Coll Cardiol. 2019; 73(24):3168-209.
6. Enas E, Varkey B. Chapter 15. Management of dyslipidemia in Indians: implications of cholesterol guidelines and practical applications. In: Gundu Rao (Ed). Textbook of Coronary Artery Disease. Bombay: Jaypee Brothers; 2019.
7. Randomized trial of cholesterol lowering in 4444 patients with coronary heart disease: The Scandinavian Simvastatin Survival Study (4S). Lancet. 1994;344(8934):1383-9.
8. Shepherd J, Cobbe SM, Ford I, Isles CG, Lorimer AR, MacFarlane PW, et al. Prevention of coronary heart disease with pravastatin in men with hypercholesterolemia. West of Scotland Coronary Prevention Study Group. N Engl J Med. 1995;333(20):1301-7.
9. Ford I, Murray H, McCowan C, Packard CJ. Long-term safety and efficacy of lowering low-density lipoprotein cholesterol with statin therapy: 20-year follow-up of West of Scotland Coronary Prevention Study. Circulation. 2016;133(11):1073-80.
10. McConnachie A, Walker A, Robertson M, Marchbank L, Peacock J, Packard CJ, et al. Long-term impact on healthcare resource utilization of statin treatment, and its cost effectiveness in the primary prevention of cardiovascular disease: a record linkage study. Eur Heart J. 2014;35(5):290-8.
11. Ridker PM, Pradhan A, MacFadyen JG, Libby P, Glynn RJ. Cardiovascular benefits and diabetes risks of statin therapy in primary prevention: an analysis from the JUPITER trial. Lancet. 2012;380(9841):565-71.
12. Ridker PM, MacFadyen JG, Fonseca FA, Genest J, Gotto AM, Kastelein JJ, et al. Number needed to treat with rosuvastatin to prevent first cardiovascular events and death among men and women with low low-density lipoprotein cholesterol and elevated high-sensitivity C-reactive protein: justification for the use of statins in prevention: an intervention trial evaluating rosuvastatin (JUPITER). Circ Cardiovasc Qual Outcomes. 2009;2(6):616-23.
13. Ridker PM, Danielson E, Fonseca FA, Genest J, Gotto AM Jr, Kastelein JJ, et al. Rosuvastatin to prevent vascular events in men and women with elevated C-reactive protein. N Engl J Med. 2008;359(21): 2195-207.
14. Virani SS, Newby LK, Arnold SV, Bittner V, Brewer LC, Demeter SH, et al. 2023 AHA/ACC/ACCP/ASPC/NLA/PCNA Guideline for the Management of Patients With Chronic Coronary Disease: A Report of the American Heart Association/American College of Cardiology Joint Committee on Clinical Practice Guidelines. Circulation. 2023;148(9):e9-e119.
15. LaRosa JC, Grundy SM, Waters DD, Shear C, Barter P, Fruchart JC, et al. Intensive lipid lowering with atorvastatin in patients with stable coronary disease. N Engl J Med. 2005;352(14):1425-35.
16. Domanski MJ, Fuster V, Diaz-Mitoma F, Grundy S, Lloyd-Jones D, Mamdani M, et al. Next steps in primary prevention of coronary heart disease: rationale for and design of the ECAD trial. J Am Coll Cardiol. 2015;66(16):1828-36.
17. Cholesterol Treatment Trialists C, Mihaylova B, Emberson J, Blackwell L, Keech A, Simes J, Barnes EH, et al. The effects of lowering LDL cholesterol with statin therapy in people at low risk of vascular disease: meta-analysis of individual data from 27 randomised trials. Lancet. 2012; 380(9841):581-90.
18. Ference BA, Yoo W, Alesh I, Mahajan N, Mirowska KK, Mewada A, et al. Effect of long-term exposure to lower low-density

lipoprotein cholesterol beginning early in life on the risk of coronary heart disease: a mendelian randomization analysis. J Am Coll Cardiol. 2012;60(25):2631-9.
19. Cholesterol Treatment Trialists' (CTT) Collaboration; Baigent C, Blackwell L, Emberson J, Holland LE, Reith C, Bhala N, Peto R, et al. Efficacy and safety of more intensive lowering of LDL cholesterol: a meta-analysis of data from 170 000 participants in 26 randomised trials. Lancet. 2010; 376(9753):1670-81.
20. Patel AP, Wang M, Kartoun U, Ng K, Khera AV. Quantifying and understanding the higher risk of atherosclerotic cardiovascular disease among south asian individuals: results from the uk biobank prospective cohort study. Circulation. 2021;144(6): 410-22.
21. Healthdata.org. The Institute of Health Metrics and Evaluation. IHME/GHDx/GBD compare. [online] Available from www.healthdata.org [Last accessed May, 2025].
22. Ference BA, Bhatt DL, Catapano AL, Packard CJ, Graham I, Kaptoge S, et al. Association of genetic variants related to combined exposure to lower low-density lipoproteins and lower systolic blood pressure with lifetime risk of cardiovascular disease. JAMA. 2019;322(14):1381-91.
23. Cohen JC, Boerwinkle E, Mosley TH, Jr, Hobbs HH. Sequence variations in PCSK9, low LDL, and protection against coronary heart disease. N Engl J Med. 2006; 354(12):1264-72.
24. Navar-Boggan AM, Peterson ED, D'Agostino RB Sr, Neely B, Sniderman AD, Pencina MJ. Hyperlipidemia in early adulthood increases long-term risk of coronary heart disease. Circulation. 2015;131(5):451-8.
25. Zhang Y, Vittinghoff E, Pletcher MJ, Allen NB, Zeki Al Hazzouri A, et al. Associations of Blood Pressure and Cholesterol Levels During Young Adulthood With Later Cardiovascular Events. J Am Coll Cardiol. 2019;74(3):330-41.
26. Pencina M, Pencina K, Lloyd-Jones D, Catapano AL, Thanassoulis G, Sniderman AD. The expected 30-year benefits of early versus delayed primary prevention of cardiovascular disease by lipid lowering. Circulation. 2020;142(9):827-37.
27. Singh A, Collins BL, Gupta A, Fatima A, Qamar A, Biery D, et al. Cardiovascular risk and statin eligibility of young adults after an MI: Partners YOUNG-MI registry. J Am Coll Cardiol. 2018;71(3):292-302.
28. Singh A, Gupta A, Collins BL, Qamar A, Monda KL, Biery D, et al. Familial Hypercholesterolemia among young adults with myocardial infarction. J Am Coll Cardiol. 2019;73(19):2439-50.
29. Zeitouni M, Clare RM, Chiswell K, Abdulrahim J, Shah N, Pagidipati NP, et al. Risk factor burden and long-term prognosis of patients with premature coronary artery disease. J Am Heart Assoc. 2020;9(24): e017712.
30. Collet JP, Zeitouni M, Procopi N, Hulot JS, Silvain J, Kerneis M, et al. Long-term evolution of premature coronary artery disease. J Am Coll Cardiol. 2019;74(15):1868-78.
31. Law MR, Wald NJ, Rudnicka AR. Quantifying effect of statins on low density lipoprotein cholesterol, ischaemic heart disease, and stroke: systematic review and meta-analysis. BMJ. 2003;326(7404):1423.
32. Lloyd-Jones DM, Huffman MD, Karmali KN, Sanghavi DM, Wright JS, Pelser C, et al. Estimating longitudinal risks and benefits from cardiovascular preventive therapies among medicare patients: The Million Hearts Longitudinal ASCVD Risk Assessment Tool: A Special Report From the American Heart Association and American College of Cardiology. J Am Coll Cardiol. 2017;69(12): 1617-36.
33. Sniderman AD, Furberg CD. Age as a modifiable risk factor for cardiovascular disease. Lancet. 2008;371(9623):1547-9.
34. Mach F, Baigent C, Catapano AL, Koskinas KC, Casula M, Badimon L, et al. 2019 ESC/EAS Guidelines for the management of dyslipidaemias: lipid modification to reduce cardiovascular risk. Eur Heart J. 2020; 41(1):111-88.
35. Ke C, Gupta R, Xavier D, Prabhakaran D, Mathur P, Kalkonde YV, et al. Divergent

trends in ischaemic heart disease and stroke mortality in India from 2000 to 2015: a nationally representative mortality study. Lancet Glob Health. 2018;6(8):e914-23.
36. Beernink JM, Oosterwijk MM, van Boven JFM, Heerspink HJL, Bakker SJL, Navis G, et al. Adherence to Statin Therapy and Attainment of LDL Cholesterol Targets in an Outpatient Population of Type 2 Diabetes Patients: Analysis in the DIAbetes and LifEstyle Cohort Twente (DIALECT). Front Pharmacol. 2022;13:888110.
37. Cannon CP, Blazing MA, Giugliano RP, McCagg A, White JA, Theroux P, et al. Ezetimibe added to statin therapy after acute coronary syndromes. N Engl J Med. 2015; 372(25):2387-97.
38. Cannon CP. Low-density lipoprotein cholesterol: Lower is totally better. J Am Coll Cardiol. 2020;75(17):2119-21.
39. Szarek M, Amarenco P, Callahan A, DeMicco D, Fayyad R, Goldstein LB, et al. Atorvastatin reduces first and subsequent vascular events across vascular territories: The SPARCL Trial. J Am Coll Cardiol. 2020; 75(17):2110-8.
40. Biccire FG, Haner J, Losdat S, Ueki Y, Shibutani H, Otsuka T, et al. Concomitant coronary atheroma regression and stabilization in response to lipid-lowering therapy. J Am Coll Cardiol. 2023;82(18): 1737-47.
41. Mazhar F, Hjemdahl P, Clase CM, Johnell K, Jernberg T, Sjölander A, et al. Intensity of and adherence to lipid-lowering therapy as predictors of major adverse cardiovascular outcomes in patients with coronary heart disease. J Am Heart Assoc. 2022;11(14): e025813.
42. Chiavaroli L, Nishi SK, Khan TA, Braunstein CR, Glenn AJ, Mejia SB, et al. Portfolio dietary pattern and cardiovascular disease: a systematic review and meta-analysis of controlled trials. Prog Cardiovasc Dis. 2018; 61(1):43-53.
43. Vazquez-Manjarrez N, Guevara-Cruz M, Flores-Lopez A, Pichardo-Ontiveros E, Tovar AR, Torres N. Effect of a dietary intervention with functional foods on LDL-C concentrations and lipoprotein subclasses in overweight subjects with hypercholesterolemia: results of a controlled trial. Clin Nutr. 2021;40(5):2527-34.
44. Laffin LJ, Bruemmer D, Garcia M, Brennan DM, McErlean E, Jacoby DS, et al. Comparative effects of low-dose rosuvastatin, placebo, and dietary supplements on lipids and inflammatory biomarkers. J Am Coll Cardiol. 2023;81(1):1-12.
45. Agarwala A, Ballantyne C, Stone NJ. Primary prevention management of elevated lipoprotein(a). JAMA Cardiol. 2023;8(1):96-7.
46. Enas EA, Varkey B, Gupta R. Expanding statin use for prevention of ASCVD in Indians: Reasoned and simplified proposals. Indian Heart J. 2020;72(2):65-9.
47. Lloyd-Jones DM, Braun LT, Ndumele CE, Smith SC Jr, Huo Y, Fonarow GC, et al. Use of risk assessment tools to guide decision-making in the primary prevention of atherosclerotic cardiovascular disease: A Special Report From the American Heart Association and American College of Cardiology. Circulation. 2019;139(25): e1162-77.
48. Ference BA, Graham I, Tokgozoglu L, Catapano AL. Impact of lipids on cardiovascular health: JACC health promotion series. J Am Coll Cardiol. 2018;72(10): 1141-56.
49. An J, Zhang Y, Zhou H, Zhou M, Safford MM, Muntner P, et al. Incidence of atherosclerotic cardiovascular disease in young adults at low short-term but high long-term risk. J Am Coll Cardiol. 2023;81(7):623-32.
50. Enas EA, Dharmarajan TS, Varkey B. Consensus statement on the management of dyslipidemia in Indian subjects: a different perspective. Indian Heart J. 2015;67(2): 95-102.
51. Gupta R, Rao RS, Misra A, Sharma SK. Recent trends in epidemiology of dyslipidemias in India. Indian Heart J. 2017;69(3):382-92.
52. Akintoye E, Afonso L, Bengaluru Jayanna M, Bao W, Briasoulis A, Robinson J. Prognostic Utility of Risk Enhancers and Coronary Artery Calcium Score Recommended in the 2018 ACC/AHA Multisociety Cholesterol

53. Malik S, Zhao Y, Budoff M, et al. Coronary artery calcium score for long-term risk classification in individuals with type 2 diabetes and metabolic syndrome from the multi-ethnic study of atherosclerosis. JAMA Cardiol. 2017;2(12):1332-40.
54. Pencina MJ, D'Agostino RB, Sr., Larson MG, Massaro JM, Vasan RS. Predicting the 30-year risk of cardiovascular disease: the Framingham heart study. Circulation. 2009; 119(24):3078-84.
55. Pencina MJ, Navar AM, Wojdyla D, Sanchez RJ, Khan I, Elassal J, et al. Quantifying importance of major risk factors for coronary heart disease. Circulation. 2019; 139(13):1603-11.
56. Gill EA, Blaha MJ, Guyton JR. JCL roundtable: coronary artery calcium scoring and other vascular imaging for risk assessment. J Clin Lipidol. 2019;13(1):4-14.
57. Carr JJ, Jacobs DR, Jr, Terry JG, Shay CM, Sidney S, Liu K, et al. Association of coronary artery calcium in adults aged 32 to 46 years with incident coronary heart disease and death. JAMA Cardiol. 2017;2(4):391-9.
58. Gallone G, Elia E, Bruno F, Angelini F, Franchin L, Bocchino PP, et al. Impact of lipid-lowering therapies on cardiovascular outcomes according to coronary artery calcium score: a systematic review and meta-analysis. Rev Esp Cardiol (Engl Ed). 2022;75(6):506-14.
59. Budoff MJ, Young R, Burke G, Jeffrey Carr J, Detrano RC, Folsom AR, et al. Ten-year association of coronary artery calcium with atherosclerotic cardiovascular disease (ASCVD) events: the multi-ethnic study of atherosclerosis (MESA). Eur Heart J. 2018; 39(25):2401-8.
60. Peng AW, Dardari ZA, Blumenthal RS, Dzaye O, Obisesan OH, Iftekhar Uddin SM, et al. Very high coronary artery calcium (>/=1000) and association with cardio-vascular disease events, non-cardiovascular disease outcomes, and mortality: results from MESA. Circulation. 2021;143(16): 1571-83.
61. Razavi AC, Uddin SMI, Dardari ZA, Berman DS, Budoff MJ, Miedema MD, et al. Coronary artery calcium for risk stratification of sudden cardiac death: The Coronary Artery Calcium Consortium. JACC Cardiovasc Imaging. 2022;15(7):1259-70.
62. Razavi AC, Wong N, Budoff M, Bazzano LA, Kelly TN, He J, et al. Predicting long-term absence of coronary artery calcium in metabolic syndrome and diabetes: The MESA study. JACC Cardiovasc Imaging. 2021;14(1):219-29.
63. Khan SS, Matsushita K, Sang Y, Ballew SH, Grams ME, Surapaneni A, et al. Development and validation of the American Heart Association's PREVENT equations. Circulation. 2024;149(6):430-49.
64. Martin SS, Aday AW, Almarzooq ZI, Anderson CAM, Arora P, Avery CL, et al. 2024 heart disease and stroke statistics: A report of US and global data from the American Heart Association. Circulation. 2024;149(8):e347-e913.
65. Gupta R, Khedar RS, Gaur K, Xavier D. Low quality cardiovascular care is important coronary risk factor in India. Indian Heart J. 2018;70 Suppl 3:S419-S430.
66. Armitage J. The safety of statins in clinical practice. Lancet. 2007;370(9601):1781-90.
67. Coste J, Billionnet C, Rudnichi A, Pouchot J, Dray-Spira R, Giral P, et al. Statins for primary prevention and rhabdomyolysis: A nationwide cohort study in France. Eur J Prev Cardiol. 2019;26(5):512-21.
68. Cholesterol Treatment Trialists C; Emberson JR, Kearney PM, Blackwell L, Newman C, Reith C, Bhala N, et al. Lack of effect of lowering LDL cholesterol on cancer: meta-analysis of individual data from 175,000 people in 27 randomised trials of statin therapy. PLoS One. 2012;7(1):e29849.
69. Cheung BM, Lam KS. Is intensive LDL-cholesterol lowering beneficial and safe? Lancet. 2010;376(9753):1622-4.
70. Sattar N, Preiss D, Murray HM, Welsh P, Buckley BM, de Craen AJ, et al. Statins and risk of incident diabetes: a collaborative

meta-analysis of randomised statin trials. Lancet. 2010;375(9716):735-42.
71. Cholesterol Treatment Trialists' Collaboration. Electronic address cnoau, Cholesterol Treatment Trialists C. Effects of statin therapy on diagnoses of new-onset diabetes and worsening glycaemia in large-scale randomised blinded statin trials: an individual participant data meta-analysis. Lancet Diabetes Endocrinol. 2024;12(5):306-19.
72. Emerging Risk Factors C, Sarwar N, Gao P, Seshasai SR, Gobin R, Kaptoge S, Di Angelantonio E, et al. Diabetes mellitus, fasting blood glucose concentration, and risk of vascular disease: a collaborative meta-analysis of 102 prospective studies. Lancet. 2010;375(9733):2215-22.
73. Kashef MA, Giugliano G. Legacy effect of statins: 20-year follow up of the West of Scotland Coronary Prevention Study (WOSCOPS). Glob Cardiol Sci Pract. 2016; 2016(4):e201635.
74. Heart Protection Study Collaborative G. Effects on 11-year mortality and morbidity of lowering LDL cholesterol with simvastatin for about 5 years in 20,536 high-risk individuals: a randomised controlled trial. Lancet. 2011;378(9808):2013-20.
75. Cheeley MK, Saseen JJ, Agarwala A, Ravilla S, Ciffone N, Jacobson TA, et al. NLA scientific statement on statin intolerance: a new definition and key considerations for ASCVD risk reduction in the statin intolerant patient. J Clin Lipidol. 2022;16(4):361-75.
76. Goldstein LB, Toth PP, Dearborn-Tomazos JL, Giugliano RP, Hirsh BJ, Peña JM, et al. Aggressive LDL-C lowering and the brain: Impact on risk for dementia and hemorrhagic stroke: A scientific statement from the American Heart Association. Arterioscler Thromb Vasc Biol. 2023;43(10):e404-42.
77. Zhou Z, Ryan J, Ernst ME, Zoungas S, Tonkin AM, Woods RL, et al. Effect of statin therapy on cognitive decline and incident dementia in older adults. J Am Coll Cardiol. 2021;77(25):3145-56.
78. Swerdlow DI, Preiss D, Kuchenbaecker KB, Holmes MV, Engmann JE, Shah T, et al. HMG-coenzyme A reductase inhibition, type 2 diabetes, and bodyweight: evidence from genetic analysis and randomised trials. Lancet. 2015;385(9965):351-61.
79. Benn M, Nordestgaard BG, Frikke-Schmidt R, Tybjaerg-Hansen A. Low LDL cholesterol, PCSK9 and HMGCR genetic variation, and risk of Alzheimer's disease and Parkinson's disease: Mendelian randomisation study. BMJ. 2017;357:j1648.
80. Richardson K, Schoen M, French B, Umscheid CA, Mitchell MD, Arnold SE, et al. Statins and cognitive function: a systematic review. Ann Intern Med. 2013;159(10):688-97.
81. Newman CB, Preiss D, Tobert JA, Jacobson TA, Page RL 2nd, Goldstein LB, et al. Statin safety and associated adverse events: A scientific statement from the American Heart Association. Arterioscler Thromb Vasc Biol. 2019;39(2):e38-e81.
82. Engelen SE, van der Graaf Y, Stam-Slob MC, Grobbee DE, Cramer MJ, Kappelle LJ, et al. Incidence of cardiovascular events and vascular interventions in patients with type 2 diabetes. Int J Cardiol. 2017;248:301-7.

CHAPTER 14

Nonstatins: Powerful Drugs to Fight Heart Disease

■ INTRODUCTION

Statins, as elaborated in the previous chapter, are very effective in lowering low-density lipoprotein cholesterol (LDL-C) level and thereby reducing major adverse cardiovascular events (MACEs) in patients with and without heart disease. While statins continue to be the bedrock of treatment, the need for newer drugs have become clearer with our increased understanding on two fronts: Firstly, as we have alluded to previously, the lower the LDL-C level, the better the protection in patients with high risk and secondly, statin by itself does not always bring down LDL-C to the target level.

Prospective and observational studies have shown a direct and significant relationship between LDL-C level and atherosclerosis progression and MACE, and that the absolute reduction in LDL-C directly correlates with risk reduction.[1-4] Notably, in the US in 2019, 24 million coronary artery disease (CAD) patients [31% at "very high risk" (VHR)] were treated with statins to get to an LDL-C goal of <70 mg/dL.[5] Of these very high-risk patients, only 35% met their LDL-C goal of 70 mg/dL and even a much lower percentage (18%) achieved the level of <55 mg/dL. Hence, the important need for nonstatin drugs to achieve the optimal level of LDL-C to maximize risk reduction.

Risk Definitions

The 2018 American College of Cardiology/American Heart Association (ACC/AHA) guidelines recognize a new category of atherosclerotic cardiovascular disease (ASCVD) patients at "VHR" who have a history of multiple major ASCVD events or one major ASCVD event and multiple high-risk conditions.[6] However, they did not endorse a lower LDL-C target pending several cardiovascular outcome trials (CVOTs). Since then, many of these CVOTs have been completed.[2,4,7] Based on these, the 2022 ACC Expert Consensus Decision Pathway (ECDP) on the Role of Nonstatin Therapies for LDL-C Lowering in the Management of ASCVD risk was released recently,[8] prior to the next iteration of cholesterol guideline expected in 2025. The ACC EDCP recommended a lower LDL-C target of <55 mg/dL (or non-HDL-C of 85 mg/dL) for ASCVD patients at VHR **(Table 1)**. This recommendation is based on the documented net clinical benefit of achieving very low levels of LDL-C from adding nonstatin drug(s) on top of high-intensity statin therapy and lifestyle management.

Table 1 shows the risk definitions and states and the LDL-C goals that match the respective risks. The major risk factors and risk enhancing factors for ASCVD were explained in **Chapter 3**. Furthermore, it is our considered judgment and recommendation,

TABLE 1: Expert Consensus Decision Pathway (ECDP) on the Role of Nonstatin Therapies for lowering low-density lipoprotein cholesterol (LDL-C) in the Management of Atherosclerotic Cardiovascular Disease (ASCVD) Risk.[8]

High risk (HR) states	• Age >65 • Heterozygous familial hypercholesterolemia • History of CABG or PCI outside of major ASCVD events • Diabetes • Hypertension • CKD (eGFR 15–59 mL/min/1.73 m^2) • Current smoking • Persistently elevated LDL-C (>100 mg/dL) despite maximally tolerated statin therapy and ezetimibe • History of heart failure	LDL-C goal <70 mg/dL
Very high risk (VHR) states	Multiple major ASCVD events • Recent ACS (within the past 12 months) • History of MI (other than recent ACS) • History of ischemic stroke • Symptomatic PAD (claudication with ABI <0.85 or previous revascularization or amputation) • One major ASCVD event (listed above) and multiple high-risk conditions	LDL-C goal <55 mg/dL

(ABI: ankle brachial index; ACS: acute coronary syndrome; CABG: coronary artery bypass; CKD: chronic kidney disease; eGFR: estimated glomerular filtration rate; MI: myocardial infarction; PAD: peripheral artery disease; PCI: percutaneous coronary intervention)

based on decades of study on the prevalence, premature onset, and increased morbidity and mortality, that in Indians who are at a very high-risk state (as defined in **Table 1**) the goal of LDL-C goal should be lower than 50 mg/dL (range 30–50 mg/dL). Parenthetically, it should be noted that lifelong LDL-C in the range of 15–30 mg/dL in patients with hypobetalipoproteinemia or proprotein convertase subtilisin-kexin type 9 (PCSK9) loss-of-function mutations and in shorter-term lipid-lowering clinical trials are associated with a lower incidence of ASCVD without causing adverse effects.[9]

CLASSES OF DRUGS: METHODS OF ACTION AND SPECIFIC INDICATIONS

Table 2 shows the mechanism(s) of action of the first three nonstatin drugs listed on **Table 3** (also lists all other drugs). Short descriptions of these nonstatins follow.

Ezetimibe

Ezetimibe is a cost-effective drug that when added to a statin lowers LDL-C a further (16 mg/dL) by decreasing the absorption of cholesterol from the intestines. Studies have shown that adding ezetimibe to a lower dose of stain can achieve target LDL-C.[3] A large CVOT has shown a reduction in MACE with ezetimibe. This medication has become generic, (meaning low cost in the US), and has become a valuable, preferred second tier of lipid lowering medication (LLM) in high-risk patients to reduce their LDL-C to a target level appropriate to their risk.[5]

Bempedoic Acid (Nexletol)

Bempedoic acid (Nexletol) is a new and welcome alternative to statins for patients

TABLE 2: Drugs that lower cholesterol and their mechanisms of action.

Drug(s)	Bile acid sequestrants	Bempedoic acid	Ezetimibe
Mechanism of action	Increased bile synthesis	Decreased cholesterol synthesis	Decreased intestinal cholesterol absorption
Effect	• Decrease in hepatic cholesterol • Increase in hepatic low-density lipoprotein cholesterol (LDL-C) receptors	• Decrease in hepatic cholesterol • Increase in hepatic LDL-C receptors	• Decrease in hepatic cholesterol • Increase in hepatic LDL-C receptors
Result	Decrease in LDL-C	Decrease in LDL-C	Decrease in LDL-C

TABLE 3: Types of nonstatins, method of actions, and indications.

Ezetimibe	• A cholesterol absorption inhibitor and the first nonstatin drug of choice • Lowers the risk of MACE and is inexpensive in the US
Bempedoic acid	• ATP citrate lyase inhibitor • Lowers LDL-C and lowers risk for MACE but expensive • An acceptable alternative but not an ideal substitute for patients with SAMS
Bile acid sequestrants	• An optional alternative for ezetimibe intolerance and triglyceride (TG) <300 mg/dL • Numerous gastrointestinal side effects and cumbersome to consume
PCSK9 inhibitors	Monoclonal antibody and small interfering RNA (siRNA)
Inclisiran	Ideally suited for patients with poor medication adherence
Evinacumab	Indicated for FH
Lomitapide	Indicated for FH
LDL-C apheresis	Limited to patients with FH
Fibrates	Limited to patients with elevated TG
Icosapent ethyl	Limited to patients with elevated TG and is expensive

(FH: familial hypercholesterolemia; LDL-C: low-density lipoprotein cholesterol; MACE: major adverse cardiovascular events; PCSK9: Proprotein convertase subtilisin-kexin type 9; SAMS: statin associated muscle symptoms)

with statin-associated muscle symptoms (SAMS). An inhibitor of adenosine triphosphate citrate lyase, bempedoic acid upregulates LDL receptors in the liver, thereby reducing cholesterol synthesis.[10] Bempedoic acid 180 mg/day lowers LDL-C by 17–18% as monotherapy and 40% when used in combination with ezetimibe 10 mg (Nexlizet).[8] This combination lowers LDL-C by their complimentary mechanisms—inhibition of cholesterol synthesis in the liver **(Table 2)** and absorption in the intestine.[11,12]

A large (n = 13,970) international double-blinded randomized CVOT on subjects who were statin-intolerant or were unwilling to take statins showed a 22 mg/dL decrease in LDL-C and 13% reduction in MACE with bempedoic acid vs. placebo.[13,14] In primary prevention patients (n = 4,206) bempedoic acid was associated with a reduction in MACE (39%), nonfatal myocardial infarction (MI) (39%), and coronary artery revascularization procedures (CARP 36%).[15] Treatment was also associated with significant reductions in cardiovascular mortality (CVM) and all-cause mortality.[13] Despite these results, bempedoic acid is not the preferred first choice among lipid lowering drugs for preventing heart disease. Use it cautiously in people with joint pain, gout, or high tendon rupture risk (e.g., over 60-year-olds on corticosteroids or on fluoroquinolones). New attacks of gout developed in 1% of study participants.[14]

Bile Acid Sequestrants (BAS)

BAS lower LDL-C by 10–30% but are difficult to use due to side effects such as constipation and potential interference with other medications. Triglycerides (TG) may increase with BAS use. They can improve blood sugar control in diabetics. BAS are an option for pregnant women because of their safety profile.[16]

Proprotein Convertase Subtilisin-kexin Type 9 Inhibitors

The PCSK9 is a protein that interferes with the LDL receptors' ability to remove LDL-C from blood and consequently to elevated LDL-C levels. Statin therapy, while effective in lowering LDL-C, can paradoxically increase PCSK9 levels, limiting their effectiveness in some individuals. PCSK9 inhibitors, either monoclonal antibodies (MABs) or small interfering RNA (SiRNA), lower LDL-C by 50–60% and Lp(a) levels by 30%.[17-20] These agents also significantly lower intermediate-density lipoprotein (IDL) in patients with familial dysbetalipoproteinemia. This rare genetic dyslipidemia is associated with a VHR of CVD, due to accumulation of highly atherogenic remnant cholesterol (Chapter 7), despite having very low concentration of LDL-C. PCSK9 inhibitors do not lower C-reactive protein (CRP) levels. Angiographic studies have shown greater decrease in plaque volume with evolocumab, a PCSK9 inhibitor, compared with placebo.[21,22] PCSK9 inhibitors are particularly useful in patients with statin intolerance or familial dysbeta-lipoproteinemia.

Two large CVOTs involving nearly 30,000 participants showed PCSK9 inhibitors could reduce LDL-C to previously unimaginable levels.[2,4,9,23] The largest decrease in MACE with progressive decline in LDL-C was in those who achieved LDL-C <20 mg/dL **(Table 4)**.[9]

Thus, PCSK9 inhibitors are especially indicated in very high-risk ASCVD patients with an LDL-C goal of <55 mg/dL. While PCSK9 inhibitors are effective in reducing atherosclerotic plaque buildup and progression and are without major side effects and drug-drug interactions. However, their

TABLE 4: Achieved low-density lipoprotein cholesterol (LDL-C) level and relative risk reduction (RRR) in FOURIER Trial (*n* = 25,982).[9]

Achieved LDL-C	Number of participants	Percentage of participants	Relative risk reduction (RRR)
>100 mg/dL	4,395	17%	Reference
62–100 mg/dL	7,471	29%	3%
59–61	3,444	13%	6%
20–54	8,003	31%	15%
<20 mg/dL	2,669	10%	24%
<10 mg/dL	500	2%	Fewest events

TABLE 5: Salient features of PCSK9 inhibitor therapy.[9,23-27]

Profound LDL-C reduction	PCSK9 inhibitors (evolocumab, alirocumab) significantly lower LDL-C (50–60%) on top of statins and ezetimibe. The lower the LDL-C level and the longer it is maintained at that level, the greater the reduction in MACE. Particularly useful in secondary prevention after a heart attack (AMI)
Double advantage in individuals with high LDL-C and high Lp(a)	PCSK9 inhibitors are more efficacious in lowering LDL-C levels (50–60%) compared to statins vs. (30–50% reduction). Unlike statins, which may increase Lp(a) levels, PCSK9 inhibitors also lower Lp(a) by around 30%. This make PCSK9 inhibitors especially beneficial for patients with high Lp(a) (Chapter 8) and high LDL-C
Diabetes concern	PCSK9 inhibitors, like statins, may carry a slight risk of increasing new-onset diabetes, but this risk seems to be concentrated in people who already have prediabetes or a family history of diabetes. Further research is ongoing to definitively determine the impact of PCSK9 inhibitors on diabetes risk
Protection against hemorrhagic stroke	PCSK9 inhibitors, while effective at lowering LDL-C, do not increase the risk of hemorrhagic stroke and in fact, reduce the risk of ischemic stroke and therefore are good choices for those at risk for hemorrhagic stroke
Improving cost effectiveness	• PCSK9 inhibitors are a powerful tool for managing high cholesterol, but their high cost of ~$5,000/year in the US is a barrier to widespread use. Here is how targeting specific patient groups can improve their cost effectiveness • Targeting very high-risk ASCVD patients whose LDL-C goal is <55 mg/dL • Prioritizing patients with high LDL-C levels >100–130 mg/dL; they require an additional >50% reduction in LDL-C • Using ezetimibe as the first nonstatin therapy taking advantage of its lower cost ($100/year) but at a lower efficacy (16% reduction in LDL-C)

(ASCVD: atherosclerotic cardiovascular disease AMI: acute myocardial infarction; PCSK9: Proprotein convertase subtilisin-kexin type 9; LDL-C: low-density lipoprotein cholesterol; MACE: major adverse cardiovascular events)

high-cost limits widespread use.[8] The salient features of PCSK9 inhibitor therapy are tabulated in **Table 5**.

Inclisiran

Inclisiran is a promising new twice-yearly intravenous infusion treatment for millions struggling with their LDL-C control. It offers a breakthrough 50% reduction in LDL-C and the potential to reduce MACE by 26% by silencing PCSK9. The convenience in dosing frequency and route of administration may improve adherence compared to other medications. Inclisiran is ideal for those who are unable to tolerate orally administered PCSK9 inhibitors or have side effects. However, it is quite expensive and on par with PCSK9 inhibitors. Large ongoing trials (ORION-4) with results expected in 2025 will shed more light on inclisiran's long-term impact.[28,29]

FAMILIAL HYPERCHOLESTEROLEMIA

Familial hypercholesterolemia (FH) is a genetic disorder caused by a gene variant on chromosome 19. There are two types of FH—homozygous and heterozygous. The former is rare, affecting one in 300,000 people, while the latter is more common affecting one in 250 people. Those who inherit the variant gene from both parents develop homozygous type (HoFH) while those who inherit it from one parent develop heterozygous type (HeFH).

HoFH causes extremely high LDL-C (4–10 times normal) and very early heart disease (childhood to teenage). Those with HeFH also are at higher risk (3x normal) of premature heart disease that often go undiagnosed and untreated. Family history of very early heart disease, physical examination (xanthelasmas, xanthomas, and corneal arcus) and laboratory findings (markedly elevated LDL-C) are integral to the diagnosis. Early diagnosis is important as earlier the treatment is started the benefits are more in preventing MACE and prolonging life. Besides lifestyle modifications that include a healthy diet, regular exercise, maintenance of normal weight, and avoidance of tobacco smoking, new medications are now available to reduce LDL-C.[30,31]

Evinacumab

Evinacumab drastically reduces LDL-C by up to 135 mg/dL, allowing over half of HoFH patients to achieve optimal levels (<70 mg/dL). Evinacumab is approved for use for children as young as 10 and can potentially add 12 years or more to their lifespan. However, its high cost (over $450,000 annually) is a major hurdle.[8,32-34]

Lomitapide (Juxtapid)

Lomitapide (Juxtapid) offers substantial (40–50%) LDL-C reduction by targeting microsomal triglyceride transfer protein, hindering fat absorption and LDL-C production in the liver. However, it is very expensive and requires strict monitoring due to safety concerns that include a "Black Box" warning on liver health.[8]

LDL Apheresis

LDL apheresis is a powerful but expensive procedure used as a last resort for people with extremely high LDL-C (often >200–500 mg/dL).[8,35] Apheresis removes LDL particles directly from the bloodstream and achieves significant reductions (50–60% per treatment). While promising, large-scale studies are limited. The cost is prohibitive (up to $250,000 annually) and it requires specialized equipment and expertise.[35]

According to the HoFH International Registry (n = 751 patients from 38 countries), pretreatment LDL-C was nearly 4 times higher in low-middle-income countries (LMICs) (568 vs. 153 mg/dL) and on-treatment LDL-C was more than double in LMICs (363 vs. 153 mg/dL), compared to high-income countries (HICs), indicating inadequate treatment in LMICs. Only 3% of those from LMIC reached the LDL-C goal of <100 mg/dL compared to 21% in HICs. The first MACE occurred 10 years earlier in LMICs (24.5 vs. 37.0 years in HICs). These data underscore the limited access and affordability to advanced therapies in LMICs.[30]

■ HYPERTRIGLYCERIDEMIA

Triglycerides are fats made by the liver and contribute to plaque buildup in arteries, increasing heart disease risk. Very high TG (>500 mg/dL) is associated with pancreatitis but not acute myocardial infarction (AMI), because only 20% of the TG is atherogenic (remnant cholesterol).[36] The treatment goal when the TGs are very high is to lower it to <500 mg with diet, statins, and fenofibrate and in VHR patients **(Table 1)** to aim for a nonhigh-density cholesterol (NHDL-C) of ≤85 mg/dL. LDL-C levels decrease as the remnant cholesterol level increases thereby the actual risk may be underestimated.[37]

Medications that lower both TGs (remnant cholesterol) and LDL-C are effective in reducing heart disease risk. In fact, lowering remnant cholesterol seems to be as important as lowering LDL-C and therefore for optimal heart disease prevention, both remnant cholesterol and LDL-C needs to be targeted. The overall benefit of reducing these atherogenic lipids is linked to the total reduction in apolipoprotein B (ApoB).[38,39] Studies show lowering ApoB by 10 mg/dL has an equal benefit regardless of whether the reduction was achieved in LDL-C or very low density lipoprotein (VLDL)-C. This aligns with updated Canadian guidelines recommending use of ApoB/non-HDL-C alongside LDL-C as treatment targets.[36,39,40]

A fasting test is needed to confirm high TGs (>400 mg/dL) as a recent meal can affect the level. Liver derived VLDL particles dominate TG <1,000 mg/dL while dietary fat or chylomicrons dominate TG >1,000 mg/dL mainly. The management of hypertriglyceridemia varies depending on the TG level and the underlying pathophysiological factors but always begins with lifestyle management. TG over 500 mg/dL and especially a level over 1,000 mg/dL, raises the risk of pancreatitis, a potentially life-threatening condition. Once the TG is lowered to <500 mg/dL, further lowering should be based on NHDL-C, which might contain a disproportionately large proportion of highly atherogenic remnant cholesterol.

Lifestyle Changes

Lifestyle changes are essential to the management of hypertriglyceridemia **(Table 6)** and when combined with medications they effectively lower the TGs and reduce the risk of pancreatitis.[41]

Individuals with elevated TG are more likely to have high body mass index (BMI)

TABLE 6: Lifestyle management of patients with hypertriglyceridemia.[37,42]	
Strategy	*Comments*
Triglyceride (TG) levels	• Normal: <150 mg/dL (1.7 mmol/L); Borderline:150–199 mg/dL (1.7–2.2 mmol/L) • High TG (HTG): 200–499 mg/dL (2.3–5.6 mmol/L); very high TG: ≥500 mg/dL (≥5.6 mmol/L)
Exercise more	Regular physical activity boosts TG clearance
Limit alcohol	• Heavy drinking elevates TG and poses pancreatitis risk, especially when TG >1,000 mg/dL • Complete alcohol abstinence is essential for such cases
Eat less	Refined carbohydrates, sugar, sugar sweetened beverages, dairy desserts, saturated fats, and trans fats. 3–4 servings of fruit are allowed except for those with TG >1,000 mg/dL
Eat more	Unsaturated fats (like seafood), whole grains and whole fruits (avoid fruit juices when possible)
Manage weight	Lowering body mass index (BMI) is important when associated with high TG
Protein matters	A higher-protein diet (25% of energy) with moderate carbohydrates (45% carbohydrates) helps to lower TG
Diet extremes	Temporary very low-carb diets (20% carbohydrates) under medical supervision can be effective

TABLE 7: Helpful guides to the management of hypertriglyceridemia in Indians.[37-39,43,49-53]

Do not prioritize triglycerides over LDL-C	While managing TGs is important, focusing solely on them can be misleading. For instance, a person with a high TG (300 mg/dL) might only have a small portion (20%) contributing to bad cholesterol (atherogenic remnant-C), compared to someone with a high total cholesterol level (300 mg/dL) where two-thirds (200 mg/dL) is directly linked to bad cholesterol (atherogenic LDL-C). Thus, understanding the composition of cholesterol and TG is essential to accurately assess ASCVD risk
Contrasting heart disease risk from high TG and high TC	High triglycerides (TG >500 mg/dL) raise pancreatitis risk but not necessarily heart attack risk because they contain less harmful ApoB protein (Chapter 7). On the other hand, very high total cholesterol (TC >500 mg/dL) is a major red flag for heart attack risk at an early age (<30 years)
Limit added sugar and total fat intake	Those with persistently high (>175 mg/dL) TG, should limit the consumption of added sugar (especially sugary drinks) to < 5% of your total daily calories (TDC) and reduce overall fat intake to 20–25% of your TDC. For extremely high TG (>1,000 mg/dL), even stricter fat restriction (10–15% of daily calories) is necessary. Strongly recommend avoiding alcohol altogether in both cases
Statins trump fibrates for preventing heart attacks	Statins are more effective than fibrates in reducing the risk of MACE because they directly target ApoB, the protein believed to be a major culprit in heart attacks. While fibrates can lower triglycerides, their effect on ApoB is inconsistent. For example, Pemafibrate, a new fibrate, lowered triglycerides but failed to reduce MACE events and even raised ApoB levels in a recent trial, raising safety concerns
The STRENGTH trial poured cold water on omega-3 fish oil	Large studies testing omega-3 fatty acids for heart disease prevention have not shown a clear benefit. For instance, the STRENGTH trial showed a significant reduction in TG in but no decrease in MACE, leading to the early termination of the study
REDUCE-IT showed reduction in MACE with icosapent ethyl (IPE)	The REDUCE-IT trial with IPE (4 g/day) showed a significant decrease in MACE, despite only a modest TG reduction. For ASCVD patients with persistently high fasting TG (150–500 mg/dL) despite optimal lifestyle changes and statins, consider: • IPE if LDL-C is well-controlled (<70 mg/dL)[31,48] • High cost (~$3,000/year) and cumbersome dosing (4 g/day) hinder IPE's wider use in the US for managing high triglycerides • Ezetimibe or Nexletol if LDL-C remains high (>100 mg/dL)
Using CAC score as a tie breaker	For patients with high TG but no ASCVD or statin indications, consider CAC scoring, to refine ASCVD risk estimation[30]
TG > 1,000 mg/dL	• *Very high TG (>1,000 mg/dL):* Fenofibrate or icosapent ethyl (IPE) are preferred • *Moderate TG (150–499 mg/dL):* Focus on addressing underlying causes and consider starting statins[45-47]

(ASCVD: atherosclerotic cardiovascular disease; AMI: acute myocardial infarction; ApoB: apolipoprotein B; CAC: coronary artery calcium; HIST: high-intensity statin therapy; IPE: Icosapent ethyl; LDL-C: low-lipoprotein density cholesterol; LSM: lifestyle modification; MACE: major adverse cardiovascular events; REDUCE-IT: Reduction of Cardiovascular Events with Icosapent Ethyl-Intervention Trial; remnant-c = remnant cholesterol; TC: total cholesterol; TDC: total daily calories; TG: triglycerides; TG-RLP: triglyceride-rich lipoprotein; VLDL: very-low density lipoprotein) that needs lowering with diet, exercise, and medications. A case history of the management lowering TG level 4,000 mg/dL to 290 mg/dL over years has been reported.[41] The management consisted of: a low-fat, low-glycemic load diet, focusing on vegetables, whole grains, low-fat dairy, and poultry; regular exercise in the form of running 12–16 kilometers (7–10 miles) per week; smaller, consistent meals and statin, and fibrate therapy.[41] As hypertriglyceridemia is a problem that many Indians and their physicians contend with, a few helpful guides on management are provided in **Table 7**.

Fibrates

Fibrates (gemfibrozil, fenofibrate, and pemafibrate) may be considered in high-risk ASCVD patients, but their modest benefits must be balanced against side effects. Studies show minimal reduction in MACE with gemfibrozil but there is an increased risk of muscle breakdown (rhabdomyolysis) when combined with statins. Therefore, fibrates are generally not recommended for reducing ASCVD risk in patients already on statins.[37,43]

Icosa Pentyl Ether (IPE)

Icosa pentyl ether (IPE) (Vascepa), unlike other omega-3 fatty acids has shown benefit in reducing heart disease risk: (1) In the REDUCE-IT (Reduction of Cardiovascular Events With Icosapent Ethyl–Intervention Trial), IPE significantly lowered the risk of MACE by 18%, outperforming combined docosahexaenoic acid (DHA) and eicosapentaenoic acid (EPA) regimens used in many other studies and (2) This benefit seems to be linked to increased levels of IPE not just lower TG. Notably, half of the MACE reduction was associated with a decrease in remnant cholesterol (part of TG). However, IPE as a single therapy comes with increased risks of bleeding (49%) and atrial fibrillation (35%). There is some debate on whether a slight LDL-C increase in the control group might have influenced the positive IPE results. Overall, IPE offers a promising new approach for managing heart disease risk, but its safety risks demand a cautious approach.[44-48]

Omega-3 Supplements (Over the Counter Fish Oils)

Despite their popularity, omega-3 supplements have not been proven to have cardiovascular benefits regardless of statin use. There are conflicting results in recent trials possibly due to variations in supplement type, dosage, and subject populations. Current guidelines advise against relying solely on omega-3 fish oil for heart health. A worthwhile subject of future research is specific omega-3 formulations and their effectiveness and safety in targeted populations.[48,54]

■ KEY TAKEAWAYS

- Stricter LDL-C goals (<70 mg/dL for high-risk and <55 mg/dL for VHR) and the rise of non-statin therapies alongside statins are paving the way for strategies personalized to individuals and tailored to ethnic groups, such as Indians, at increased risks.
- Statins are the first line of treatment to lower LDL-C due to their proven benefits, safety, and affordability. Nonstatin drugs have an important role to reduce LDL-C to optimally low targets in high and VHR patients and they work well with statins. They not only lower LDL-C but may also impact ApoB lipoprotein levels to provide clinical benefits comparable to statins.
- Ezetimibe is the preferred nonstatin to add to statin for its efficacy (additional reduction of LDL-C <20%), excellent safety profile and is inexpensive. These attributes make ezetimibe especially suited for use in India.

- Bempedoic acid, a relatively more expensive drug, fills an important niche in those with statin-related muscle symptoms. It can be used alone or combined with ezetimibe to effectively lower LDL-C.
- PCSK9 inhibitors are powerful (an additional 50% reduction in LDL-C) but very pricey. While highly effective in lowering LDL-C, they are typically reserved for high risk and VHR patients. PCSK9 is also an appropriate addition to high-intensity statin therapy (HIST) in patients with a coronary artery calcium (CAC) score >1,000 and LDL-C >70 mg/dL.
- Inclisiran, an injectable medication requiring only a dose every 6 months, offers a promising solution for those struggling with adherence. However, the cost is prohibitive in low- and middle-income countries.
- Dietary and other lifestyle changes are essential to treat all cases of hypertriglyceridemia. HIST addresses both LDL-C and TG and is the first line of medication. Patients with high TG (>500 mg/dL) or very high TG (>1,000 mg/dL) despite lifestyle changes require fibrate (fenofibrate) or IPE. An important caveat: Do not prioritize TG level over LDL-C level.

■ REFERENCES

1. Cholesterol Treatment Trialists' (CTT) Collaboration; Baigent C, Blackwell L, Emberson J, Holland LE, Reith C, Bhala N, et al. Efficacy and safety of more intensive lowering of LDL cholesterol: a meta-analysis of data from 170,000 participants in 26 randomised trials. Lancet. 2010;376(9753): 1670-81.
2. Sabatine MS, Giugliano RP, Keech AC, Honarpour N, Wiviott SD, Murphy SA, et al. Evolocumab and Clinical Outcomes in Patients with Cardiovascular Disease. N Engl J Med. 2017;376(18):1713-22.
3. Cannon CP, Blazing MA, Giugliano RP, McCagg A, White JA, Theroux P, et al. Ezetimibe Added to Statin Therapy after Acute Coronary Syndromes. N Engl J Med. 2015;372(25):2387-97.
4. Schwartz GG, Steg PG, Szarek M, Bhatt DL, Bittner VA, Diaz R, et al. Alirocumab and cardiovascular outcomes after acute coronary syndrome. N Engl J Med. 2018;379(22): 2097-107.
5. Tsao CW, Aday AW, Almarzooq ZI, Anderson CAM, Arora P, Avery CL, et al. Heart disease and stroke statistics-2023 update: A report from the American Heart Association. Circulation. 2023;147(8): e93-e621.
6. Grundy SM, Stone NJ, Bailey AL, Beam C, Birtcher KK, Blumenthal RS, et al. 2018 AHA/ACC/AACVPR/AAPA/ABC/ACPM/ADA/AGS/APhA/ASPC/NLA/PCNA Guideline on the Management of Blood Cholesterol: Executive Summary: A Report of the American College of Cardiology/American Heart Association Task Force on Clinical Practice Guidelines. J Am Coll Cardiol. 2019; 73(24):3168-209.
7. Lloyd-Jones DM, Huffman MD, Karmali KN, Sanghavi DM, Wright JS, Pelser C, et al. Estimating longitudinal risks and benefits from cardiovascular preventive therapies among medicare patients: The million hearts longitudinal ASCVD risk assessment tool: A special report from the American Heart Association and American College of Cardiology. J Am Coll Cardiol. 2017;69(12): 1617-36.
8. Writing Committee; Lloyd-Jones DM, Morris PB, Ballantyne CM, Birtcher KK, Covington AM, DePalma SM et al. 2022 ACC Expert Consensus Decision Pathway on the Role of Nonstatin Therapies for LDL-Cholesterol Lowering in the Management of Atherosclerotic Cardiovascular Disease Risk: A Report of the American College of Cardiology Solution Set Oversight Committee. J Am Coll Cardiol. 2022;80(14): 1366-418.
9. Giugliano RP, Pedersen TR, Park JG, De Ferrari GM, Gaciong ZA, et al. Clinical efficacy and safety of achieving very low LDL-cholesterol concentrations with the PCSK9 inhibitor evolocumab: a prespecified secondary analysis of the FOURIER trial. Lancet. 2017;390(10106):1962-71.
10. Ferri N, Colombo E, Corsini A. Bempedoic acid, the first-in-class oral atp citrate

lyase inhibitor with hypocholesterolemic activity: clinical pharmacology and drug-drug interactions. Pharmaceutics. 2024; 16(11):1371.
11. Feingold K. Endotext 2022. Cholesterol lowering drugs. [online] Available from https://www.ncbi.nlm.nih.gov/books/NBK395573/ [Last accessed May, 2025].
12. Marazzi G, Caminiti G, Perrone MA, Campolongo G, Cacciotti L, Giamundo DM, et al. Addition of bempedoic acid to statin-ezetimibe versus statin titration in patients with high cardiovascular risk: A single-centre prospective study. J Cardiovasc Dev Dis. 2024;11(9):286.
13. Ballantyne CM, Laufs U, Ray KK, Leiter LA, Bays HE, Goldberg AC, et al. Bempedoic acid plus ezetimibe fixed-dose combination in patients with hypercholesterolemia and high CVD risk treated with maximally tolerated statin therapy. Eur J Prev Cardiol. 2020;27(6):593-603.
14. Nissen SE, Lincoff AM, Brennan D, Ray KK, Mason D, Kastelein JJP, et al. Bempedoic acid and cardiovascular outcomes in statin-intolerant patients. N Engl J Med. 2023; 388(15):1353-64.
15. Nissen SE, Menon V, Nicholls SJ, Brennan D, Laffin L, Ridker P, et al. Bempedoic acid for primary prevention of cardiovascular events in statin-intolerant patients. JAMA. 2023;330(2):131-40.
16. LRCCPTT. The lipid research clinics coronary primary prevention trial results. I. Reduction in incidence of coronary heart disease. JAMA. 1984;251(3):351-64.
17. Xiao G, Gao S, Xie Y, Wang Z, Shu M. Efficacy and safety of evolocumab and alirocumab as PCSK9 inhibitors in pediatric patients with familial hypercholesterolemia: A systematic review and meta-analysis. Medicina (Kaunas). 2024;60(10):1646.
18. Blanchard V, Chemello K, Hollstein T, Hong-Fong CC, Schumann F, Grenkowitz T, et al. The size of apolipoprotein (a) is an independent determinant of the reduction in lipoprotein (a) induced by PCSK9 inhibitors. Cardiovasc Res. 2022;118(9):2103-11.
19. Hu E, Wan M. Effect of PCSK9 inhibitors on major cardiac adverse events and lipoprotein-a in patients with coronary heart disease: a meta-analysis. Coron Artery Dis. 2024;36(3):200-10.
20. Sabatine MS, De Ferrari GM, Giugliano RP, Huber K, Lewis BS, Ferreira J, et al. Clinical benefit of evolocumab by severity and extent of coronary artery disease: An analysis from FOURIER. Circulation. 2018;138(8):756-66.
21. Nicholls SJ, Puri R, Anderson T, Ballantyne CM, Cho L, Kastelein JJ, et al. Effect of evolocumab on progression of coronary disease in statin-treated patients: The GLAGOV randomized clinical trial. JAMA. 2016;316(22):2373-84.
22. Raber L, Ueki Y, Otsuka T, Losdat S, Häner JD, Lonborg J, et al. Effect of alirocumab added to high-intensity statin therapy on coronary atherosclerosis in patients with acute myocardial infarction: The PACMAN-AMI randomized clinical trial. JAMA. 2022; 327(18):1771-81.
23. Sabatine MS, Leiter LA, Wiviott SD, Giugliano RP, Deedwania P, De Ferrari GM, et al. Cardiovascular safety and efficacy of the PCSK9 inhibitor evolocumab in patients with and without diabetes and the effect of evolocumab on glycaemia and risk of new-onset diabetes: a prespecified analysis of the FOURIER randomised controlled trial. Lancet Diabetes Endocrinol. 2017;5(12): 941-50.
24. Ference BA, Cannon CP, Landmesser U, Luscher TF, Catapano AL, Ray KK. Reduction of low density lipoprotein-cholesterol and cardiovascular events with proprotein convertase subtilisin-kexin type 9 (PCSK9) inhibitors and statins: an analysis of FOURIER, SPIRE, and the Cholesterol Treatment Trialists Collaboration. Eur Heart J. 2018;39(27):2540-5.
25. Sabatine MS, Wiviott SD, Im K, Murphy SA, Giugliano RP. Efficacy and safety of further lowering of low-density lipoprotein cholesterol in patients starting with very low levels: A meta-analysis. JAMA Cardiol. 2018; 3(9):823-8.
26. Wiviott SD, Giugliano RP, Morrow DA, De Ferrari GM, Lewis BS, Huber K, et al. Effect of

evolocumab on type and size of subsequent myocardial infarction: A prespecified analysis of the FOURIER randomized clinical trial. JAMA Cardiol. 2020;5(7):787-93.
27. Rosoff DB, Bell AS, Jung J, Wagner J, Mavromatis LA, Lohoff FW. Mendelian Randomization Study of PCSK9 and HMG-CoA Reductase Inhibition and Cognitive Function. J Am Coll Cardiol. 2022;80(7): 653-62.
28. Soffer D, Stoekenbroek R, Plakogiannis R. Small interfering ribonucleic acid for cholesterol lowering - Inclisiran: Inclisiran for cholesterol lowering. J Clin Lipidol. 2022; 16(5):574-82.
29. Ray KK, Raal FJ, Kallend DG, Koenig W, Leiter LA, Landmesser U, et al. Inclisiran and cardiovascular events: a patient-level analysis of phase III trials. Eur Heart J. 2023; 44(2):129-38.
30. Tromp TR, Hartgers ML, Hovingh GK, Vallejo-Vaz AJ, Ray KK, Soran H, et al. Worldwide experience of homozygous familial hypercholesterolaemia: retrospective cohort study. Lancet. 2022;399(10326):719-28.
31. Fahed AC, Wang M, Patel AP, Ajufo E, Maamari DJ, Aragam KG, et al. Association of the interaction between familial hypercholesterolemia variants and adherence to a healthy lifestyle with risk of coronary artery disease. JAMA Netw Open. 2022;5(3): e222687.
32. Rosenson RS, Burgess LJ, Ebenbichler CF, Baum SJ, Stroes ESG, Ali S, et al. Longer-term efficacy and safety of evinacumab in patients with refractory hypercholesterolemia. JAMA Cardiol. 2023;8(11):1070-6.
33. Kosmas CE, Bousvarou MD, Sourlas A, Papakonstantinou EJ, Peña Genao E, Echavarria Uceta R, et al. Angiopoietin-like protein 3 (ANGPTL3) inhibitors in the management of refractory hypercholesterolemia. Clin Pharmacol. 2022;14:49-59.
34. Schludi B, Giugliano RP, Sabatine MS, Raal FJ, Teramoto T, Koren MJ, et al. Time-averaged low-density lipoprotein cholesterol lowering with evolocumab: Pooled analysis of phase 2 trials. J Clin Lipidol. 2022;16(4):538-43.

35. Gianos E, Duell PB, Toth PP, Moriarty PM, Thompson GR, Brinton EA, et al. Lipoprotein apheresis: utility, outcomes, and implementation in clinical practice: A scientific statement from the American Heart Association. Arterioscler Thromb Vasc Biol. 2024;44(12):e304-e321.
36. Sniderman AD, Couture P, Martin SS, DeGraaf J, Lawler PR, Cromwell WC, et al. Hypertriglyceridemia and cardiovascular risk: a cautionary note about metabolic confounding. J Lipid Res. 2018;59(7):1266-75.
37. Virani SS, Morris PB, Agarwala A, Ballantyne CM, Birtcher KK, Kris-Etherton PM, et al. 2021 ACC expert consensus decision pathway on the management of ASCVD risk reduction in patients with persistent hypertriglyceridemia: A report of the American College of Cardiology Solution Set Oversight Committee. J Am Coll Cardiol. 2021;78(9):960-93.
38. Langsted A, Madsen CM, Nordestgaard BG. Contribution of remnant cholesterol to cardiovascular risk. J Intern Med. 2020;288(1): 116-127.
39. Ference BA, Kastelein JJP, Ray KK, Ginsberg HN, Chapman MJ, Packard CJ, et al. Association of triglyceride-lowering LPL variants and LDL-C-lowering LDLR variants with risk of coronary heart disease. JAMA. 2019;321(4):364-73.
40. Johannesen CDL, Mortensen MB, Langsted A, Nordestgaard BG. Apolipoprotein B and Non-HDL cholesterol better reflect residual risk than LDL cholesterol in statin-treated patients. J Am Coll Cardiol. 2021;77(11): 1439-50.
41. Patel J, Sharma T, Allan C, Curnew G. Use of lifestyle modifications for management of a patient with severely high total cholesterol (>14 mmol/L) and triglycerides (>40 mmol/L). J Lifestyle Med. 2021;11(1): 43-6.
42. Virani SS. The Fibrates Story - A Tepid End to a PROMINENT Drug. N Engl J Med. 2022; 387(21):1991-2.
43. Das Pradhan A, Glynn RJ, Fruchart JC, MacFadyen JG, Zaharris ES, Everett BM,

et al. Triglyceride lowering with pemafibrate to reduce cardiovascular risk. N Engl J Med. 2022;387(21):1923-34.

44. Khan SU, Lone AN, Khan MS, Virani SS, Blumenthal RS, Nasir K, et al. Effect of omega-3 fatty acids on cardiovascular outcomes: A systematic review and meta-analysis. EClinicalMedicine. 2021;38:100997.

45. Skulas-Ray AC, Wilson PWF, Harris WS, Brinton EA, Kris-Etherton PM, Richter CK, et al. Omega-3 fatty acids for the management of hypertriglyceridemia: A science advisory from the American Heart Association. Circulation. 2019;140(12):e673-91.

46. Bhatt DL, Steg PG, Miller M, Brinton EA, Jacobson TA, Ketchum SB, et al. Cardiovascular risk reduction with icosapent ethyl for hypertriglyceridemia. N Engl J Med. 2019; 380(1):11-22.

47. Castaner O, Pinto X, Subirana I, Amor AJ, Ros E, Hernáez Á, et al. Remnant cholesterol, not LDL cholesterol, is associated with incident cardiovascular disease. J Am Coll Cardiol. 2020;76(23):2712-24.

48. Mason RP, Libby P, Bhatt DL. Emerging mechanisms of cardiovascular protection for the omega-3 fatty acid eicosapentaenoic acid. Arterioscler Thromb Vasc Biol. 2020;40(5): 1135-47.

49. Boden WE, Baum S, Toth PP, Fazio S, Bhatt DL. Impact of expanded FDA indication for icosa pent ethyl on enhanced cardiovascular residual risk reduction. Future Cardiol. 2021;17(1):155-74.

50. Mason RP, Eckel RH. Mechanistic insights from REDUCE-IT STRENGTHen the case against triglyceride lowering as a strategy for cardiovascular disease risk reduction. Am J Med. 2021;134(9):1085-90.

51. Marston NA, Giugliano RP, Im K, Silverman MG, O'Donoghue ML, Wiviott SD, et al. Association between triglyceride lowering and reduction of cardiovascular risk across multiple lipid-lowering therapeutic classes: A systematic review and meta-regression analysis of randomized controlled trials. Circulation. 2019;140(16):1308-17.

52. Accord Study Group, Ginsberg HN, Elam MB, Cushman WC, Evans GW, Byington RP, Goff DC Jr, et al. Effects of combination lipid therapy in type 2 diabetes mellitus. N Engl J Med. 2010;362(17):1563-74.

53. Doi T, Langsted A, Nordestgaard BG. A possible explanation for the contrasting results of REDUCE-IT vs. STRENGTH: cohort study mimicking trial designs. Eur Heart J. 2021;42(47):4807-17.

54. Virani SS, Nambi V, Ballantyne CM. Has the 'strength' of fish oil therapy been 'reduced'? Reconciling the results of REDUCE-IT and STRENGTH. Eur Heart J Cardiovasc Pharmacother. 2021;7(3):e7-e8.

CHAPTER 15

Prevention of Heart Disease: Focus on Primordial and Primary Prevention

■ INTRODUCTION

This is the first in a trio of chapters on the prevention of heart disease. The other two deal with a heart-healthy diet and Life's Essential 8. In this chapter, we focus on two of the three tiers of preventive care **(Fig. 1)** and highlight how action on all these tiers have dramatically reduced the incidence, prevalence, and impact of heart disease in some countries thereby providing a clear road map for India to follow. We also appraise the state of primary preventive heart care in India and list some of the barriers to high-quality preventive care and end on a positive note for a better future.

■ PRIMORDIAL PREVENTION

Primordial prevention aims to prevent or reduce the development of cardiovascular risk factors (CVRFs) through optimizing health behaviors and societal conditions.[1] As represented on the bottom tier of **Figure 1**, the wide base indicates its wide scope at individual, community, state, and country

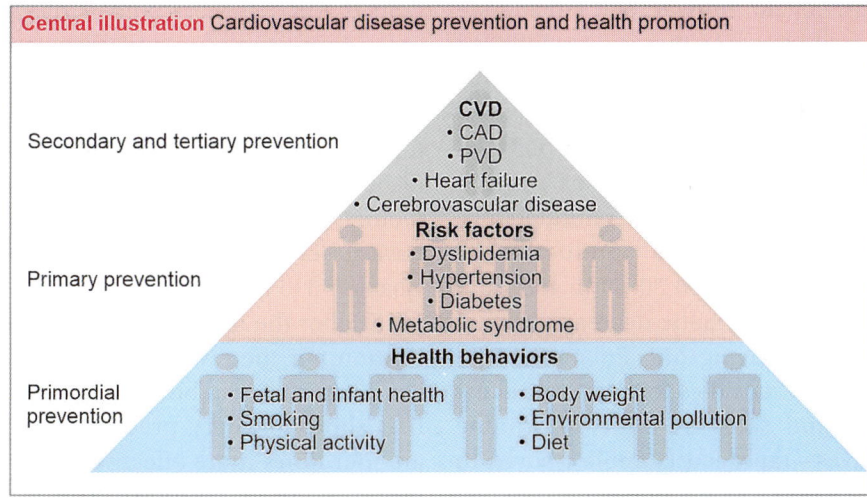

Fig. 1: Tiered approach to prevent cardiovascular disease (CVD). Primordial prevention makes up the base and optimizes health behaviors to reduce the development of CVD risk factors. The second tier is primary prevention, which targets CVD risk factors to prevent the development of CVD. Last, the apex is secondary and tertiary prevention, where CVD is targeted to prevent progression and development of additional CVD. (CAD: coronary artery disease; PVD: peripheral vascular disease)
Source: Reproduced with permission from Hong et al.[1]

levels. The roots of heart disease run deep; hence preventive aspects are important even before birth. Healthy eating, abstaining from tobacco smoking, and physical activity are basic good habits to be cultivated from childhood through youth and adulthood.[2,3]

At a community and state level much can be done to create environments that promote healthy choices—where fresh fruits and vegetables are available at affordable prices locally, where parks and green spaces abound for exercise and where the air is not polluted. Public policies on a state and national level can influence and change dietary practices, institute universal health care with emphasis on prevention, aid in urban farming subsidies, provide infrastructure for walking/cycling, and importantly address the social determinants of health like poverty. Many countries have enacted laws that ban smoking in public places and cigarette sales to minors.[1]

Successful Examples

Mauritius, Poland, Norway, and Finland are examples of countries that successfully led changes in dietary patterns of their people toward reduced heart disease and deaths.[4] Mauritius, in 1987, swapped palm oil (high in saturated fats) commonly used cooking oil for soybean oil, rich in unsaturated fats. Cross-sectional surveys conducted on over 5,000 subjects aged 30–64 in 1987 and 1992 revealed a dramatic decrease in total cholesterol by 31 mg/dL.[5] Poland, in the late 1980s, cut subsidies for dairy and meat products and sales of more affordable alternatives—rapeseed (Canola), soybean products, and vegetables increased resulting in reduced consumption (19%) of saturated fatty acids and increased consumption (32%) of unsaturated fatty acids. This is believed to be a key factor in the remarkable drop of ~40% (3% annually) in Poland's heart disease deaths (HDDs) rate between 1990 and 2002.[6] Norway, over the years 1975 to 1993, implemented a comprehensive nutrition strategy with incentives and subsidies for whole grains, vegetables, low-fat milk, and disincentives of higher prices on sugar and butter. Saturated fat intake decreased by 18% and cholesterol decreased by 10%; concomitantly, HDDs in middle-aged men were approximately halved.[7] Finland developed and encouraged the consumption of low-fat dairy and yogurts, and also increased the supply of berries, fruits, and vegetables. Primordial and primary prevention at the national levels reduced the risk factors and strikingly reduced HDDs by >80%.[8]

■ PRIMARY PREVENTION

Primary preventive measures (middle tier in **Figure 1**) target CVRFs to prevent major adverse cardiovascular events (MACEs) such as heart attacks, percutaneous coronary intervention (PCI), coronary artery bypass graft (CABG) surgery, and strokes,[9] while secondary preventive measures are those taken after a MACE to prevent another MACE (Chapter 11). Each of the major/established CVRFs (tobacco smoking, hypertension, diabetes, and cholesterol) and risk-enhancing factors (including metabolic syndrome) have deservedly received our attention in Chapters 3 to 7.

Neither the importance of primary prevention nor the rewards (reducing MACE) can be overstated as brought home in **Table 1** that shows primary prevention measures are four times more effective in preventing mortality from coronary artery disease (CAD) than secondary prevention.[10] Primary prevention measures that target established CVRFs and risk-enhancing factors are discussed in several of the previous chapters and the role of statins in Chapter 13.

TABLE 1: Primary prevention of three major risk factors markedly more impactful than secondary prevention in reducing deaths from coronary artery disease (CAD) in the US (1980–2000).

	Tobacco use	Systolic blood pressure	Cholesterol	All three risk factors
Primary prevention	46,315	97,315	107,300	64,930 (21%)
Secondary prevention	8,390	34,330	22,210	251,170 (79%)
Total	54,705	131,645	129,510	316,100 (100%)

Nearly four times as many CAD deaths were averted from primary prevention than from secondary prevention.[10]

Lessons from the United States

The 20th century in the US (and also in the UK, Finland, and Japan) saw a dramatic shift in the landscape of heart disease from its early and mid-decades to the last decades and has continued on to the 21st century.[11] Early decades witnessed a rising number of MACEs and deaths fueled by smoking, high cholesterol, and uncontrolled blood pressure. However, 1968 marked a turning point—public health initiatives that targeted the major CVRFs informed by the groundbreaking Framingham Heart Study.[12-14] Successful antismoking campaigns and policies, healthier lifestyle, advances in hypertension treatment, and other measures together reduced risks. HDDs dropped 68% from 1970 to 2013.[15,16]

This success story was largely, but not solely, due to primary prevention as this era also marked significant advances in treatment and changes in lifestyle (diet, activity, and tobacco abstinence). The contribution of lifestyle factors to CAD is further buttressed by the comparison of young American soldiers who died in the Korean war and the Iraq war as coronary atherosclerosis was found in 70% of the former and 9% in the latter.[17] The lessons on successfully combating CAD from the US are of practical value to countries grappling with this major health problem.[17]

Though the importance of major risk factors in the decline of CAD and related mortality is well established, it is harder to establish the relative contribution of the role of primordial, primary, and secondary prevention in that decline.[15,18] Ford et al.[15] used a previously validated statistical model to examine contributions to the decline in age-adjusted mortality rate for CAD in the US from 1980 through 2000 and reported that approximately 44% was attributed to changes in risk factors, including reductions in total cholesterol (24%), systolic blood pressure (20%), smoking prevalence (12%), and physical inactivity (5%).

Scandinavian Studies

Mannsverk et al.[19] in a 15-year prospective study (1994–2008) in Norway showed that changes in risk factors contributed to almost two-thirds of the change in CAD events. The prevalence of most risk factors decreased during that period, except for increases in body mass index (BMI) and diabetes. The major cause of the observed decline in HDDs was a cholesterol decrease of about one-third that accounted for about half of the observed decline. Changes in systolic blood pressure, smoking, resting heart rate, and physical activity each accounted for 9–14% of the decrease in risk of heart disease.

It is also cautionary that increases in BMI and diabetes prevalence accounted for a 7% and 2% increase, respectively. Björck et al.[20] used a previously validated model to quantify the relative contribution of primary and secondary prevention and the part played by medical treatment on the reduced cardiovascular mortality recorded in Sweden between 1986 and 2002. They reported that 75% of the mortality reduction was accounted for by the reduction of the major risk factors (cholesterol, blood pressure, and smoking) and concluded that the "largest effects on mortality came from primary prevention". They also gave recognition to the role of primordial prevention—specifically dietary changes—as the use of statins at that time was very low in Sweden.

Lessons from Finland

Finland is a standout, achieving an 82% decline in HDDs (men: 82%, women: 84%). This remarkable feat is a testament to the power of aggressive public health initiatives focused on smoking cessation and control of blood pressure and cholesterol as shown in **Figure 2**.

Cholesterol reduction, mainly through dietary changes, played a weighty role, as 37% of the decrease in HDDs was attributed to a 57 mg/dL drop in average cholesterol levels from 267 to 210 mg/dL between 1972 and 2007.[21] Notably, the overall decline in MACE was more than what could be expected from the control of the risk factors, suggesting there were additional benefits from improved acute coronary syndrome (ACS) management and secondary prevention measures.[8,21-24]

A Cautionary Lesson from China

Unlike the laudable successes in prevention in the US, Finland, and others, China's increase in heart disease is a cautionary lesson for India and other countries with fast growing economies. China with its impressive economic growth lifted many millions—more than one half of their population, out of poverty. However, along with

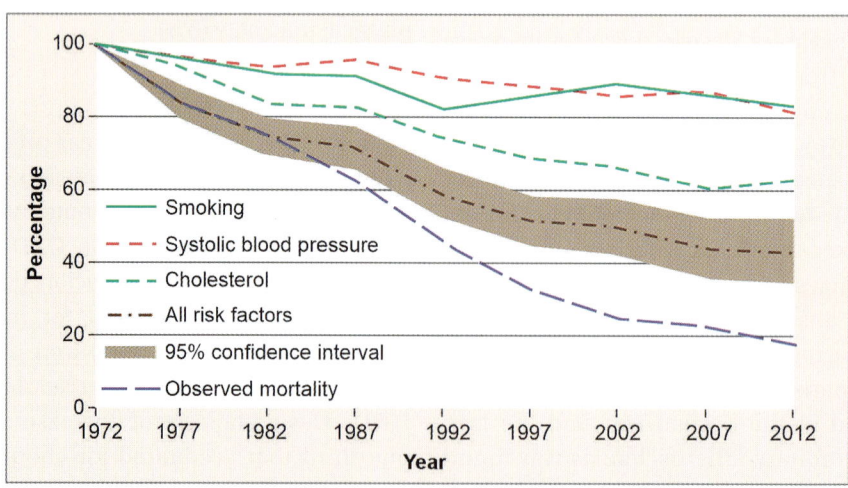

Fig. 2: Decrease in age-standardized heart disease death rates from 1972 to 2012 (logarithmic scale) for working aged men and women (age 35–64 years) in eastern Finland and the contribution of three major risk factors.
Source: Reproduced with permission from Jousilahti et al.[8]

this economic boom there came a marked shift in diet toward meat, sugary drinks, and eggs. Cholesterol levels rose by 40 mg/dL and so did multiple other risk factors such as salt intake, hypertension, and diabetes (19%), and tobacco use was already high. As a result, HDDs increased markedly (77%). Air pollution further threatens China's population—especially the vulnerable at extremes of age and those with heart and lung diseases. Even the marked advances in treatment were not capable of keeping up with the pace of increased heart disease and therefore, a holistic plan to curb this onslaught is of paramount importance for its citizens.[25-28] The clear lesson to be learned from China is that economic growth must be balanced with public health initiatives that promote healthy diets and lifestyles.

APPRAISAL OF HEART DISEASE PREVENTION IN INDIA

The axiom that to successfully wage a war one must know the enemy holds true in the war against heart disease. There is poor awareness of the major CVRFs among the populace (urban and rural) in India as Gupta and associates[29] reported in their review of population-based studies in 2018. **Figure 3** depicts the poor awareness of three of the major CVRFs: Hypertension: 42% in urban areas and 25% in rural areas; diabetes 72%; and hypercholesterolemia 15% in urban areas. Not surprisingly, those who were treated were less in number and those who were controlled on treatment were even less. Only 20% (11% in rural areas) of those with hypertension, 40% of those with diabetes, and a dismal 4% of those with hypercholesterolemia achieved control. A state-wide study by Sarma et al.,[30] from Kerala in 2019, found a lower rate of control for hypertension at 12% and diabetes 15% without a significant difference between urban and rural areas (cholesterol was not measured in this study).

Bleak but with Reasons for Hope

In spite of these bleak numbers there are reasons for optimism and hope for better years ahead for India. Firstly, even though

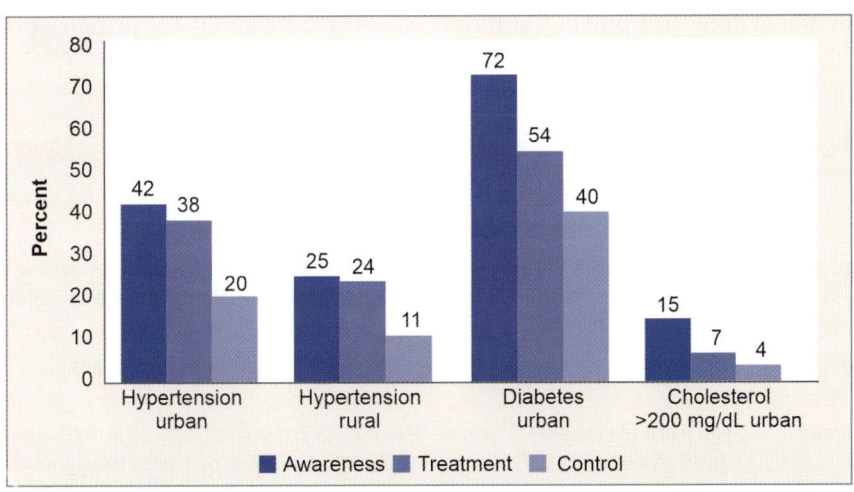

Fig. 3: Poor awareness and treatment of hypertension, diabetes, high cholesterol in India.
Source: Reproduced with permission Gupta et al.[29]

the record on primary prevention is poor, India's age-standardized deaths from heart disease decreased 12% in 30 years according to The Institute for Health Metrics and Evaluation (IHME). Secondly, the current barriers—cultural, costs, governmental—to implement primary prevention measures are not insurmountable. These barriers include individual (lack of knowledge, passive acceptance of health issues, expense involved, access to good quality care), physician/health care provider (lack of knowledge and interest in preventive cardiology that is not very remunerative), and governmental [low priority and low spending—3-4% of GDP on health care (compared to 17% in US and 9.8% in UK), lack of policies that promote physical activity and healthy eating]. Thirdly, and importantly, India has already shown what it can accomplish in markedly reducing tobacco smoking (one of the major heart disease risk factors). Currently, only 15% of men and 2% of women are smokers, with an overall prevalence of 9%.[31,32] India's success in curbing the scourge of tobacco smoking is a testament to the power of concerted, multifront educational, media, public policy, governmental actions and provides a blueprint for the control of the other CVRFs.

DRUGS USED IN PRIMARY PREVENTION

Statins, with their proven record and impressive safety profile, remain the bedrock of prevention and are covered in detail in Chapter 13.

Aspirin

Aspirin merits further discussion as its conventional role in primary prevention has come under scrutiny. The rationale for its use and efficacy are not the issue but the question is whether aspirin's benefits outweigh its risks. Large studies of aspirin involving over 134,000 participants found: 10% reduction in MACE, 44% increase in bleeding complications, and no significant impact on overall death rates.[33-36] Based on these findings recent guidelines reflect a restricted role for aspirin in primary prevention of heart disease **(Table 2)**. Aspirin is now recommended only for those with a high risk of heart disease, low risk of bleeding, and within a specific age range. Thankfully, with advancements in blood pressure management, smoking cessation, and widespread statin use, the overall need for aspirin in healthy individuals for primary prevention has decreased.[37-39]

TABLE 2: Aspirin's redefined role in primary prevention of heart disease.[33-40]	
For all	Not recommended as potential benefit of reduced heart attack risk is outweighed by increased risk of bleeding (predominantly gastrointestinal)
Men aged 40–59	Aspirin may be an option selectively in adults with a 10-year atherosclerotic cardiovascular disease (ASCVD) risk exceeding 10% after the physician weighs benefits and risks
Men over 60 years of age	If presently on aspirin, consult with a physician whether to stop or not
Women aged 60–69	Selectively in women (1) with a 10-year ASCVD risk over 20%, (2) with diabetes and ASCVD risk over 10%, if the benefits outweigh the risk of aspirin therapy
European guidelines	Aspirin for individuals with a 10-year ASCVD risk of >20%; in contrast, statin therapy is recommended for individuals with a 10-year ASCVD risk exceeding 10%

Note that these guidelines pertain only to primary prevention and not to secondary prevention. Aspirin continues to be indicated in patients who have had a stroke or a heart attack as in these patients the benefits outweigh the risks.

Blood Pressure-lowering Medications

Diuretic, angiotensin-converting enzyme inhibitor (ACE-I), angiotensin receptor blocker (ARB), beta blocker and calcium channel blocker are the main drugs alone or in combinations used to treat hypertension (Chapter 5).

Polypill

Polypill is the term applied to fixed-combination medication that has generated much interest and increasing acceptance in primary prevention of heart disease. Most common ingredients of a polypill are a statin, two blood pressure-lowering medication(s), and aspirin. Polypill has been found to be remarkably effective in reducing the incidence of fatal and nonfatal cardiovascular events in patients with intermediate and high cardiovascular risk as well as in secondary prevention in three meta-analyses.[41-43]

In the meta-analysis of primary prevention trials by Joseph et al. (n = 18,612), polypill was associated with a significant 38% reduction in primary outcome (which included heart attack, stroke, revascularization, and cardiovascular deaths).[41] Reductions were also observed for the separate components of the primary outcome: Myocardial infarction (48%), revascularization (46%), stroke (41%), and cardiovascular death (35%) with greater reductions for strategies that included aspirin. In another meta-analysis of eight randomized controlled trials representing (n = 25,584 and 3 of 8 were of primary prevention). Rao and co-authors[43] found that polypill achieved a 30% decrease in the risk of MACE in primary prevention trials. A similar 30–40% reduction in MACE has also been reported in secondary prevention trials.

The advantages of a single pill with ingredients directed at the major risk factors over multiple drugs in ease, expense, and adherence are particularly relevant in low- and middle-income countries where control of risk factors is low.[44] The polypill has only a very small risk of aspirin-induced bleeding.[44] The latest and important recognition of polypill is that the World Health Organization (WHO) has included polypill on its model list of essential medicines. WHO defines essential medicine as one intended to be available in functioning health systems at all times, in appropriate dosage forms, of assured quality, and at prices individuals and health systems can afford.

The overarching benefits of preventive cardiac care for all, regardless of the degree of risk, cannot be overstressed. Though it is appropriate to prioritize high-risk patients for preventive treatments, it must be understood that heart disease and heart attacks are not limited to them. Enlarging the focus of preventive care to include populations at low and moderate risk for heart disease is the right strategy to decrease the overall burden of heart disease.[45,46]

■ KEY TAKEAWAYS

- Primordial prevention—the prevention of CVRFs through dietary policy changes have been successful in Mauritius, Poland, Norway, and other countries.
- Though all three tiers of prevention (primordial, primary, and secondary) are important, primary prevention (control of major CVRFs) pays the highest dividend (~4 times more deaths prevented compared to secondary prevention).

- Multiple countries, especially the US, Norway, Sweden, and Finland, have seen a marked reduction in cardiovascular disease and MACE to a large extent from focusing on management of three major CVRFs—smoking, hypertension, and high cholesterol.
- In contrast, China as its economy boomed experienced an increase in the major CVRFs and heart disease and MACE. This is a cautionary lesson to countries with improving economies.
- In India, primary prevention of heart disease is low **(Fig. 3)** as hypertension, diabetes, and high cholesterol are often not recognized, and when recognized are not treated and when treated are not well controlled.
- However, India has made commendable progress in curbing tobacco smoking and therefore there is hope that similar multilevel efforts on smoking if applied to other CVRFs—hypertension, diabetes, and high cholesterol—and to lifestyle factors like unhealthy diet and physical inactivity would reduce heart disease, MACE, and cardiovascular deaths.
- Among the drugs useful for primary prevention, statins remain preeminent. Aspirin's role in primary prevention has been reassessed and is no longer considered for use in all but limited to those with a high risk of heart disease, a low risk of bleeding, and within a specific age range.
- The benefits of preventive care are overarching as they benefit apparently healthy people with unknown or low risk factors for heart disease besides those with known CVRFs at intermediate or high risk for heart disease.

■ REFERENCES

1. Hong KN, Fuster V, Rosenson RS, Rosendorff C, Bhatt DL. How low to go with glucose, cholesterol, and blood pressure in primary prevention of CVD. J Am Coll Cardiol. 2017;70(17):2171-85.
2. D'Ascenzi F, Sciaccaluga C, Cameli M, Cecere A, Ciccone MM, Di Francesco S, et al. When should cardiovascular prevention begin? The importance of antenatal, perinatal and primordial prevention. Eur J Prev Cardiol. 2021;28(4):361-9.
3. Chiou A, Hermel M, Chai Z, Eiseman A, Jeschke S, Mehta S, et al. Going from primary to primordial prevention: is the juice worth the squeeze? Curr Cardiol Rep. 2024;26(10):1135-43.
4. CADI Research Foundation USA. [online] Available from https://cadiresearch.org/ [Last accessed May 2025].
5. Uusitalo U, Feskens EJ, Tuomilehto J, Dowse G, Haw U, Fareed D, et al. Fall in total cholesterol concentration over five years in association with changes in fatty acid composition of cooking oil in Mauritius: cross sectional survey. BMJ. 1996;313(7064):1044-6.
6. Zatonski WA, Willett W. Changes in dietary fat and declining coronary heart disease in Poland: population based study. BMJ. 2005;331(7510):187-8.
7. Norum KR, Johansson L, Botten G, Bjørneboe GE, Oshaug A. Nutrition and food policy in Norway: effects on reduction of coronary heart disease. Nutr Rev. 1997;55(11 Pt 2):S32-9.
8. Jousilahti P, Laatikainen T, Peltonen M, Borodulin K, Männistö S, Jula A, et al. Primary prevention and risk factor reduction in coronary heart disease mortality among working aged men and women in eastern Finland over 40 years: population based observational study. BMJ. 2016;352:i721.
9. Arnett DK, Blumenthal RS, Albert MA, Buroker AB, Goldberger ZD, Hahn EJ, et al. 2019 ACC/AHA Guideline on the Primary Prevention of Cardiovascular Disease: Executive Summary: A Report of the American College of Cardiology/American Heart Association Task Force on Clinical Practice Guidelines. J Am Coll Cardiol. 2019;74(10):1376-414.
10. Young F, Capewell S, Ford ES, Critchley JA. Coronary mortality declines in the U.S. between 1980 and 2000 quantifying the contributions from primary and secondary prevention. Am J Prev Med. 2010;39(3):228-34.
11. Cooney MT, Dudina A, D'Agostino R, Graham IM. Cardiovascular risk-estimation systems in primary prevention: do they differ? Do they make a difference? Can we

see the future? Circulation. 2010;122(3): 300-10.
12. Kannel WB, Dawber TR, Kagan A, Revotskie N, Stokes J, 3rd. Factors of risk in the development of coronary heart disease—six year follow-up experience. The Framingham Study. Ann Intern Med. 1961;55:33-50.
13. Kannel WB. The Framingham Study: historical insight on the impact of cardiovascular risk factors in men versus women. J Gend Specif Med. 2002;5(2):27-37.
14. Kannel WB. Fifty years of Framingham Study contributions to understanding hypertension. J Hum Hypertens. 2000;14(2):83-90.
15. Ford ES, Ajani UA, Croft JB, Critchley JA, Labarthe DR, Kottke TE, et al. Explaining the decrease in U.S. deaths from coronary disease, 1980-2000. N Engl J Med. 2007; 356(23):2388-98.
16. Ma J, Ward EM, Siegel RL, Jemal A. Temporal Trends in Mortality in the United States, 1969-2013. JAMA. 2015;314(16):1731-9.
17. Dalen JE, Alpert JS, Goldberg RJ, Weinstein RS. The epidemic of the 20(th) century: coronary heart disease. Am J Med. 2014; 127(9):807-12.
18. Mensah GA, Wei GS, Sorlie PD, Fine LJ, Rosenberg Y, Kaufmann PG, et al. Decline in cardiovascular mortality: possible causes and implications. Circ Res. 2017; 120(2):366-80.
19. Mannsverk J, Wilsgaard T, Mathiesen EB, Løchen ML, Rasmussen K, Thelle DS, et al. Trends in modifiable risk factors are associated with declining incidence of hospitalized and nonhospitalized acute coronary heart disease in a population. Circulation. 2016;133(1):74-81.
20. Björck L, Rosengren A, Bennett K, Lappas G, Capewell S. Modelling the decreasing coronary heart disease mortality in Sweden between 1986 and 2002. Eur Heart J. 2009; 30(9):1046-56.
21. Vartiainen E, Laatikainen T, Peltonen M, Juolevi A, Männistö S, Sundvall J, et al. Thirty-five-year trends in cardiovascular risk factors in Finland. Int J Epidemiol. 2010;39(2):504-18.
22. Puska P, Jaini P. The North Karelia Project: Prevention of Cardiovascular Disease in Finland Through Population-Based Lifestyle Interventions. Am J Lifestyle Med. 2020;14(5):495-499.
23. Salomaa V, Ketonen M, Koukkunen H, Immonen-Räihä P, Jerkkola T, Kärjä-Koskenkari P, et al. Decline in out-of-hospital coronary heart disease deaths has contributed the main part to the overall decline in coronary heart disease mortality rates among persons 35 to 64 years of age in Finland: the FINAMI study. Circulation. 2003;108(6):691-6.
24. Salomaa V, Pietila A, Peltonen M, Kuulasmaa K. Changes in CVD Incidence and Mortality Rates, and Life Expectancy: North Karelia and the Nationl. Glob Heart. 2016;11(2): 201-5.
25. Wang CR, Meng XF, Wang CP, Liu SW. [Trends of burden on ischemic heart disease and epidemiological transition of related risk factors in China, 1990-2017]. Zhonghua Liu Xing Bing Xue Za Zhi. 2020;41(10):1703-9.
26. Chen Z, Peto R, Collins R, MacMahon S, Lu J, Li W. Serum cholesterol concentration and coronary heart disease in populations with low cholesterol concentrations. BMJ. 1991;303:276-82.
27. Critchley J, Liu J, Zhao D, Wei W, Capewell S. Explaining the increase in coronary heart disease mortality in Beijing between 1984 and 1999. Circulation. 2004;110(10):1236-44.
28. Wu Y, Benjamin EJ, MacMahon S. Prevention and Control of Cardiovascular Disease in the Rapidly Changing Economy of China. Circulation. 2016;133(24):2545-60.
29. Gupta R, Khedar RS, Gaur K, Xavier D. Low quality cardiovascular care is an important coronary risk factor in India. Indian Heart J. 2018;70(Suppl 3):S419-S430.
30. Sarma PS, Sadanandan R, Thulaseedharan JV, Soman B, Srinivasan K, Varma RP, et al. Prevalence of risk factors of non-communicable diseases in Kerala, India: results of a cross-sectional study. BMJ Open. 2019;9(11):e027880.
31. Suliankatchi Abdulkader R, Sinha DN, Jeyashree K, Rath R, Gupta PC, Kannan S,

et al. Trends in tobacco consumption in India 1987-2016: impact of the World Health Organization Framework Convention on Tobacco Control. Int J Public Health. 2019; 64(6):841-51.
32. Mishra S, Joseph RA, Gupta PC, Pezzack B, Ram F, Sinha DN, et al. Trends in bidi and cigarette smoking in India from 1998 to 2015, by age, gender and education. BMJ Glob Health. 2016;1(1):e000005.
33. Nudy M, Cooper J, Ghahramani M, Ruzieh M, Mandrola J, Foy AJ. Aspirin for primary atherosclerotic cardiovascular disease prevention as baseline risk increases: a meta-regression analysis. Am J Med. 2020; 133(9):1056-64.
34. Guirguis-Blake JM, Evans CV, Perdue LA, Bean SI, Senger CA. Aspirin use to prevent cardiovascular disease and colorectal cancer: updated evidence report and systematic review for the US preventive services task force. JAMA. 2022;327(16): 1585-97.
35. Shah R, Khan B, Latham SB, Khan SA, Rao SV. A meta-analysis of aspirin for the primary prevention of cardiovascular diseases in the context of contemporary preventive strategies. Am J Med. 2019;132(11): 1295-304.e3.
36. Brett AS. Should patients take aspirin for primary cardiovascular prevention?: Updated recommendations from the US preventive services task force. JAMA. 2022; 327(16):1552-4.
37. Enas EA, Kuruvila A, Khanna P, Pitchumoni CS, Mohan V. Benefits & risks of statin therapy for primary prevention of cardiovascular disease in Asian Indians—a population with the highest risk of premature coronary artery disease & diabetes. Indian J Med Res. 2013;138(4):461-91.
38. Taylor F, Huffman MD, Macedo AF, Moore TH, Burke M, Davey Smith G, et al. Statins for the primary prevention of cardiovascular disease. Cochrane Database Syst Rev. 2013; (1):CD004816.
39. Khan SU, Lone AN, Kleiman NS, Arshad A, Jain V, Al Rifai M, et al. Aspirin with or without statin in individuals without atherosclerotic cardiovascular disease across risk categories. JAAC Adv. 2023;2(2): 100197.
40. Shufelt CL, Mora S, Manson JE. Aspirin for the primary prevention of atherosclerotic cardiovascular disease in women. JAMA. 2022;328(7):672-3.
41. Joseph P, Roshandel G, Gao P, Pais P, Lonn E, Xavier D, et al.; Polypill Trialists' Collaboration. Fixed-dose combination therapies with and without aspirin for primary prevention of cardiovascular disease: an individual participant data meta-analysis. Lancet. 2021;398(10306):1133-46.
42. Kandil OA, Motawea KR, Aboelenein MM, Shah J. Polypills for primary prevention of cardiovascular disease: a systematic review and meta-analysis. Front Cardiovasc Med. 2022;9:880054.
43. Rao S, Jamal Siddiqi T, Khan MS, Michos ED, Navar AM, Wang TJ, et al. Association of polypill therapy with cardiovascular outcomes, mortality, and adherence: a systematic review and meta-analysis of randomized controlled trials. Prog Cardiovasc Dis. 2022;73:48-55.
44. Bahiru E, de Cates AN, Farr MR, Jarvis MC, Palla M, Rees K, Ebrahim S, et al. Fixed-dose combination therapy for the prevention of atherosclerotic cardiovascular diseases. Cochrane Database Syst Rev. 2017;3:CD009868.
45. Rose G. Strategy of prevention: lessons from cardiovascular disease. Br Med J (Clin Res Ed). 1981;282(6279):1847-51.
46. Raza SA, Salemi JL, Zoorob RJ. Historical perspectives on prevention paradox: When the population moves as a whole. J Family Med Prim Care. 2018;7(6):1163-5.

Prime Importance of a Healthy Diet

CHAPTER 16

■ INTRODUCTION

What types of food should I eat? What should I reduce, modify, or avoid? These questions are often asked by people who have heart disease and by those who want to prevent it. In the past, these direct and seemingly easy questions seldom received a direct and actionable answer from their doctors for several reasons: Nutrition was not taught in medical schools, knowledge was limited, and importantly there was no evidence-based information. This is no longer the case as well-done studies have shown consistent patterns of diet that can reduce the risk of cardiovascular disease (CVD) and must be an integral part of management in those with CVD.[1-3] Best known among the healthy diets are the Mediterranean diet that reduces the risk of CVDs and major adverse cardiovascular events (MACE)[4] and the more recent diet that emanated from the Prospective Urban Rural Epidemiology (PURE) study.[5]

Though the importance of a healthy diet in preventing cardiometabolic diseases and the components of such a diet are now known, the dietary pattern of South Asians has not substantially changed. The MASALA study, a prospective study of South Asians in the US, identified three key dietary patterns:[6] (1) Animal protein-rich diet associated with higher body mass index (BMI), total cholesterol, and low-density lipoprotein (LDL) cholesterol that may be linked to frequent eating out in fast food places and restaurants; (2) unhealthy high-fat vegetarian diet of fried snacks, sweets, and high-fat dairy, rich in saturated fat acid (SAFA) and refined carbohydrate, which leads to increased insulin resistance and lower high-density lipoprotein cholesterol (HDL-C); and (3) low-fat vegetarian with ample fruits, vegetables, nuts, and legumes associated with a favorable metabolic profile and reduced hypertension risk. As each of these three patterns has a fairly similar number of adherents it follows that the majority of South Asians eat an unhealthy diet. Simple steps of modifying the first two patterns by reducing SAFA and refined carbohydrates in diet would pay rich dividends to improve cardiometabolic health and therefore health education, dietary information, and support for promoting healthy eating habits are needed.[6]

■ HEALTHY DIET: COMPONENTS AND BENEFITS

A healthy diet is one with macronutrients (carbohydrates, proteins, fat) in appropriate proportions and quantity, and trace amounts of micronutrients (vitamins, minerals) and adequate hydration that meets the physiological needs of the body. Carbohydrates from grains, fruits, and legumes are the primary source of energy. Whole grains are better than processed ones that have been stripped of germ and bran the sources of fiber and micronutrients as prospective cohort studies have shown its benefit in reducing the risk of CVD and deaths from CVD.[7] Fresh fruits and vegetables are rich in fiber and phytochemicals (polyphenols, phytosterols, carotenoids) and decrease the risk of CVD.[5] Proteins from animal source (meat, dairy, fish, and eggs) and plant source (legumes, soya products, grains, nuts, and seeds) provide energy and amino acids (importantly essential amino acids). Proteins sourced from animals are rich in amino acids but contain saturated fatty acids linked to CVD (more later in this chapter). Adequate dietary protein intake is needed to maintain lean body mass throughout the lifespan and is particularly important in older adults.[8]

Fats (lipids) are essential for the structural integrity of cell membranes and also provide cellular energy. Among the four types of dietary fat, the "good fats", unsaturated fats—found in fish, many but not all plant-derived oils, nuts, and seeds are associated with reduced CVD risk and mortality and polyunsaturated fatty acids, particularly omega-3 and omega-6, likely protect the cardiovascular system.[9-11] In contrast, the "bad fats", SAFAs and trans fat acids (TFAs), increase CVD risk. A large prospective dietary fat study with over 24 years of follow-up (8 million person-years) showed that replacement of 5% energy from animal fat (red meat, dairy fat, egg) with 5% energy from plant fat, particularly from grains or vegetable oils, was associated with a 4–24% reduction in overall mortality and 5–30% reduction in cardiovascular mortality.[8]

The health benefits of the Mediterranean diet for noncommunicable diseases in general and CVDs in particular have been shown in several research studies.[12-14] The Mediterranean eating pattern prioritizes a variety of fruits and vegetables, whole grains, legumes, healthy fats from olive oil, nuts, seeds, and fatty fish and low amounts of dairy and red meat.[15] This pattern is mostly similar to the results of other major studies that followed.

The Prospective Urban Rural Epidemiology (PURE) Study

Most notable is the massive PURE study of individuals, 35–70 years of age, from the general population in 21 low-, middle-, and high-income countries in five continents between 2003 and 2018. From the analysis of the complete dietary information and outcome events in 147,642 participants a healthy diet score (PURE diet score) was developed.[5]

Besides the sheer and breadth of this study, its results are of added importance to people of low- and middle-income countries (LMICs) and in particular to Indians. The mean PURE healthy diet score was 2.95 (SD 1.50). A higher healthy diet score was associated with higher per capita gross national income (P trend <0.0001) **(Fig. 1)**.

The highest median diet scores and intake of food components in the diet score were found in North America and Europe, Middle East, and South America; while South Asia, China, Southeast Asia, and Africa had lower scores and intake of their component foods as shown in **Figure 2**. The higher diet scores were associated with lower risks of CVD, heart attack, and death. A diet with higher amounts of fruit, vegetables, nuts, legumes, fish, and whole-fat dairy was associated with lower CVD and mortality in all world regions.

How can we translate the healthy PURE diet of six healthy groups of food to the kitchen table of each household? **Table 1** breaks it down to a user-friendly format.

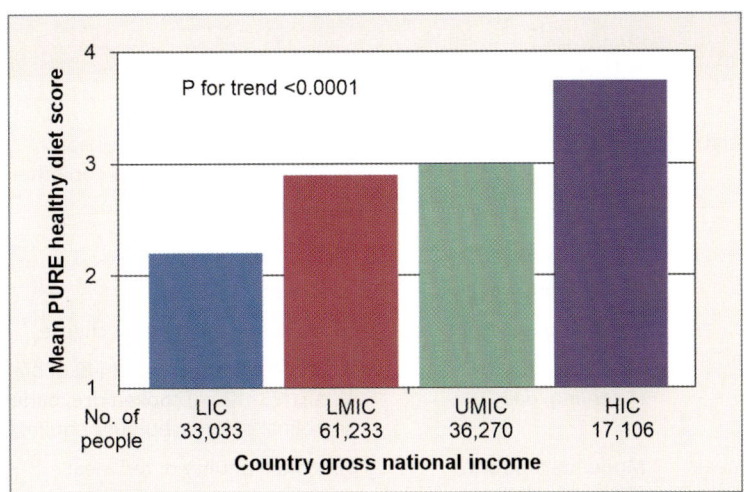

Fig. 1: Mean PURE (Prospective Urban Rural Epidemiology) healthy diet score increase relates to gross national income.[5] (HIC: high-income countries; LIC: low-income countries; LMIC: low- and middle-income countries; UMIC: upper middle-income countries)

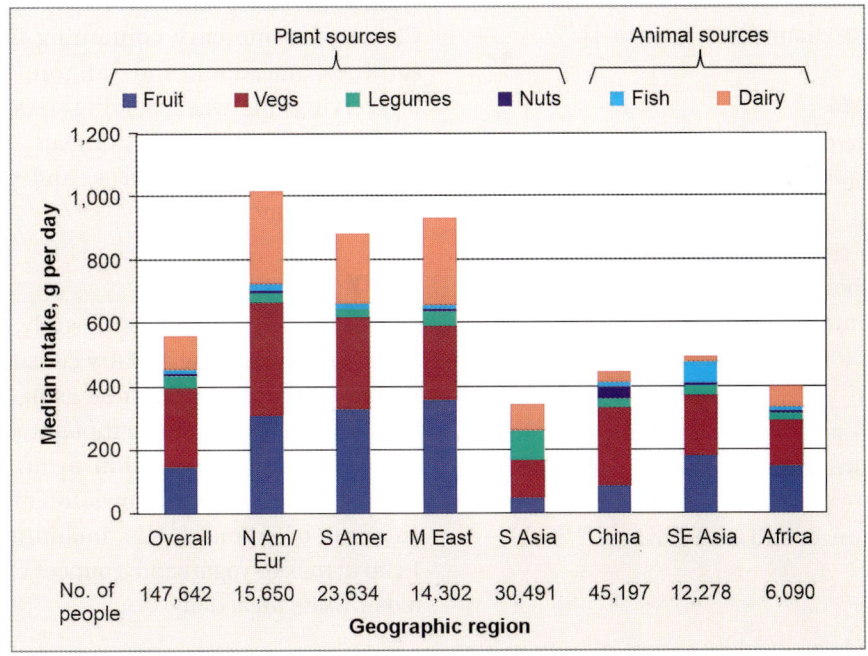

Fig. 2: PURE diet median score variations in different regions/countries of the world.[5]

Fruits and Vegetables

Besides their known benefits in increasing bulk through fiber and providing vitamins and minerals, polyphenols in fruits and vegetables are shown to improve inflammatory biomarkers related to atherosclerosis [i.e., interleukin 6 (IL)-6, tumor necrosis factor-alpha, soluble intercellular adhesion molecule-1,

TABLE 1: The PURE (Prospective Urban Rural Epidemiology) study healthy diet score translated into a healthy eating pattern.

Eat more	Amount	What counts as a serving
Fruits and vegetables	4–5 servings daily	• 1 medium apple, banana, pear • 1 cup leafy vegetables; ½ cup other vegetables
Legumes	3–4 servings daily	½ cup beans or lentils
Nuts	7 servings weekly	1 oz tree nuts or peanuts
Fish	2–3 servings weekly	3 oz cooked
Dairy	14 servings weekly	1 cup milk or yogurt, 1½ oz cheese
Whole grains	Moderate amount (1 serving) daily	• 1 slice (40 g) bread, ½ flat (40 g) bread • ½ cup (75–120 g) cooked rice, barley, buckwheat, semolina, polenta, bulgur or quinoa
Unprocessed meats	Moderate amount (1 serving) daily	3 oz cooked poultry or red meat

Source: Adapted from Mente et al.[5]

vascular cell adhesion molecule-1, and monocyte chemotactic protein-1].[16]

Legumes

Legumes (beans, lentils, peas) are packed with protein and fiber, they keep you feeling full and aid weight management. They are also rich in vitamins and minerals and besides being heart-healthy they aid in blood sugar control.[17,18]

Nuts

Nuts and seeds are healthy sources for protein, fiber, nutrients, and healthy fats **(Table 2)**. These are good as snacks and in salads and satisfy hunger and food cravings.[18,19]

Fish

Fish is a heart-healthy source of protein and provides omega-3 fatty acids that combat inflammation and helps to keep blood vessels from hardening. Baking or grilling (rather than frying) unlocks the full potential of the nutrients. Studies show incorporating fish into a diet can reduce heart disease death risk (36%) and overall mortality (17%).[20,21] Choose low-mercury containing fish, like sardines, mackerel, and salmon, aim for 2-3 servings per week. Serving sizes vary by age: Adults and teens 3-4 ounces, children 8-11 years of age 3 ounces, and younger children 2 ounces.[21,22]

Dairy

Recent studies, like the PURE study, suggest a more nuanced view of dairy consumption. Whole-fat dairy might not be as harmful to heart health as previously thought and may even offer some protection against CVD. The PURE diet score allows for moderate amounts of animal foods, including up to 1 cup of milk or yogurt and 3 ounces of cooked red or white meat daily.[4,23]

Whole Grains

Embrace whole grains and ditch refined grains. Not all carbohydrates are equal. Refined (processed) carbohydrates found in white bread, pastries, and sugary drinks are to be avoided as they spike blood sugar,

TABLE 2: Composition of monounsaturated fat acid (MUFA) polyunsaturated fat acid (PUFA), and saturated and fats (SAFA) in 100 grams (g) of commonly used nuts.

Type of nuts	Calories	Total fat (g)	MUFA (g)	PUFA (g)	SAFA (g)
Pecan	710	74	44	21	6
Almond	597	53	34	13	4
Cashew	574	46	27	8	9
Pistachio	567	44	25	13	6
Flaxseed	492	34	7	22	5
Peanut	630	50	25	18	7
Walnut	618	59	15	35	3

Source: Enas et al.[10]

contribute to weight gain, and increase heart disease risk. Instead, choose complex carbohydrates found in whole grains—brown rice, quinoa, oats, and whole-wheat options. They provide sustained energy, fiber, and essential nutrients. Additionally, as they are rich in fiber, they keep you feeling fuller for a longer time, and deter overeating. While some traditionally consume 200–250 g of carbohydrates daily, 130–150 g of whole grains is a more heart-healthy quantity.[24-26]

Unprocessed Meats

Lean meats in moderate quantities offer proteins (along with essential amino acids), monounsaturated fat acid (MUFA) and nutrients that are healthy. Choose cuts of meat labeled "choice" or "lean" that have lower SAFA. For example, a 3-ounce serving of trimmed loin steak has around 6–7 g of total fat, with only 2–3 g SAFA.[10,22]

In contrast, processed meats are treated through processes like smoking, salting, curing, drying, or canning and some common examples of these are salami, pepperoni, hot dogs, corned beef, jerky, ham, bacon, and sausages. These are staples of fast food restaurants, delis, and convenience stores that cater to our fast-paced life. Consumption of these meats should at best be avoided or at least minimized. Be wary of ground beef in fast food (hamburgers, tacos) often high in SAFA. Regular ground meat (80% lean/20% fat) can contain a concerning 6 g of SAFA fat per 3 ounces. A typical taco with ground beef, cheese, lettuce, and a hard shell can contain around 8–18 g of total fat and 3–6 g of SAFA depending on the leanness of the ground beef and the amount of cheese used.[22]

Thus, while the plant kingdom offers a bounty of heart-healthy options, incorporating some animal-based foods can be beneficial as well. Fish rich in omega-3 fatty acids, lean meats with moderate fat content, low-fat dairy products, and eggs can all contribute to a balanced diet. To maximize benefits combine them with avocados, nuts, and olive oil (rich in MUFA) to create a heart-healthy diet.

UNDERSTANDING FATS FOR A HEALTHY HEART

As depicted in **Flowchart 1**, dietary fats fall into four categories: Two of them trans fat (TFA) and saturated fats (SAFA)—are unhealthy and the other two fats [MUFA and polyunsaturated (PUFA)] are healthy. The fat content of food is generally an admixture

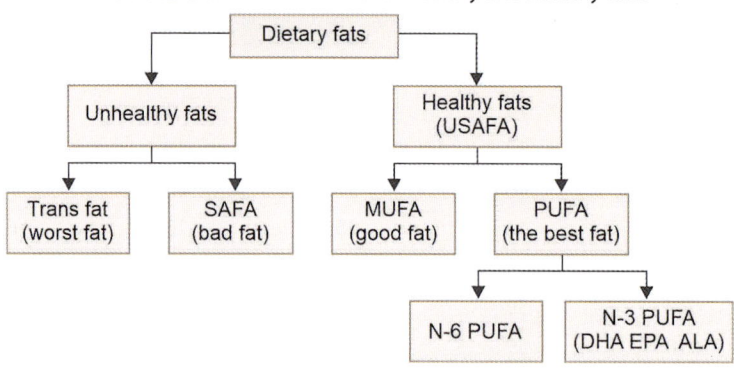

Flowchart 1: Classification of unhealthy and healthy fats.

(ALA: alpha-linolenic acid; DHA: docosahexaenoic acid; EPA: eicosapentaenoic acid; MUFA: monounsaturated fat acid; PUFA: polyunsaturated fat acid; SAFA: saturated fat; USAFA: unsaturated fats)

of these different types.[22] Unsaturated fats are found in a variety of foods, including fish, many plant-derived oils, nuts, and seeds. Avocado is a rich source of healthy unsaturated fats and may lower low-density lipoprotein-cholesterol (LDL-C) of particular benefit to those with high LDL-C.[27] Animal products (and some plant-derived oils) contribute a larger proportion of SAFAs.[28,29] TFAs found in foods are predominantly the result of processing vegetable oils but are also present in small quantities in animal products (i.e., ruminant TFAs from cows, sheep, and goats). Among the types of dietary fats, unsaturated fats are associated with reduced cardiovascular and mortality risks, whereas TFAs and SAFAs are associated with negative impacts on health, including increased mortality risk.[22]

Two families of polyunsaturated fatty acids, omega-3 and omega-6 are described as essential fatty acids, because they are required for normal growth and reproduction but are not produced by the body and, therefore, must be obtained from dietary sources.[30] Omega-3 fatty acids, in particular, eicosapentaenoic acid (EPA), and docosahexaenoic acid (DHA), have been widely studied for their potential health benefits, with evidence suggesting positive effects including cardioprotection, preventing cognitive decline, reducing inflammation, sustaining muscle mass, and improving systemic insulin resistance.[31] Seafood, especially oily fish, provides EPA and DHA, and supplements are widely available for those not meeting recommended intakes with diet alone.[32] Nuts and some seeds and plant oils provide alpha-linolenic acid, the major plant omega-3 fatty acid.[33]

Monounsaturated Fats

MUFAs can lower bad cholesterol and increase good cholesterol, while PUFAs can also lower bad cholesterol and potentially reduce heart disease risk.[22] Studies show that replacement of 5% of energy from SAFA with unsaturated fatty acids lowers LDL-C by 5–10% and CVD risk by 25%.[34] Two major sources of healthy fats (MUFAs, PUFAs) are nuts **(Table 2)** and cooking oils **(Table 3)**.[10]

Cooking Oils

As shown in **Table 3**, olive oil and almond oil have the highest MUFAs, sunflower oil and safflower oil have the highest PUFAs, and canola oil has the healthiest profile of fats (93% unsaturated fats) and has omega-3 also.[10,35] Note these aforementioned

TABLE 3: Monounsaturated fat acid (MUFA), polyunsaturated fat acid (PUFA), and saturated fat acid (SAFA) in grams (g) per 100 g of cooking oil.

Type of oil	MUFA (g)	PUFA (g)	SAFA (g)
Olive oil	74	8	14
Almond oil	70	17	8
Mustard oil	59	21	12
Canola	59	30	7
Peanut oil	46	32	17
Sesame oil	40	42	14
Palm oil	37	9	49
Palm kernel oil	11	2	82
Coconut oil	6	2	92
Corn oil	24	59	13
Sunflower oil	19	69	12
Safflower oil	13	78	9
Soybean oil	23	58	14

Source: Adapted from Enas et al.[10]

TABLE 4: Major dietary sources of saturated fats.[1,3,10,22,36]

Category	Examples
Tropical oils	Coconut and palm oil; liberal amounts of grated coconut, coconut milk, and coconut cream are used extensively for vegetable dishes (e.g., Thoran) and staples like Palappam, Kallappam, Vattayappam, etc.
Full-fat dairy products	Butter, ghee, paneer, cheese, curd, ice cream, milk shakes, etc.
Desserts and commercial dairy products	Cake, pie, biscuits, cookies, donuts, halwas, ladu, gulab jamun, breakfast pastries, etc.
Red meat	Fatty cuts of beef, lamb, pork, bacon, sausage, ribs, taco, poultry with skin
Fast foods	Kentucky Fried Chicken, McDonalds, Pizza, etc.
Chips fried in tropical oils	Banana fries, potato chips, etc.

beneficial oils have not only high unsaturated fats but also have low SAFA. On the other end of the spectrum the worst oils are coconut oil, cocoa butter, and palm oil with very high SAFAs. Despite their plant-based origin some of the tropical oils have a high content of SAFA as shown in **Tables 3 and 4**.

MAJOR DIETARY SOURCES OF SATURATED FATS

The harmful effect of SAFAs in diet through dyslipidemia was discussed in Chapter 3 on the risk factors for heart disease and showed the substantial benefit of substituting PUFAs for SAFAs. For children over 2 years of age with high cholesterol, limiting SAFA intake to <7% of total daily calories which amounts to around 12–15 g/day is crucial.[1,37,38] Limiting SAFAs in diet is important for Indians because of their propensity for heart attacks at lower LDL-C levels than Whites.[39]

Coconut Oil

Coconut oil, a flavorful oil, gained prominence a decade ago in haute cuisine in the US and other western countries as a finishing oil and the fad has largely ebbed. But in coconut-producing countries in Asia, Africa, and South America this oil is popular for consumption and export. India produces over 14 million metric tons of coconuts per year, and it is not only a source of food but is also a source of livelihood for millions of its people. Nowhere is coconut more popular than in Kerala, the southernmost state in India, where the name, Keralam, is derived from "land of the coconut trees". All parts of a coconut tree are put to use in various forms (e.g., thatching, cooking fuel, toddy, coir manufacturing, hair oils). Coconuts in one form or another or in combination—coconut oil, coconut milk, and coconut flesh (grated, sliced, diced)—are staples of the daily diet of a Keralite. It is therefore understandable that Keralites, fiercely loyal to coconuts, may not readily accept any negative remarks on coconut oil. However, the bond we have with the coconut tree that symbolizes our native state and its products would not deter us from presenting the facts here as well as on a controversy that continues to linger.[11]

Facts

Coconut oil contains 92% SAFA and a portion size of 100 g contains 82.5 g of SAFA. The major fatty acids in coconut oil are lauric acid (32–51%), myristic acid (17–21%), and palmitic acid (6.9–14%). The American Heart Association (AHA) Presidential Advisory Report suggests the replacement of 5% of energy intake derived from SAFAs with PUFAs or MUFAs to lower the incidence or risk of coronary artery disease (CAD) by 25 and 15%, respectively, according to a recent presidential advisory from the AHA.[3,40] Multiple studies over the past decades have shown the cholesterol-raising effect of coconut oil on the cardiovascular system starting with the very early study by Ahrens and colleagues.[41,42] **Figure 3** depicts the drop in cholesterol on a corn oil diet and rise on a coconut oil diet in the same patient.

In 2010, Waqar et al.[43] demonstrated that rabbits fed a high-fat diet of 10% coconut oil had anatomic evidence of increased atherosclerosis. A comprehensive review in 2016 by Eyres et al.[44] of 8 clinical trials and 13 observational studies, concluded that coconut oil raised cholesterol (and LDL-C) compared to other plant oils. Two recent systematic reviews found that coconut oil consumption significantly increased LDL-C level and also HDL-C level.[45,46]

Controversy

While there is total agreement on the SAFA content of coconut oil and its constituents, there are differing views on the individual constituents and their cardiovascular effects. Specifically, the focus is on lauric acid, the main constituent that has 12 carbon atoms—upper range for a medium-chain fatty acid (MCFA)—compared to capric acid and caprylic acid with 8 and 10 carbon atoms. MCFAs are healthier than long-chain fatty acids (12–18 carbon atoms) and do not affect total cholesterol and LDL-C but cause a small increase in triglycerides. Though lauric acid is often classified as an MCFA, the fact is with 12 carbon atoms it straddles both MCFA and long-chain fatty acids. The other constituents

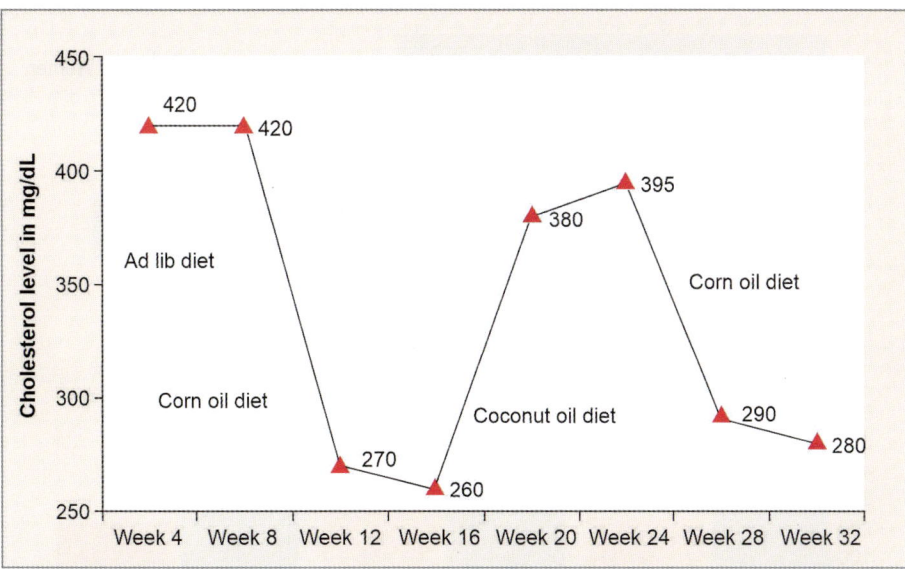

Fig. 3: Decrease in total cholesterol on a 40% corn oil diet and increase in cholesterol on a 40% coconut oil diet at 8-week intervals.
Source: Adapted from Ahrens et al.[41]

of coconut oil are long-chain fatty acids, myristic and palmitic with 14 and 16 carbon atoms respectively.[47]

CHOLESTEROL LEVELS AND CARDIOVASCULAR MORTALITY IN KERALA

The abundant use of coconut products practically in every meal is in all likelihood a factor in the higher cholesterol levels (>200 mg/dL) of Keralites in comparison to the rest of India (52% vs. 25%).[48] A personal observation—Just one Palappam, a popular breakfast item—contains 2.1 grams of SFA.[49]

As shown in the figure the age-standardized cardiovascular mortality rates In India are strikingly different than in the US (325 vs. 190 in men and 225 vs. 140 in women) **(Fig. 4)**. Of particular note is the difference in cardiovascular mortality within India: Mumbai city and Kerala more than Andhra Pradesh. Mortality rate in Kerala is markedly higher than in the US and India (with the exception of Mumbai city). One of the important steps to improve heart health in Kerala is to change dietary habits to incorporate MUFAs and PUFAs found in various plants and marine sources in the diet. This step of replacing SAFAs with healthy fats lowers LDL-C by upregulating LDL receptors and improving LDL-C clearance from the bloodstream.[37,51-53] An informed public, patients with heart disease and healthcare providers should work together to reduce and replace SAFA-rich coconut dishes with healthier alternatives rich in MUFAs and PUFAs (refer to **Table 3** for options).

INDIAN DIET

The PURE study investigators emphasized the need to increase consumption of natural foods including whole-fat dairy, fruits, vegetables, nuts, legumes, and fish in countries with lower gross national income (where

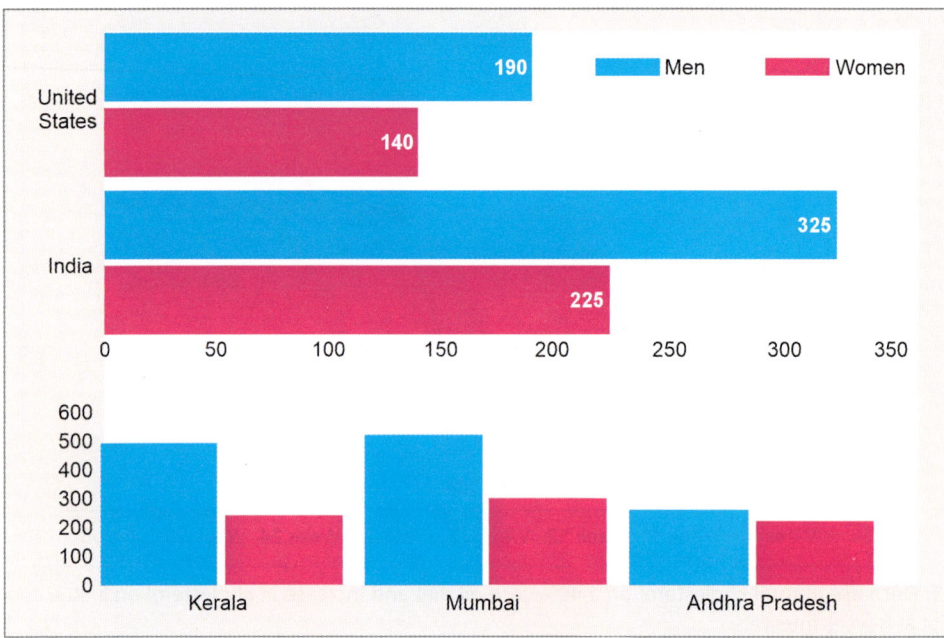

Fig. 4: Comparison of age-standardized cardiovascular mortality per 100,000 in the US and India for men and women are shown in the horizontal bars on top. Below in the vertical bars is a comparison of age-standardized cardiovascular mortality in Kerala, Mumbai, and Andhra Pradesh.
Source: Adapted from Prabhakaran et al.[50]

these food intakes are low due to cultural and economic factors) to improve heart health and reduce CVD and deaths. In spite of regional variations in diet and cooking patterns in India some common conclusions can be made based on the PURE study (30,491 participants from South Asia). The mean PURE diet score, an indicator of a healthy diet, was the lowest, 2.1 in South Asia compared to 3.1 in China and 6.7 in North America/Europe.[5] Meat consumption is low and vegetarianism is high in India and the diet is deficient in healthy foods—very low fruits and nuts, low in vegetables as shown in **Figure 2**. Vegetarians in India are mostly lacto-vegetarians and unlike their western counterparts do not get their protein and nutrients from fish. Indians also have an affinity for sweet treats (picture of a sampler plate shown in **Figure 5**).

Hydrogenated vegetable oil, such as margarine and Crisco, was produced as a substitute for animal and saturated fats. However, the process of hydrogenation as well as deep frying produces large amounts of TFAs that are more harmful than SFAs. TFAs increase LDL-C more than SFAs and increase the risk of heart disease.[54] Estimated to cause up to 500,000 deaths per year globally,[22,55] TFAs are banned in the US and several other countries have curtailed the consumption of TFAs. Earlier studies in India showed TFA consumption as high as 40% of total fat energy intake.[56] Vanaspati, a popular plant-based ghee substitute, in India harbors a large amount (~40%) of TFA. Generous use of ghee (shelf-stable clarified butter), refined flours, and fried snacks can elevate unhealthy fats and carbohydrates, leading to a phenomenon called "contaminated

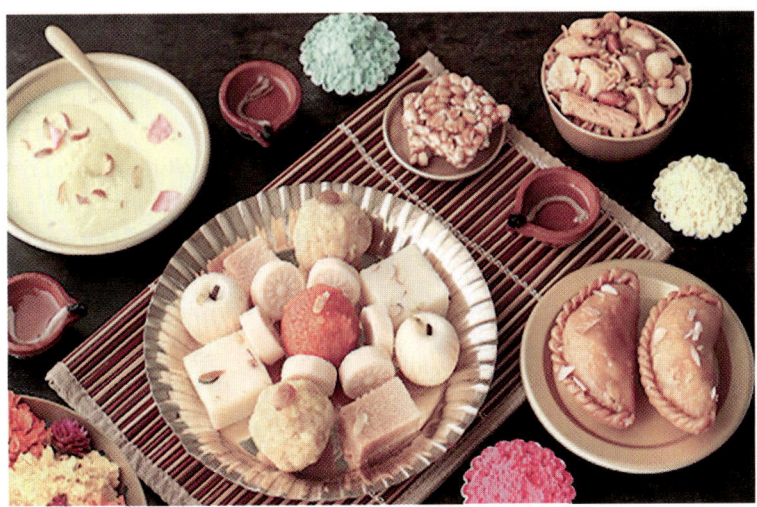

Fig. 5: Indian sweets are loaded with unhealthy fats and refined carbohydrates.

vegetarianism". The good news is that the Food Safety and Standards Authority of India (FSSAI) has aligned with the World Health Organization (WHO) to eliminate TFAs. India has passed legislation to lower consumption to 10% in 2013, 5% in 2015, and 2% in 2022.[55]

Two other accouterments deserve a few short comments: (1) Salt: 3–4 g of salt daily is acceptable for most adults.[57] Excessive salt intake can contribute to hypertension (Chapter 5), a major risk factor for heart disease and stroke. Make use of other healthy ingredients—fresh herbs, lemon juice, and vinegar to boost the flavor of food. (2) Alcohol, a part of celebrations at times, has no health benefits and can be harmful and binge drinking (four or more drinks) in particular should be avoided.

TABLE 5: Portfolio diet for lowering LDL-C and estimated reduction in LDL-C.[58-61]

Nutrition intervention	Daily dose	Reduction in LDL-C
Replacement of energy	5% of the TDC from SAFA to USAFA	Reduce LDL by 5–10%
Viscous fiber	7.5 g/day	6–9%
Plant sterols/stanols	2 g/day	5–8%
Plant protein	30 g/day	3–5%
Weight loss if excess adiposity is present	Loss of 5% of body weight	3–5%
	Total expected effect	22–37%

(LDL-C: low-density lipoprotein cholesterol; SAFA: saturated fat; TDC: total daily calories; USAFA: unsaturated fats)

DIETS THAT LOWER LOW-DENSITY LIPOPROTEIN-C AND TRIGLYCERIDES

Portfolio Diet

The portfolio diet is a dietary strategy designed to target and lower LDL-C levels. This diet combines several dietary components known to have cholesterol-lowering effects. A breakdown of its key aspects is given in **Table 5**.[58-61]

Oatmeal, beans, fruits, and vegetables and other fiber-rich foods act like tiny sponges trapping cholesterol and taking it out of the body.[22,37,62] Plant sterols and stanols lower LDL-C in youth unable to achieve their lipid-lowering goals with dietary modification alone.[38,63] Limited studies in those 5–16 years of age have demonstrated 6–15% lowering of LDL-C, and Apo B in individuals with familial combined hyperlipidemia.[37,64,65] The recommended dose for those aged 2 and above is 2 g/day, typically incorporated as a replacement for usual dietary fats.

Plant sterols and stanols are often available in fortified foods like margarines or come in capsule or chewable supplement form. Plant proteins (legumes, beans, nuts, seeds, whole grains) are a versatile option for vegetarians and flexitarians and are packed with fiber, vitamins, and minerals and are lower in SAFA than animal proteins. In addition to following the portfolio diet, one must refrain from fast foods and limit dietary cholesterol. Unlike SAFA, dietary cholesterol's effect on blood cholesterol levels is generally considered modest. Individual absorption rates of dietary cholesterol vary markedly, from 5 to 95%. While most people absorb around 20–25%, those with high cholesterol are often "high absorbers" and among these individuals it is advisable to limit daily dietary cholesterol to <200 mg.[22]

Hypertriglyceridemia

For those with very high triglycerides (above 500 mg/dL), a short-term, very-low-fat diet can be highly effective. This initial approach typically restricts dietary fat to <10% of daily calories. Long-term management strategies vary as some people may require a chronically low-fat diet (<20% of calories) to prevent triglyceride levels from rising again while others may be able to consume a moderate-fat intake (20–40% of calories) while maintaining healthy cholesterol levels.[66] Besides markedly reducing fat intake, limiting added sugars is highly important. This means limiting processed foods and sugary drinks to <10% of daily calories. While natural fruit sugars are not a primary concern, packaged or bottled fruit juice should be consumed in moderation due to its concentrated sugar content. This focus on limiting added sugars plays a vital role in preventing heart disease, stroke, and type 2 diabetes—all potential complications of very high triglycerides.

We conclude this chapter with three summary statements and a few key takeaways:

1. The marked rise in noncommunicable diseases (CVD is the prime one) has a causal link to global dietary patterns that are becoming increasingly westernized—characterized by high levels of fatty and processed meats, SAFAs, refined grains, salt, and sugars but lacking in fresh fruits and vegetables.
2. Inadequate consumption of key healthy foods is a very important factor for increased CVD risk and mortality around the world.
3. When calories from carbohydrates exceed about 60% of the caloric intake, the total mortality begins to rise, as do cardiovascular events.

■ KEY TAKEAWAYS

- The PURE healthy diet score from a study of the dietary patterns of >140,000 adults from 21 countries found that the mean score was 2.95 (South Asians had the lowest score and North Americans and Europeans had the highest). **Table 1** translates this into six groups and quantifies each of them for practical use. The Indian diet is deficient in intake of healthy groups, especially in fruits and vegetables, nuts and fish.

- The Indian diet also has a surplus of refined carbohydrates, sugars, and SAFA (mostly from plant sources) and TFAs (ghee substitutes) that increases risk factors for heart disease and other CVDs.
- Partial replacement of SAFAs with unsaturated fats (MUFAs and PUFAs) from sources like avocados, nuts, and healthy oils reduces LDL-C and CVD risk.
- Some plant-based diets (e.g., coconut oil and coconut products) carry an underappreciated risk as they share characteristics of SAFA and increase CVD risk as may be happening in Kerala.
- The portfolio diet: Combining a low-SAFA diet with unsaturated fats, fiber, soy protein, and nuts can effectively lower LDL-C by 30% for long-term heart health benefits.
- Very high triglyceride states require markedly restricted dietary fat and restricted sugars and refined carbohydrates.

REFERENCES

1. Lichtenstein AH, Appel LJ, Vadiveloo M, Hu FB, Kris-Etherton PM, Rebholz CM, et al. 2021 Dietary Guidance to Improve Cardiovascular Health: A Scientific Statement From the American Heart Association. Circulation. 2021;144(23):e472-e487.
2. Thorndike AN, Gardner CD, Kendrick KB, Seligman HK, Yaroch AL, Gomes AV, et al.; American Heart Association Advocacy Coordinating Committee. Strengthening US Food Policies and Programs to Promote Equity in Nutrition Security: A Policy Statement From the American Heart Association. Circulation. 2022;145(24):e1077-e1093.
3. Sacks FM, Lichtenstein AH, Wu JHY, Appel LJ, Creager MA, Kris-Etherton PM, et al.; American Heart Association. Dietary Fats and Cardiovascular Disease: A Presidential Advisory From the American Heart Association. Circulation. 2017;136(3):e1-e23.
4. Dehghan M, Mente A, Rangarajan S, Sheridan P, Mohan V, Iqbal R, et al.; Prospective Urban Rural Epidemiology (PURE) study investigators. Association of dairy intake with cardiovascular disease and mortality in 21 countries from five continents (PURE): a prospective cohort study. Lancet. 2018; 392(10161):2288-97.
5. Mente A, Dehghan M, Rangarajan S, O'Donnell M, Hu W, Dagenais G, et al. Diet, cardiovascular disease, and mortality in 80 countries. Eur Heart J. 2023;44(28):2560-79.
6. Gadgil MD, Anderson CA, Kandula NR, Kanaya AM. Dietary patterns are associated with metabolic risk factors in South Asians living in the United States. J Nutr. 2015; 145(6):1211-7.
7. Zong G, Gao A, Hu FB, Sun Q. Whole Grain Intake and Mortality From All Causes, Cardiovascular Disease, and Cancer: A Meta-Analysis of Prospective Cohort Studies. Circulation. 2016;133(24):2370-80.
8. Zhao B, Gan L, Graubard BI, Männistö S, Fang F, Weinstein SJ, et al. Plant and Animal Fat Intake and Overall and Cardiovascular Disease Mortality. JAMA Intern Med. 2024; 184(10):1234-45.
9. Enas EA, Dharmarajan TS. Dietary fats and cardiovascular disease: Current evidence and practical recommendations. In: Rao G (Ed). Clinical Handbook of Coronary Artery Disease. Bombay: Jaypee Brothers Medical Publishers; 2021.
10. Enas EA, Senthilkumar A, Chennikkara H, Bjurlin MA. Prudent diet and preventive nutrition from pediatrics to geriatrics: current knowledge and practical recommendations. Indian Heart J. 2003;55(4):310-38.
11. Enas EA. Cooking oil, cholesterol and coronary artery disease. Indian Heart J. 1996; 48:423-8.
12. Godos J, Guglielmetti M, Ferraris C, Frias-Toral E, Domínguez Azpíroz I, Lipari V, et al. Mediterranean Diet and Quality of Life in Adults: A Systematic Review. Nutrients. 2025; 17(3):577.
13. Naik RG, Purcell SA, Gold SL, Christiansen V, D'Aloisio LD, Raman M, et al. From Evidence to Practice: A Narrative Framework for Integrating the Mediterranean Diet into Inflammatory Bowel Disease Management. Nutrients. 2025;17(3):470.
14. Kontele I, Panagiotakos D, Yannakoulia M, Vassilakou T. Socio-Demographic Determinants of Mediterranean Diet Adherence:

Results of the EU-National Health Interview Survey (EHIS-3). J Hum Nutr Diet. 2025; 38(1):e70023.
15. Scaglione S, Di Chiara T, Daidone M, Tuttolomondo A. Effects of the Mediterranean Diet on the Components of Metabolic Syndrome Concerning the Cardiometabolic Risk. Nutrients. 2025;17(2):358.
16. Chiarioni G, Popa SL, Ismaiel A, Pop C, Dumitrascu DI, Brata VD, et al. The Effect of Polyphenols, Minerals, Fibers, and Fruits on Irritable Bowel Syndrome: A Systematic Review. Nutrients. 2023;15(18):4070.
17. Mendes V, Niforou A, Kasdagli MI, Ververis E, Naska A. Intake of legumes and cardiovascular disease: A systematic review and dose-response meta-analysis. Nutr Metab Cardiovasc Dis. 2023;33(1):22-37.
18. Jin S, Je Y. Nuts and legumes consumption and risk of colorectal cancer: a systematic review and meta-analysis. Eur J Epidemiol. 2022;37(6):569-85.
19. Afshin A, Micha R, Khatibzadeh S, Mozaffarian D. Consumption of nuts and legumes and risk of incident ischemic heart disease, stroke, and diabetes: a systematic review and meta-analysis. Am J Clin Nutr. 2014;100(1):278-88.
20. Tong TYN, Appleby PN, Bradbury KE, Perez-Cornago A, Travis RC, Clarke R, et al. Risks of ischaemic heart disease and stroke in meat eaters, fish eaters, and vegetarians over 18 years of follow-up: results from the prospective EPIC-Oxford study. BMJ. 2019;366:l4897.
21. Mozaffarian D, Rimm EB. Fish intake, contaminants, and human health: evaluating the risks and the benefits. JAMA. 2006;296(15): 1885-99.
22. U.S. Department of Agriculture and U.S. Department of Health and Human Services. (2020). Dietary Guidelines for Americans 2020-2025. [online] Available from https://www.dietaryguidelines.gov [Last accessed June 9, 2025].
23. Ros E, Martinez-Gonzalez MA, Estruch R, et al. Mediterranean diet and cardiovascular health: Teachings of the PREDIMED study. Adv Nutr. 2014;5(3):330S-6S.
24. Ying T, Zheng J, Kan J, Li W, Xue K, Du J, et al. Effects of whole grains on glycemic control: a systematic review and dose-response meta-analysis of prospective cohort studies and randomized controlled trials. Nutr J. 2024;23(1):47.
25. Hu H, Zhao Y, Feng Y, Yang X, Li Y, Wu Y, et al. Consumption of whole grains and refined grains and associated risk of cardiovascular disease events and all-cause mortality: a systematic review and dose-response meta-analysis of prospective cohort studies. Am J Clin Nutr. 2023;117(1):149-59.
26. Ghanbari-Gohari F, Mousavi SM, Esmaillzadeh A. Consumption of whole grains and risk of type 2 diabetes: A comprehensive systematic review and dose-response meta-analysis of prospective cohort studies. Food Sci Nutr. 2022;10(6):1950-60.
27. James-Martin G, Brooker PG, Hendrie GA, Stonehouse W. Avocado Consumption and Cardiometabolic Health: A Systematic Review and Meta-Analysis. J Acad Nutr Diet. 2024;124(2):233-248.e4.
28. Mendis S, Samarajeewa U, Thattil RO. Coconut fat and serum lipoproteins: effects of partial replacement with unsaturated fats. Br J Nutr. 2001;85(5):583-9.
29. Mendis S, Kumarasunderam R. The effect of daily consumption of coconut fat and soya-bean fat on plasma lipids and lipoproteins of young normolipidaemic men. Br J Nutr. 1990;63(3):547-52.
30. Farvid MS, Ding M, Pan A, Sun Q, Chiuve SE, Steffen LM, et al. Dietary linoleic acid and risk of coronary heart disease: a systematic review and meta-analysis of prospective cohort studies. Circulation. 2014;130(18): 1568-78.
31. Manuelli M, Della Guardia L, Cena H. Enriching Diet with n-3 PUFAs to Help Prevent Cardiovascular Diseases in Healthy Adults: Results from Clinical Trials. Int J Mol Sci. 2017;18(7):1552.
32. Calder PC. Very long-chain n-3 fatty acids and human health: fact, fiction and the future. Proc Nutr Soc. 2018;77(1):52-72.
33. Baker EJ, Miles EA, Burdge GC, Yaqoob P, Calder PC. Metabolism and functional

effects of plant-derived omega-3 fatty acids in humans. Prog Lipid Res. 2016;64:30-56.

34. Li Y, Hruby A, Bernstein AM, Ley SH, Wang DD, Chiuve SE, et al. Saturated Fats Compared with Unsaturated Fats and Sources of Carbohydrates in Relation to Risk of Coronary Heart Disease: A Prospective Cohort Study. J Am Coll Cardiol. 2015; 66(14):1538-48.

35. Enas EA. Cooking oils, cholesterol and CAD: facts and myths. Indian Heart J. 1996; 48(4):423-7.

36. Sacks FM. Coconut Oil and Heart Health: Fact or Fiction? Circulation. 2020;141(10):815-7.

37. Williams L, Baker-Smith CM, Bolick J, Carter J, Kirkpatrick C, Ley SL, et al. Nutrition interventions for youth with dyslipidemia: a National Lipid Association clinical perspective. J Clin Lipidol. 2022;16(6):776-96.

38. Expert Panel on Integrated Guidelines for Cardiovascular Health, Risk Reduction in Children Adolescents; National Heart L, Blood Institute. Expert panel on integrated guidelines for cardiovascular health and risk reduction in children and adolescents: summary report. Pediatrics. 2011; 128(Suppl 5):S213-56.

39. Karthikeyan G, Teo KK, Islam S, et al. Lipid profile, plasma apolipoproteins, and risk of a first myocardial infarction among Asians: an analysis from the INTERHEART Study. J Am Coll Cardiol. 2009;53(3):244-53.

40. Writing Committee; Lloyd-Jones DM, Morris PB, Ballantyne CM, Birtcher KK, Covington AM, DePalma SM, et al. 2022 ACC Expert Consensus Decision Pathway on the Role of Nonstatin Therapies for LDL-Cholesterol Lowering in the Management of Atherosclerotic Cardiovascular Disease Risk: A Report of the American College of Cardiology Solution Set Oversight Committee. J Am Coll Cardiol. 2022;80(14):1366-418.

41. Ahrens EHJ, Insull W Jr, Blomstrand R, Hirsch J, Tsaltas TT, Peterson ML. The influence of dietary fats on serum-lipid levels in man. Lancet. 1957;272(6976):943-53.

42. Ahrens EH Jr, Blankenhorn DH, Tsaltas TT. Effect on human serum lipids of substituting plant for animal fat in diet. Proc Soc Exp Biol Med. 1954;86(4):872-8.

43. Waqar AB, Koike T, Yu Y, Inoue T, Aoki T, Liu E, et al. High-fat diet without excess calories induces metabolic disorders and enhances atherosclerosis in rabbits. Atherosclerosis. 2010;213(1):148-55.

44. Eyres L, Eyres MF, Chisholm A, Brown RC. Coconut oil consumption and cardiovascular risk factors in humans. Nutr Rev. 2016;74(4):267-80.

45. Neelakantan N, Seah JYH, van Dam RM. The Effect of Coconut Oil Consumption on Cardiovascular Risk Factors: A Systematic Review and Meta-Analysis of Clinical Trials. Circulation. 2020;141(10):803-14.

46. Teng M, Zhao YJ, Khoo AL, Yeo TC, Yong QW, Lim BP. Impact of coconut oil consumption on cardiovascular health: a systematic review and meta-analysis. Nutr Rev. 2020;78(3): 249-59.

47. Mensink RP. Effects of saturated fatty acids on serum lipids and lipoproteins: a systematic review and regression analysis. Geneva: World Health Organization; 2016.

48. Krishnamoorthy Y, Rajaa S, Murali S, Rehman T, Sahoo J, Kar SS. Prevalence of metabolic syndrome among adult population in India: A systematic review and meta-analysis. PLoS One. 2020;15(10):e0240971.

49. https://www.nutritionix.com/fr/food/palappam. [Last accessed June 9, 2025].

50. Prabhakaran D, Jeemon P, Roy A. Cardiovascular Diseases in India: Current Epidemiology and Future Directions. Circulation. 2016;133(16):1605-20.

51. Arnett DK, Blumenthal RS, Albert MA, Buroker AB, Goldberger ZD, Hahn EJ, et al. 2019 ACC/AHA Guideline on the Primary Prevention of Cardiovascular Disease: Executive Summary: A Report of the American College of Cardiology/American Heart Association Task Force on Clinical Practice Guidelines. J Am Coll Cardiol. 2019;74(10):1376-414.

52. Kris-Etherton PM, Krauss RM. Public health guidelines should recommend reducing saturated fat consumption as

much as possible: YES. Am J Clin Nutr. 2020; 112(1):13-8.
53. Krauss RM, Kris-Etherton PM. Public health guidelines should recommend reducing saturated fat consumption as much as possible: Debate Consensus. Am J Clin Nutr. 2020;112(1):25-6.
54. Rani U, Basha A, Raghavendra P, Shahida Md, Usha SA, Saritha B, et al. Trajectory of transfats in India—from regulation to realty. Insights Nutr Metab. 2022;6:1-5.
55. Steele L, Drummond E, Nishida C, Yamamoto R, Branca F, Parsons Perez C, et al. Ending Trans Fat-The First-Ever Global Elimination Program for a Noncommunicable Disease Risk Factor: JACC International. J Am Coll Cardiol. 2024;84(7):663-74.
56. Ghafoorunissa G. Role of trans fatty acids in health and challenges to their reduction in Indian foods. Asia Pac J Clin Nutr. 2008; 17(Suppl 1):212-5.
57. Mente A, O'Donnell M, Yusuf S. Sodium Intake and Health: What Should We Recommend Based on the Current Evidence? Nutrients. 2021;13(9):3232.
58. Jenkins DJ, Jones PJ, Lamarche B, Kendall CW, Faulkner D, Cermakova L, et al. Effect of a dietary portfolio of cholesterol-lowering foods given at 2 levels of intensity of dietary advice on serum lipids in hyperlipidemia: a randomized controlled trial. JAMA. 2011; 306(8):831-9.
59. Chiavaroli L, Nishi SK, Khan TA, Braunstein CR, Glenn AJ, Mejia SB, et al. Portfolio Dietary Pattern and Cardiovascular Disease: A Systematic Review and Meta-analysis of Controlled Trials. Prog Cardiovasc Dis. 2018;61(1):43-53.
60. Kirkpatrick CF, Sikand G, Petersen KS, Anderson CAM, Aspry KE, Bolick JP, et al. Nutrition interventions for adults with dyslipidemia: A Clinical Perspective from the National Lipid Association. J Clin Lipidol. 2023;17(4):428-51.
61. Jenkins DJ, Josse AR, Wong JM, Nguyen TH, Kendall CW. The portfolio diet for cardiovascular risk reduction. Curr Atheroscler Rep. 2007;9(6):501-7.
62. de Bock M, Derraik JG, Brennan CM, Biggs JB, Smith GC, Cameron-Smith D, et al. Psyllium supplementation in adolescents improves fat distribution & lipid profile: a randomized, participant-blinded, placebo-controlled, crossover trial. PLoS One. 2012; 7(7):e41735.
63. Garoufi A, Vorre S, Soldatou A, Tsentidis C, Kossiva L, Drakatos A, et al. Plant sterols-enriched diet decreases small, dense LDL-cholesterol levels in children with hypercholesterolemia: a prospective study. Ital J Pediatr. 2014;40:42.
64. Guardamagna O, Abello F, Baracco V, Federici G, Bertucci P, Mozzi A, et al. Primary hyperlipidemias in children: effect of plant sterol supplementation on plasma lipids and markers of cholesterol synthesis and absorption. Acta Diabetol. 2011;48(2):127-33.
65. Jones PJH, Shamloo M, MacKay DS, Rideout TC, Myrie SB, Plat J, et al. Progress and perspectives in plant sterol and plant stanol research. Nutr Rev. 2018;76(10):725-46.
66. Virani SS, Morris PB, Agarwala A, Ballantyne CM, Birtcher KK, Kris-Etherton PM, et al. 2021 ACC Expert Consensus Decision Pathway on the Management of ASCVD Risk Reduction in Patients With Persistent Hypertriglyceridemia: A Report of the American College of Cardiology Solution Set Oversight Committee. J Am Coll Cardiol. 2021;78(9):960-93.

Life's Essential 8 and Modifications for Indians

INTRODUCTION

In 2010, the American Heart Association (AHA) shifted its focus from disease-specific treatment to overall population health with the introduction of Life's Simple 7.[1] This marked a paradigm shift in defining cardiovascular health (CVH) as a comprehensive measure encompassing multiple lifestyle factors and health metrics with the aim to reduce the burden of heart disease. In the ensuing years, AHA specifically recognized the social determinants of health (SDOH)—conditions in which people are born, grow, live, work, and age—that directly affect people's CVH, and are particularly relevant to low- and middle-income countries (LMICs). In their most recent update, AHA added an 8th element, sleep, and renamed their presidential advisory as "Life's Essential 8" (LE8).[2] These essential 8 are comprised of 4 behavioral factors and 4 health factors depicted in **Table 1** with comments. LE8 is also presented as a figure **(Fig. 1)** as it would be a useful patient education aid.

HEALTHY SLEEP

Sleep is a recent addition to the previous Life's Simple 7 based on evidence that linked sleep with health—in particular with CVH. Healthy sleep is not just adequate duration of sleep but is multidimensional. The other dimensions of timing, regularity, efficiency, and impact on daytime alertness are also of importance. Sleep metrics have independent predictive value for cardiovascular (CV) events.[9]

TABLE 1: Life's Essential 8 (LE8).[2-7]

#	Health behaviors (1–4) and health factors (5–8)	Comments
1	Eat better	Healthy eating includes whole foods, fruits, vegetables, legumes, lean protein, nuts and seeds, and to use nontropical oils (e.g., canola, olive) for cooking (Chapter 16)
2	Quit/avoid tobacco smoking and exposure	Includes all tobacco products (cigarettes, cigars, beedis, etc.) and other nicotine delivery systems—e-cigarettes, vaping, and exposure to secondhand smoke (Chapter 4)
3	Be more active	150 minutes per week of moderate activity or 75 minutes of vigorous physical activity per week for adults; 60 minutes of play/structured activities every day for children

Contd...

Contd…

#	Health behaviors (1–4) and health factors (5–8)	Comments
4	Get healthy sleep	7–9 hours of sleep each night for adults; 8–10 hours for ages 13–18; 9–12 hours for ages 6–12; 10–16 hours (including naps) for ages 5 and younger
5	Manage blood pressure	<120/80 mm Hg (optimal); keep under <130/80 mm Hg (Chapter 5)
6	Manage blood sugar	<100 mg/dL and A1c <5.7% (optimal); (A1c <7% for those with diabetes) (Chapter 6)
7	Manage weight Body mass index (BMI)	<25 kg/m^2 (Ideal BMI) *(The ideal BMI needs to be modified for Indians as we explain later in text)*
8	Control blood lipids	NHDL-C <130 mg/dL—corresponding to TC 170 mg/dL and LDL-C 100 mg/dL (Chapter 7) *(Lipid numbers need to be modified in Indians as we explain later in text)*

(A1c: glycosylated hemoglobin; LDL-C: low-density lipoprotein cholesterol; NHDL-C: non-high-density lipoprotein cholesterol; TC: total cholesterol)

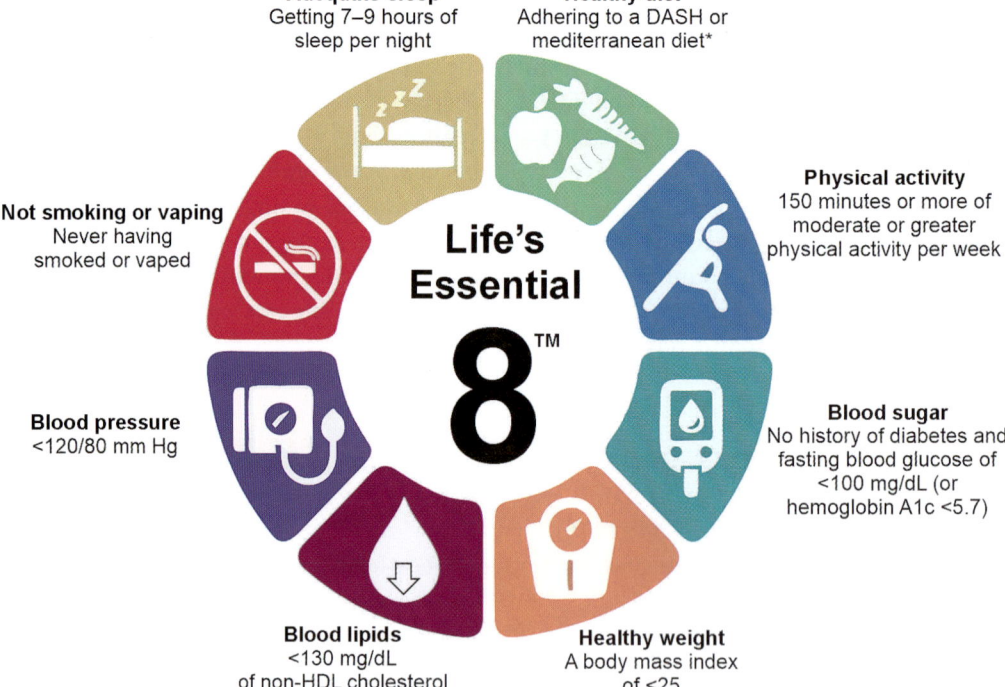

Fig. 1: Life's Essential 8. Life's essential 8 are the key measures for improving and maintaining cardiovascular health as defined by the American Heart Association. They consist of four health indicators (physical activity, healthy diet, adequate sleep, not smoking or vaping) and four health factors (blood pressure, blood lipids, healthy weight, and blood sugar). DASH indicates Dietary Approaches to Stop Hypertension.
*Healthy Eating Index Score <50.
Source: Reproduced with permission from Joynt Maddox et al.[8]

HEALTHY DIET

The US Food and Drug Administration (FDA) in December 2024 (www.fda.gov/food/nutrition-food-labeling-and-critical-foods/use-healthy-claim-food-labeling) issued an important update on specific requirements for a "healthy" claim on food items to help consumers identify those foods that are the foundation of healthy dietary patterns. A healthy diet is required to contain minimum amount of recommended food groups and subgroups (vegetables, fruits, dairy, protein foods, and whole grains) which contain an array of nutrients and recommends constructing healthy dietary patterns by eating an array of vegetables, fruits, dairy, protein foods, and whole grains to support nutrient adequacy of the diet. Examples of foods that qualify for "healthy" claim are fresh whole fruits and vegetables, frozen, chopped, dried, or canned fruits and vegetables, salmon, trail mix with nuts and dried fruit, plain low-fat or fat-free yogurt, eggs, water, and 100% olive oil. Added ingredients must meet a minimum food group amount and required limits for saturated fat, sodium, and added sugars to qualify to bear the "healthy" claim under the updated definition.

Caution on dieting: One popular measure for those who diet to bring their weight down is to skip breakfast. Results of newer studies strike a strong cautionary note to this practice as skipping breakfast was associated with an increased odds of prevalent noncoronary and generalized atherosclerosis independently of the presence of conventional CV risk factors. A cross-sectional study within the PESA (Progression of Early Subclinical Atherosclerosis) study of a prospective cohort of asymptomatic (free of CV events at baseline) 4,052 participants showed three breakfast patterns: High-energy breakfast, when contributing to >20% of total daily energy intake (27% of the population); low-energy breakfast, when contributing between 5 and 20% of total daily energy intake (70% of the population); and skipping breakfast, when consuming <5% of total daily energy (3% of the population). Independent of the presence of traditional and dietary CV risk factors, and compared with high-energy breakfast, habitual skipping breakfast was associated with a higher prevalence of noncoronary (odds ratio: 1.55; 95% confidence interval: 0.97–2.46) and generalized (odds ratio: 2.57; 95% confidence interval: 1.54–4.31) atherosclerosis.[10]

PHYSICAL ACTIVITY

Physical activity of moderate or greater intensity for 150 minutes or more per week is clearly stated and the benefit of adherence to this element of LE8 is well established. The opposite side of the coin—inactivity—and its effects has also been studied. Among 89,530 participants (age 62 ± 8 years, 56.4% women) in a prospective cohort study, sedentary behavior was associated with major adverse cardiovascular events (MACE) and CV mortality with an inflection of risk at 10.6 hours/day. Another important finding was that reducing sedentary time was important to all, even to those who are active and adhere to the guideline recommended physical activity.[11]

VALIDATION OF LIFE'S ESSENTIAL 8 USING CARDIOVASCULAR HEALTH SCORE

Validation of LE8 using CVH score is a quantitative tool that assigns a score from 0 to 100, to each component and then totaled. From this total, if medication(s) is/are used to control the major risk factors (hypertension, diabetes, cholesterol) a deduction of 20 points for each is made. The overall CVH score is then calculated by dividing the total by 8. A score above 80 is considered excellent, while a score 50–79 is moderate, and below 50 indicates poor CVH.[2]

In a large prospective cohort study of data from the National Health and Nutrition Examination Survey (NHANES) 2005–2018 at baseline, linked to the 2019 National Death Index of US adults showed that among the LE8 metrics, physical activity, nicotine exposure, and diet accounted for a large proportion of the population-attributable risks for all-cause mortality, whereas physical activity, blood pressure, and blood glucose accounted for a large proportion of cardiovascular disease (CVD)-specific mortality. The association of total CVH score to all-cause and CVD-specific mortality was approximately of a linear-dose type as illustrated in **Figure 2**.[12]

Adherence to the 8 components of LE8 and improvement in CVH score that was low at baseline is associated with reduction in 10-year and lifetime risk of stroke,[13] CVD, and all-cause mortality,[12,14,15] In addition, improving LE8 score also foretold a longer lifespan free from CVD, diabetes, cancer, and dementia.[16,17] Similar results were also reported in a large study of over 400,000 veterans that adherence to the LE8—significantly reduced the risk of CVD and death.[16] Participants who adhered to LE8 not only experienced a 64% lower risk of developing CVD, but the benefit extended also to those with existing CVD as they reduced the likelihood of heart attacks and strokes by 50%.[18]

Cardiovascular health scoring has improved the precision and usability of LE8 to assess CVH and to provide targeted advice and treatments. In a meta-analysis of nearly 2 million participants, those with high CVH score had a markedly lower risk of CVDs (82% less myocardial infarction) and cardiometabolic diseases (40% less atrial fibrillation) compared to those with low CVH score.[3-5] Even modest improvements in CVH score can lead to substantial health benefits.[4]

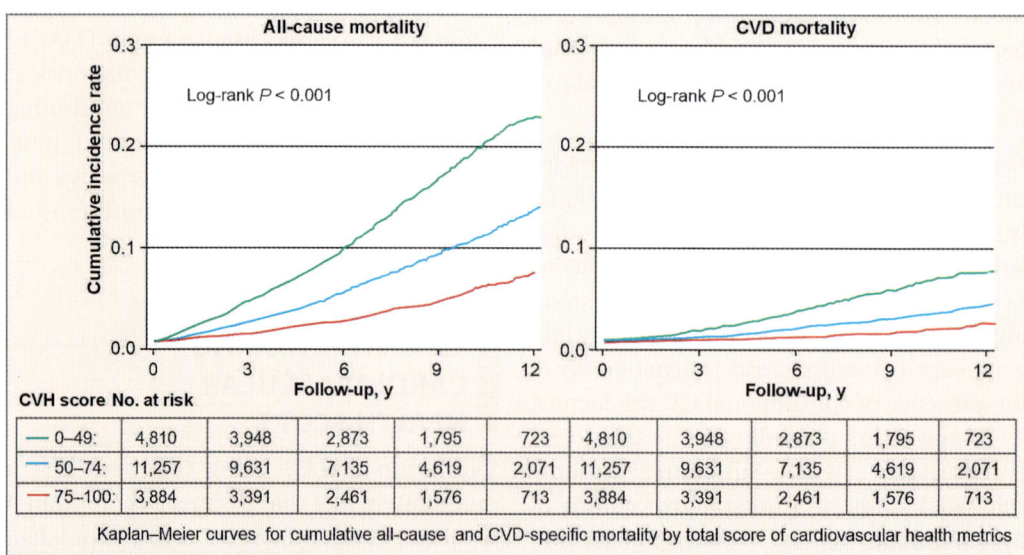

Fig. 2: Associations of Cardiovascular Health (CVH) scores to all-cause and cardiovascular disease (CVD)-specific mortality.
Source: Reproduced with permission from Sun et al.[12]

RATIONALE TO MODIFY 2 OF THE LIFE'S ESSENTIAL 8 FOR INDIANS

Life's Essential 8 provides proven standards to improve CVH and reduce the burden of heart disease for all. Six of the 8 elements of LE8 do not need any population-specific modifications. However, 2 of them (weight and lipids as noted in comments in **Table 1**) need modifications to best serve Indians who grapple with heart disease and other CVDs.

Body Mass Index and Waist Circumference

Body mass index (BMI) is the gold standard used for assessing the weight of a person—whether it is normal (healthy weight), underweight, or overweight. A healthy weight for an adult (male and female) based on height and weight is 18.5–24.9. Between 25 and 29.9 is overweight and 30 and above is obese. Obesity affects approximately 19% of women and 14% of men worldwide and is associated with increased mortality and morbidity, such as metabolic syndrome, diabetes, cancer, etc. BMI measurement (easily determined by using a widely available BMI calculator) may not accurately differentiate healthy weight and unhealthy weight in Indians because of their unfavorable distribution of fat around the abdomen.[19]

Huffman et al.[20] evaluated the differences in prevalence of overweight, obesity, and abdominal obesity using different criteria by the World Health Organization (WHO) and the International Obesity Task Force.[21,22] Overweight was defined by using the WHO criterion (BMI ≥25 kg/m^2) and for Asians (BMI ≥23 kg/m^2).[22] Obesity was defined as BMI ≥30 kg/m^2, as recommended by WHO and >25 for Indians.[23] Central obesity was defined as a waist circumference (WC) ≥90 cm for men and ≥80 cm for women, as recommended for South Asians by the International Diabetes Federation.[24] Using the WHO definition (BMI >30 kg/m^2) only 20% of Indian men and 35% of Indian women were obese. But by using the Asian criteria (BMI >25 kg/m^2) obesity rates more than doubled in Indian men and nearly doubled in Indian women **(Fig. 3)**. Besides, 80% of Indian men and women were overweight and 70% had abdominal obesity using the Asian criteria.

This data underscore the underestimation of obesity and consequently obesity-related risks by not using the Asian criteria.[20] Therefore, India (and other Asian countries) use lower BMI thresholds for overweight and obesity as follow:[25,26]

- *Optimal:* <23 kg/m^2 (metabolic risk equivalent BMI 25 in Whites)
- *Overweight:* 23–24.9 kg/m^2 (metabolic risk equivalent to BMI >25–29.9 in Whites)
- *Obese:* Over 25 kg/m^2 (metabolic risk equivalent Whites to BMI >30 in Whites).

Palaniappan et al.[27] in a large study of 43,507 patients found that Indian American men and women have a higher prevalence of metabolic syndrome in every BMI category **(Table 2)** compared to their American counterparts.

As shown on **Table 2**, Indian Americans with BMI of 20 kg/m^2 have the similar prevalence of metabolic syndrome as Whites with BMI of 25 kg/m^2, and Indian Americans with a BMI of 25 kg/m^2 have similar prevalence of metabolic syndrome as Americans with BMI 30 kg/m^2.[28] Overall, Indians develop metabolic syndrome at 5-6 units of lower BMI than Whites. Besides the lower BMI, Indians develop metabolic syndrome at lower WC compared to other populations. In recognition, national and international guidelines have lowered their metrics for Indians.[21,22,28-30]

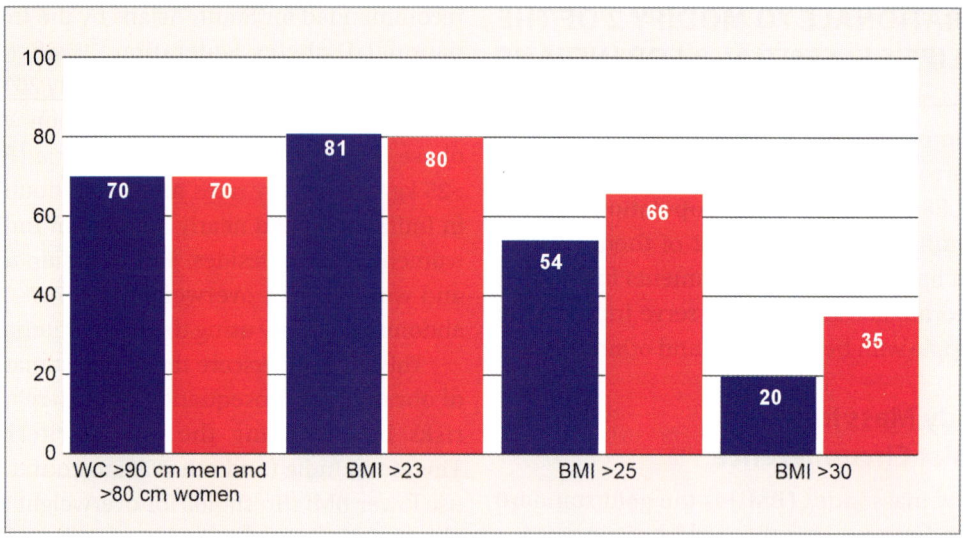

Fig. 3: Differences in central obesity measured by waist circumference (WC), overweight [body mass index (BMI) >23 kg/m^2], and obesity (>25 kg/m^2) using Asian criteria in Indian men (blue bar) and in Indian women (red bar). Note using the World Health Organization (WHO) general criteria for obesity of BMI >30 only 20% of Indian men and 30% of women would be classified as obese but by Asian criteria the obesity rate in Indian men more than doubles (20–54) and nearly doubles in women.
Source: Adapted from Huffman et al.[20]

TABLE 2: Difference in the prevalence of metabolic syndrome and body mass index (BMI) equivalence in Indian American men and women compared to White Americans.[27,28]

Prevalence of metabolic syndrome	BMI 25 kg/m^2	BMI 25 kg/m^2 equivalence	BMI 30 kg/m^2 equivalence
Indian American women	30%	19.6	23.9
White women	12%	25	30
Indian American men	43%	19.9	24.3
White men	22%	25	30

Waist circumference guidelines:[21,30]
- *Indian women:* 80 cm (31.5 inches)
- *Indian men:* 90 cm (35.4 inches)

Compared to these, the WC guidelines for Americans are significantly higher:
- *US women:* 88 cm (34.6 inches)
- *US men:* 102 cm (40 inches)

Indian women with WC of 80 cm are found to have metabolic abnormalities comparable to White women with WC of 88 cm, while Indian men with WC 90 cm develop metabolic abnormalities similar to White men with WC 102 cm.[28,31] In Indians, abdominal obesity (WC of ≥90 cm in men and ≥80 cm in women) is associated with a twofold higher risk of diabetes, hypertension, and atherosclerotic cardiovascular disease (ASCVD).[32] In a nationally representative study of 698,286 participants in India the prevalence of abdominal obesity was fourfold higher than overall obesity (57.71% vs. 13.85%).[33] A meta-analysis of prospective studies involving 669,560 participants and 25,214 CVD cases showed that each 10 cm increase of WC increased CVD risk by 3.4% in women and 4% in men.[34] This association between abdominal obesity (visceral and subcutaneous) and cardiometabolic risk is best appreciated in light of much research on the properties of accumulated fat, such as of anti- and proinflammatory adipokines, changes in free fatty acid metabolism, cellular hypoxia, and increase in size of adipocytes.[35]

Based on the information on BMI and WC presented, to assess LE8 in Indians, body weight and BMI would not suffice but WC should be incorporated to this assessment. Indians have high rates of overweight (≥70% have BMI >23 kg/m^2) and obesity which are markedly underestimated by the standard BMI calculator.[20] Consequently, increased weight (overweight and obesity)-related risks to CVH, remain hidden and therefore neglected. This situation demands change that include:

- Adoption of standards of BMI specific to Indians
- Personal awareness of BMI and WC and that WC matters more than weight
- Change in behavioral patterns (diet, physical activity)
- Public health campaigns and individual counseling
- Optimal management of LE8

Blood Lipids

Non-high-density lipoprotein cholesterol (NHDL-C) that includes LDL-C and remnant cholesterol is a proven marker of heart disease risk. NHDL-C of <130 mg/dL, one of the standards of LE8 **(Table 1)** is graded a CVH score of 100, and as NHDL-C increases the score goes lower and ends with a CVH score of zero (0) for NHDL-C of >200 mg/dL.[2]

Our rationale to modify the LE8 metric on blood lipids in Indians to a lower NHDL-C of <100 mg/dL rests on a four-legged stool: (1) Characteristics of the population, (2) LDL-C levels related to plaque buildup, (3) disease trajectories for prevention, and (4) benefits of statin treatment at high doses to reach theoretical minimum risk exposure level for LDL-C (TMREL) without adverse effects.

1. *Characteristics of the South Asian population:* In several chapters in this book, we have detailed the multiplicity of features that include increased major risk factors and poor recognition and control of these behavioral and inherited factors that make Indian ethnicity a cardiac risk-enhancing factor. Among the inherited factors, the increased risk of high lipoprotein (a) [Lp(a)], detailed in Chapter 8, is well demonstrated in a Finnish study of 3,596 young participants of ages 9–24 years: Those with both elevated Lp(a) >30 mg/dL and LDL-C >130 mg/dL were at a significantly higher risk (hazard ratio of 4.30 (3.30–5.30, p 0.00004) for earlier heart disease events (median age 47) than those who had either elevated Lp(a) or LDL-C who were also at high risk (hazard ratio of 2.45 (1.89–3.00, p 0.001).[36]

2. *LDL-C and plaque buildup and disease trajectories for prevention:* The PESA (n = 4,184) study found that even among those with an LDL-C of 60–70 mg/dL, 11% showed subclinical atherosclerosis and there was a linear increase in atherosclerosis with increasing LDL-C levels **(Fig. 4)**.[37] This questions the currently accepted LDL-C target of 70 mg/dL and legitimately raises the question whether the target should be lower to further reduce CV risk.[38]

3. *Disease trajectories for prevention:* The natural history of atherosclerosis is a

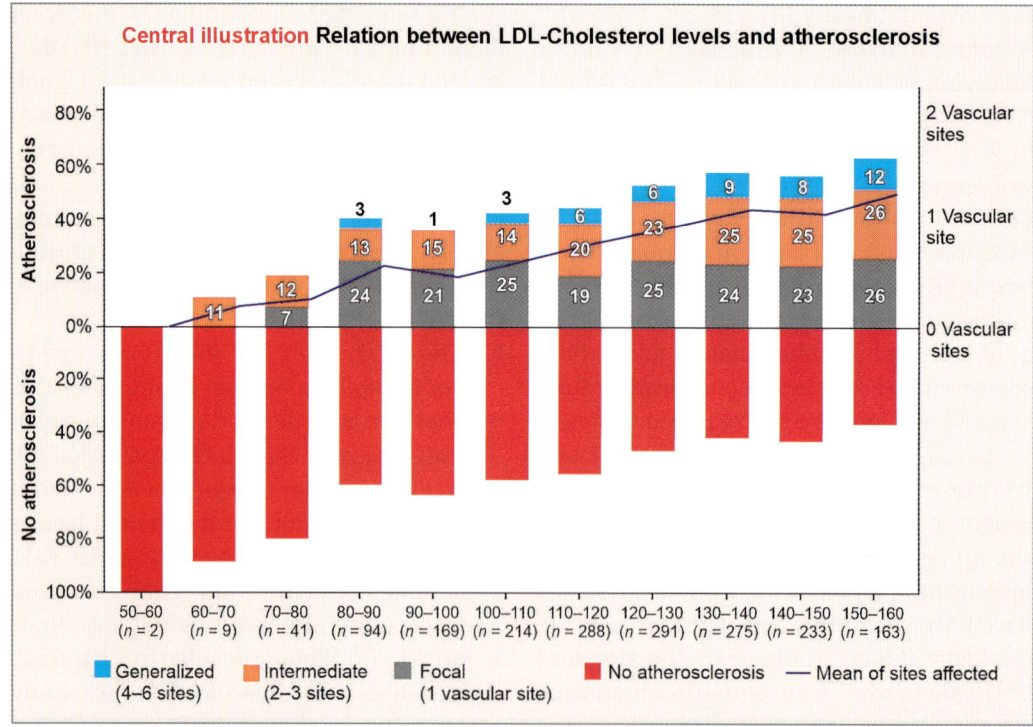

Fig. 4: 11% having subclinical atherosclerosis even at low-density lipoprotein cholesterol (LDL-C) 60–70 mg/dL and increasing with increasing LDL-C reaching 64% at LDL-C >150 mg/dL. As LDL-C levels rise, there is a linear and significant increase in the prevalence of atherosclerosis, ranging from 11% in the 60–70 mg/dL category to 64% in the 150–160 mg/dL subgroup ($p < 0.001$). A similar pattern is observed for the multiterritorial extent of atherosclerosis (focal, intermediate, or generalized disease) as well as for the mean number of vascular sites affected (blue line).
Source: Reproduced with permission from Fernández-Friera et al.[37]

lifelong one and it follows that early intervention of all modifiable and controllable risk factors hold the key to prevent heart disease and MACEs. Research suggests that initiating statin therapy as early as age 30 can prevent the progression of atherosclerosis, stabilize existing plaque[39] and delay MACEs beyond the age of 70. Combining statins with other preventive measures can further extend this protective effect **(Fig. 5)**. Studies have shown that lowering LDL-C by 40 mg/dL has a 3–5 times greater impact on reducing heart disease risk if treatment begins early.[40-42] Rosuvastatin and atorvastatin are approved for use in children as young as 10 years of age.

4. *Statins and the TMREL:* TMPREL developed by the Global Burden of Disease (GBD) study represents the lowest cholesterol level at which no adverse health effects are observed. It is a hypothetical value derived from epidemiological studies and meta-analyses and serves as a benchmark for assessing the impact of elevated cholesterol on population health. Nearly 4 million heart disease deaths and 99 million disability-adjusted life years (DALYs) are attributable to LDL-C at above the 27–50 mg/dL, a level

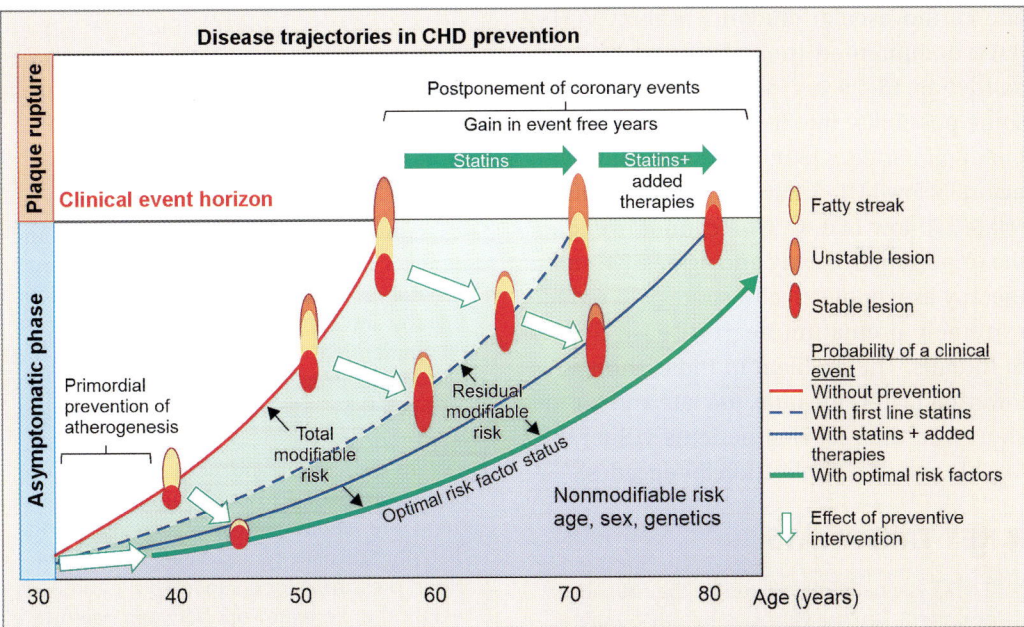

Fig. 5: Gain in cardiovascular event-free survival with statins and added therapies. (CHD: coronary heart disease)
Source: Reproduced with permission.[53]

TABLE 3: Safety and benefits of very low LDL-C.[43-52]	
Optimal LDL-C (TMREL) is 27–50 mg/dL	LDL-C 27–50 mg/dL is considered optimal with the lowest risk of ASCVD. A study linked LDL-C exceeding this range to 99 million healthy years of life lost and 4.4 deaths globally. Most newborns have LDL-C below 40 mg/dL, but it jumps to 70–80 mg/dL by age 2 years and can reach unhealthy levels by adulthood without preventative measures
Chinese adults with LDL-C 40 ng/dL have the lowest CVD risk	Recent studies, particularly from China, indicate that extremely low LDL-C levels, around 40 mg/dL, might be optimal for heart health. This could necessitate a revision of current cholesterol guidelines, potentially aiming for a total cholesterol target as low as 110–120 mg/dL
Added benefits of achieving LDL-C <50 mg/dL	Studies like JUPITER found that achieving an LDL-C level below 50 mg/dL resulted in 65% reduction in MACE compared to those with a higher LDL-C
LDL-C <60 is required to stop plaque progression	Research indicates that achieving an LDL-C level below 60 mg/dL is crucial for halting the progression of plaque buildup in arteries. This finding underscores the importance of aggressive cholesterol management in preventing heart disease
(ASCVD: atherosclerotic cardiovascular disease; LDL-C: low-density lipoprotein cholesterol; MACE: major adverse cardiovascular events; TMREL: theoretical minimum risk exposure level for LDL-C)	

currently designated as TMREL.[43] The PESA study data also support this level as TMREL.

Contrary to past thinking, very low LDL-C levels appear safe and potentially beneficial **(Table 3)**. Genetic, epidemiological studies and cardiovascular outcome trials (CVOTs) have documented the safety and benefits as low as 15–20 mg/dL.[44,45] There is even some possibility that it might regress plaque buildup in arteries. Studies show people with naturally low LDL-C have no health problems related to low LDL-C. One cannot overstate the importance of early and aggressive statin therapy as a public health strategy to reduce extremely premature heart disease deaths in Indians. The problem in India, though, is lowering LDL-C too little, too late and for too short of a time leaving patients vulnerable to CVD and its complication for decades.[52]

■ KEY TAKEAWAYS

- "Life's Essential 8", developed by the AHA, incorporates 8 key measures: 4 health behaviors and 4 health factors to reduce heart disease are effective, practical, and proven. CVH score is based on an assigned score of 0–100 for each metric and an average of all has shown excellent correlation (almost linear) with all-cause mortality and with CVD specific mortality.
- Healthy sleep is a newly added measure as sleep with its multidimensional aspects is essential for good health and has shown independent predictive value for adverse CV events.
- Physical activity ≥150 minutes of moderate or greater intensity per week is recommended. Sedentary lifestyle is associated with adverse CV events and increased CV mortality. Reducing sedentary time is important to all, even to those who are active and adhere to the guideline recommended for physical activity.
- Six of the 8 measures are applicable globally. But in 2—weight and lipids, lower targets are better for Indians and we provide our modified version and our rationale for the modifications.
- BMI does not accurately differentiate healthy and unhealthy weight in Indians because of their propensity for abdominal obesity. Abdominal obesity increases cardiometabolic risk. We propose a lower ideal BMI of <23 kg/m^2 combined with WC measurement of <80 cm for women and 90 cm for men. A waist to height ratio of >0.5 is a simple metric for obesity.
- NHDL-C of <100 mg/dL (that includes LDL-C) is our recommendation for Indians based on a multiplicity of reasons [including high Lp(a), ethnicity, poor awareness, and poor control of established risk factors].
- We recommend LDL-C <70 mg/dL in high-risk persons (primary prevention) and LDL-C of <55 mg/dL in those with ASCVD. Safety and benefits of very low LDL-C has been shown in natural states and on LDL-C lowering statin therapy and studies suggest that the present recommended target of 70 may not be low enough to prevent plaque formation. Early statin therapy in life can change the trajectory of heart disease.
- Patient education and active participation of all are needed to implement LE8 as 4 of them are behavioral—tobacco avoidance, diet, physical activity, and sleep. The other 4—blood pressure, blood sugar, lipids, and body weight require teamwork between healthcare providers and patients.

■ REFERENCES

1. Lloyd-Jones DM, Hong Y, Labarthe D, Mozaffarian D, Appel LJ, Van Horn L, et al.; American Heart Association Strategic Planning Task Force and Statistics Committee. Defining and setting national goals for cardiovascular health promotion and disease reduction: the American Heart Association's strategic Impact Goal through 2020 and beyond. Circulation. 2010;121(4):586-613.
2. Lloyd-Jones DM, Allen NB, Anderson CAM, Black T, Brewer LC, Foraker RE, et al.; American Heart Association. Life's Essential 8: Updating and Enhancing the American Heart Association's Construct of Cardiovascular Health: A Presidential Advisory From the American Heart Association. Circulation. 2022;146(5):e18-e43.
3. Te Hoonte F, Spronk M, Sun Q, Wu K, Fan S, Wang Z, et al. Ideal cardiovascular health and cardiovascular-related events: a systematic review and meta-analysis. Eur J Prev Cardiol. 2024;31(8):966-85.
4. Prugger C, Perier MC, Sabia S, Fayosse A, van Sloten T, Jouven X, et al. Association between changes in cardiovascular health

and the risk of multimorbidity: community-based cohort studies in the UK and Finland. Lancet Reg Health Eur. 2024;42:100922.

5. Radovanovic M, Jankovic J, Mandic-Rajcevic S, Dumic I, Hanna RD, Nordstrom CW. Ideal cardiovascular health and risk of cardiovascular events or mortality: a systematic review and meta-analysis of prospective studies. J Clin Med. 2023;12(13):4417.

6. Shetty NS, Parcha V, Patel N, Yadav I, Basetty C, Li C, et al. AHA Life's essential 8 and ideal cardiovascular health among young adults. Am J Prev Cardiol. 2023;13:100452.

7. Gupta B, Gupta R, Sharma KK, Gupta A, Mahanta TG, Deedwania PC. Low prevalence of AHA-defined ideal cardiovascular health factors: a study of urban indian men and women. Glob Heart. 2017;12(3):219-25.

8. Joynt Maddox KE, Elkind MSV, Aparicio HJ, Commodore-Mensah Y, de Ferranti SD, Dowd WN, et al. Forecasting the Burden of Cardiovascular Disease and Stroke in the United States Through 2050-Prevalence of Risk Factors and Disease: A Presidential Advisory From the American Heart Association. Circulation. 2024;150(4):e65-e88.

9. Makarem N, St-Onge MP, Liao M, Lloyd-Jones DM, Aggarwal B. Association of sleep characteristics with cardiovascular health among women and differences by race/ethnicity and menopausal status: findings from the American Heart Association Go Red for Women Strategically Focused Research Network. Sleep Health. 2019;5(5):501-8.

10. Uzhova I, Fuster V, Fernandez-Ortiz A, Ordovás JM, Sanz J, Fernández-Friera L, et al. The importance of breakfast in atherosclerosis disease: insights from the PESA Study. J Am Coll Cardiol. 2017;70(15):1833-42.

11. Ajufo E, Kany S, Rämö JT, Churchill TW, Guseh JS, Aragam KG, et al. Accelerometer-measured sedentary behavior and risk of future cardiovascular disease. J Am Coll Cardiol. 2025;85(5):473-86.

12. Sun J, Li Y, Zhao M, Yu X, Zhang C, Magnussen CG, et al. Association of the American Heart Association's new "Life's Essential 8" with all-cause and cardiovascular disease-specific mortality: prospective cohort study. BMC Med. 2023;21(1):116.

13. Wu S, Wu Z, Yu D, Chen S, Wang A, Wang A, et al. Life's Essential 8 and risk of stroke: a prospective community-based study. Stroke. 2023;54(9):2369-79.

14. Li X, Ma H, Wang X, Feng H, Qi L. Life's Essential 8, Genetic Susceptibility, and Incident cardiovascular disease: a prospective study. Arterioscler Thromb Vasc Biol. 2023;43(7):1324-33.

15. Yi J, Wang L, Guo X, Ren X. Association of Life's Essential 8 with all-cause and cardiovascular mortality among US adults: A prospective cohort study from the NHANES 2005-2014. Nutr Metab Cardiovasc Dis. 2023;33(6):1134-43.

16. Wang X, Ma H, Li X, Heianza Y, Manson JE, Franco OH, et al. Association of cardiovascular health with life expectancy free of cardiovascular disease, diabetes, cancer, and dementia in UK adults. JAMA Intern Med. 2023;183(4):340-9.

17. Ma H, Wang X, Xue Q, Li X, Liang Z, Heianza Y, et al. Cardiovascular health and life expectancy among adults in the United States. Circulation. 2023;147(15):1137-46.

18. Nguyen XT, Li Y, Gong Y, Houghton S, Ho YL, Pyatt M, et al.; VA Million Veteran Program. Cardiovascular health score and atherosclerotic cardiovascular disease in the million veteran program. JAMA Netw Open. 2024;7(12):e2447902.

19. Kandula NR, Tirodkar MA, Lauderdale DS, Khurana NR, Makoul G, Baker DW. Knowledge gaps and misconceptions about coronary heart disease among U.S. South Asians. Am J Prev Med. 2010;38(4):439-42.

20. Huffman MD, Prabhakaran D, Osmond C, Fall CH, Tandon N, Lakshmy R, et al.; New Delhi Birth Cohort. Incidence of cardiovascular risk factors in an Indian urban cohort results from the new delhi birth cohort. J Am Coll Cardiol. 2011;57(17):1765-74.

21. Alberti KG, Eckel RH, Grundy SM, Zimmet PZ, Cleeman JI, Donato KA, et al. Harmonizing the metabolic syndrome: a joint interim statement of the International Diabetes Federation Task Force on Epidemiology

and Prevention; National Heart, Lung, and Blood Institute; American Heart Association; World Heart Federation; International Atherosclerosis Society; and international association for the Study of Obesity. Circulation. 2009;120(16):1640-5.
22. World Health Organization, Western Pacific Regional Office. The Asia-Pacific perspective: Redefining obesity and its treatment 2000. Sydney: Health Communications Australia; 2000.
23. World Health Organization. Global Status Report on Noncommunicable Disease. Geneva: World Health Organization; 2014.
24. Alberti KG, Zimmet P, Shaw J; IDF Epidemiology Task Force Consensus Group. The metabolic syndrome—a new worldwide definition. Lancet. 2005;366(9491):1059-62.
25. Arnett DK, Blumenthal RS, Albert MA, Buroker AB, Goldberger ZD, Hahn EJ, et al. 2019 ACC/AHA Guideline on the Primary Prevention of Cardiovascular Disease: Executive Summary: A Report of the American College of Cardiology/American Heart Association Task Force on Clinical Practice Guidelines. J Am Coll Cardiol. 2019;74(10):1376-414.
26. Misra A, Chowbey P, Makkar BM, Vikram NK, Wasir JS, Chadha D, et al.; Concensus Group. Consensus statement for diagnosis of obesity, abdominal obesity and the metabolic syndrome for Asian Indians and recommendations for physical activity, medical and surgical management. J Assoc Physicians India. 2009;57:163-70.
27. Palaniappan LP, Wong EC, Shin JJ, Fortmann SP, Lauderdale DS. Asian Americans have greater prevalence of metabolic syndrome despite lower body mass index. Int J Obes (Lond). 2011;35(3):393-400.
28. Enas EA, Mohan V, Deepa M, Farooq S, Pazhoor S, Chennikkara H. The metabolic syndrome and dyslipidemia among Asian Indians: a population with high rates of diabetes and premature coronary artery disease. J Cardiometab Syndr. 2007;2(4):267-75.
29. Enas EA, Singh V, Munjal YP, Bhandari S, Yadave RD, Manchanda SC. Reducing the burden of coronary artery disease in India: challenges and opportunities. Indian Heart J. 2008;60(2):161-75.
30. World Health Organization. Cardiovascular diseases. [online] Available from https://www.who.int/health-topics/cardiovascular-diseases/#tab=tab_1 [Last accessed May 2025].
31. Grundy SM, Stone NJ, Bailey AL, Beam C, Birtcher KK, Blumenthal RS, et al. 2018 AHA/ACC/AACVPR/AAPA/ABC/ACPM/ADA/AGS/APhA/ASPC/NLA/PCNA Guideline on the Management of Blood Cholesterol: Executive Summary: A Report of the American College of Cardiology/American Heart Association Task Force on Clinical Practice Guidelines. J Am Coll Cardiol. 2019;73(24):3168-209.
32. Jayant SS, Gupta R, Rastogi A, Agrawal K, Sachdeva N, Ram S, et al. Abdominal obesity and incident cardio-metabolic disorders in Asian-Indians: A 10-years prospective cohort study. Diabetes Metab Syndr. 2022; 16(2):102418.
33. Gupta RD, Tamanna N, Siddika N, Haider SS, Apu EH, Haider MR. Obesity and Abdominal Obesity in Indian Population: Findings from a Nationally Representative Study of 698,286 Participants. Epidemiologia (Basel). 2023;4(2):163-72.
34. Xue R, Li Q, Geng Y, Wang H, Wang F, Zhang S. Abdominal obesity and risk of CVD: a dose-response meta-analysis of thirty-one prospective studies. Br J Nutr. 2021;126(9):1420-30.
35. Lee JJ, Pedley A, Hoffmann U, Massaro JM, Fox CS. Association of Changes in Abdominal Fat Quantity and Quality With Incident Cardiovascular Disease Risk Factors. J Am Coll Cardiol. 2016;68(14):1509-21.
36. Raitakari O, Kartiosuo N, Pahkala K, Hutri-Kähönen N, Bazzano LA, Chen W, et al. Lipoprotein(a) in Youth and Prediction of Major Cardiovascular Outcomes in Adulthood. Circulation. 2023;147(1):23-31.
37. Fernández-Friera L, Fuster V, López-Melgar B, Oliva B, García-Ruiz JM, Mendiguren J, et al. Normal LDL-Cholesterol Levels Are Associated With Subclinical Atherosclerosis

in the Absence of Risk Factors. J Am Coll Cardiol. 2017;70(24):2979-91.
38. Ibanez B, Fernández-Ortiz A, Fernández-Friera L, García-Lunar I, Andrés V, Fuster V. Progression of Early Subclinical Atherosclerosis (PESA) Study: JACC Focus Seminar 7/8. J Am Coll Cardiol. 2021;78(2):156-79.
39. Packard CJ, Weintraub WS, Laufs U. New metrics needed to visualize the long-term impact of early LDL-C lowering on the cardiovascular disease trajectory. Vascul Pharmacol. 2015;71:37-9.
40. Ference BA. Mendelian randomization studies: using naturally randomized genetic data to fill evidence gaps. Curr Opin Lipidol. 2015;26(6):566-71.
41. Ference BA. Interpreting the Clinical Implications of Drug-Target Mendelian Randomization Studies. J Am Coll Cardiol. 2022;80(7):663-65.
42. Cohen JC, Boerwinkle E, Mosley TH Jr, Hobbs HH. Sequence variations in PCSK9, low LDL, and protection against coronary heart disease. N Engl J Med. 2006; 354(12):1264-72.
43. Roth GA, Mensah GA, Johnson CO, Addolorato G, Ammirati E, Baddour LM, et al.; GBD-NHLBI-JACC Global Burden of Cardiovascular Diseases Writing Group. Global Burden of Cardiovascular Diseases and Risk Factors, 1990-2019: Update From the GBD 2019 Study. J Am Coll Cardiol. 2020;76(25):2982-3021.
44. Sabatine MS, Wiviott SD, Im K, Murphy SA, Giugliano RP. Efficacy and Safety of Further Lowering of Low-Density Lipoprotein Cholesterol in Patients Starting With Very Low Levels: A Meta-analysis. JAMA Cardiol. 2018;3(9):823-8.
45. Giugliano RP, Pedersen TR, Park JG, De Ferrari GM, Gaciong ZA, Ceska R, et al.; FOURIER Investigators. Clinical efficacy and safety of achieving very low LDL-cholesterol concentrations with the PCSK9 inhibitor evolocumab: a prespecified secondary analysis of the FOURIER trial. Lancet. 2017; 390(10106):1962-71.
46. Zhang X, Liu J, Wang M, Qi Y, Sun J, Liu J, et al. Twenty-year epidemiologic study on LDL-C levels in relation to the risks of atherosclerotic event, hemorrhagic stroke, and cancer death among young and middle-aged population in China. J Clin Lipidol. 2018;12(5): 1179-1189.e4.
47. Ference B A, Yoo W, Alesh I, Mahajan N, Mirowska KK, Mewada A, et al. Effect of long-term exposure to lower low-density lipoprotein cholesterol beginning early in life on the risk of coronary heart disease: a mendelian randomization analysis. J Am Coll Cardiol. 2012;60(25):2631-9.
48. Robinson JG, Williams KJ, Gidding S, Borén J, Tabas I, Fisher EA, et al. Eradicating the Burden of Atherosclerotic Cardiovascular Disease by Lowering Apolipoprotein B Lipoproteins Earlier in Life. J Am Heart Assoc. 2018;7(20):e009778.
49. Boekholdt SM, Arsenault BJ, Mora S, Pedersen TR, LaRosa JC, Nestel PJ, et al. Association of LDL cholesterol, non-HDL cholesterol, and apolipoprotein B levels with risk of cardiovascular events among patients treated with statins: a meta-analysis. JAMA. 2012;307(12):1302-9.
50. Ridker PM; JUPITER Study Group. Rosuvastatin in the primary prevention of cardiovascular disease among patients with low levels of low-density lipoprotein cholesterol and elevated high-sensitivity C-reactive protein: rationale and design of the JUPITER trial. Circulation. 2003;108(19): 2292-7.
51. Puri R, Bansal M, Mehta V, Duell PB, Wong ND, Iyengar SS, et al. Lipid Association of India 2023 update on cardiovascular risk assessment and lipid management in Indian patients: Consensus statement IV. J Clin Lipidol. 2024;18(3):e351-e373.
52. Mancini GBJ, Hegele RA. Can We Eliminate Low-Density Lipoprotein Cholesterol-Related Cardiovascular Events Through More Aggressive Primary Prevention Therapy? Can J Cardiol. 2018;34(5):546-51.
53. Packard CJ, Weintraub WS, Laufs U. New metrics needed to visualize the long-term impact of early LDL-C lowering on the cardiovascular disease trajectory. Vascul Pharmacol . 2015;71:37-9.

Epilogue

REFLECTIONS ON 50 YEARS OF RESEARCH

My journey exploring coronary artery disease (CAD) within the Indian community took a troubling turn in the early 1970s. I witnessed an alarming surge in heart attacks among young Indian physicians, including resident physicians from Kerala, India. This unsettling trend, particularly given their lack of traditional risk factors, deeply concerned me and ignited a dedicated pursuit to understand this phenomenon.

My concern deepened during my 3-year tenure as president of the Association of Kerala Medical Graduates (AKMG) in North America. This organization of physicians with roots in Kerala, India, provided a unique vantage point. Among the AKMG members, I observed a surprisingly high prevalence of heart bypass surgery scars—a mark of membership in what was then known as the "Zipper Club". This striking observation further fueled my resolve to investigate this phenomenon, despite the absence of existing research on the topic. This pursuit ultimately culminated in the establishment of the Coronary Artery Disease in Indians (CADI) Research Foundation in 1987.

The AKMG proved to be a stepping stone for national study, providing a crucial link to the vibrant community from Kerala, a state nestled along India's tropical Malabar Coast. Kerala holds the distinction of having the highest literacy rate and lowest infant mortality rate among Indian states, coupled with the highest level of epidemiological transition. Inspired by the support from AKMG and the collaborative spirit of Chicago cardiologists Michael Davidson and Isaac Thomas, I focused on identifying a representative sample of Indian Americans for a comprehensive study. Lacking a university affiliation, I sought advice and guidance from renowned cardiovascular (CV) researchers, Jeremiah Stamler (Northwestern University at Chicago, IL) and Salim Yusuf [National Institutes of Health (NIH), Bethesda, MD] on navigating this initial step.

Salim Yusuf graciously welcomed me into his home and provided invaluable advice. He facilitated connections with William Harlan, head of the noncommunicable disease (NCD) section at NIH, and Thomas Pearson, a visiting consultant with expertise in population health. Dr Harlan was vaguely aware of a study showing higher heart disease rates in Indians in Singapore. Their collective recommendation to broaden the scope of research across multiple Indian states beyond AKMG significantly influenced my research direction. As a 3-year president of AKMG and AAPI governing body member, I gained valuable insights into the diverse AAPI membership, representing Indian physicians from various regions.

THE CORONARY ARTERY DISEASE IN INDIANS STUDY UNMASKING HEART DISEASE RISK IN INDIANS

My 1985–1988 AKMG presidency was pivotal, revitalizing the organization through membership growth and large conventions, raising its profile among Indian American physician associations. This led to my election as AAPI Treasurer (representing nearly 50,000, now 100,000, Indian American physicians). Recognizing AAPI's potential for research, I prioritized heart disease research among Indian Americans over personal advancement within the organization. Leveraging connections, I secured seed money for the CADI study.

The groundbreaking CADI study, conducted at the 1990 AAPI/AKMG conventions with nearly 2,000 Indian American physicians and families, revealed a fourfold higher heart disease rate compared to the general US general population (Framingham Offspring Study). Notably, the prevalence of traditional risk factors (obesity, hypertension, cholesterol, smoking) were similar or lower. This led me to coin the term "Indian Paradox"—high heart disease rates despite lower rates of traditional risk factors.

While diabetes was more prevalent among Indian Americans, it didn't fully explain their fourfold higher heart disease rate. This contrasted with the "Caribbean Paradox" observed in the UK, where Caribbean populations, despite having three times the diabetes rate of Whites (similar to Indians), exhibited substantially lower heart disease rates. This disparity between Indians and Caribbeans, both with similarly elevated diabetes rates but drastically different heart disease outcomes, challenged the prevailing assumption that diabetes was the overarching driver of heightened heart disease in Indians.

While CADI provided valuable insights, further research exploring the interplay of genetics, lifestyle, and socioeconomic factors is crucial. Ongoing studies like the Mediators of Atherosclerosis in South Asians Living in America (MASALA; US) and the London Life Sciences Population study (LOLIPOP; UK), investigating sociocultural and dietary influences, offer hope for targeted interventions to reduce this disproportionate burden in South Asians.

A QUESTION OF IDENTITY: FROM "EAST INDIAN" TO "INDIAN"

Presenting the CADI study results brought unexpected challenges regarding terminology. Many US professors objected to the term "Indian", associating it exclusively with Native Americans, while journal editors insisted on "East Indian", a term laden with colonial baggage. This confusion stems from Christopher Columbus's misidentification of the Caribbean inhabitants as "Indians" and the subsequent colonial terms "East Indies" and "West Indies".

Mindful of these issues, I opted for "Asian Indian", which gained wider acceptance. However, with the growing number and prominence of Indian Americans (surpassing 5 million), the term "Indian" has increasingly become synonymous with people from India. Recognizing this shift, I've embraced using "Indian" in my scientific work, acknowledging its evolving acceptance and clear connection to the population. This highlights the importance of precise terminology in research. While acknowledging the shared "South Asian" heritage, it is important to recognize the distinct identity of Indians. Just as we would not group all North Americans together in research, studying Indians distinctly is essential. Understanding their unique genetic, environmental, and dietary factors is key to developing effective interventions for this vast and diverse community, especially given their high heart disease rates despite being predominantly vegetarian.

PUBLICATIONS AND EDUCATIONAL INITIATIVES

My 1990 *AAPI Journal* article with Isaac Thomas, "Immigrant Indian Men: Sitting Ducks for Heart Attack?", aimed to raise awareness about heart disease in Indian immigrants. While reaching 50,000 AAPI members, the initial response was mixed, with some cardiology leaders dismissive and others concerned about life insurance implications. However, as data accumulated, a 1992 *American Journal of Cardiology* editorial with Salim Yusuf and Jawahar Mehta, "Prevalence of Coronary Artery Disease in Asian Indians", highlighted the earlier onset and severity of heart disease in Indians, serving as a wake-up call.

POWER OF COLLABORATION

To further foster international collaboration, I organized three meetings of the International Working Group on CADI between 1996 and 1998. These meetings brought together experts from the US, UK, Canada, Singapore, and India, leading to published proceedings in the Indian Heart Journal and fostering a strong collaborative network. Many participants, including Salim Yusuf, Jawahar Mehta, Michael Davidson, Viswanath Mohan, Rajeev Gupta, CS Pitchumoni, Basil Varkey, TS Dharmarajan, Sonia Anand, Guillaume Pare, and others, became valued collaborators and co-authors in my subsequent research and publications, solidifying the lasting impact of these international efforts. I also had the honor of chairing the first two Indo-US Health Summits held in New Delhi, further contributing to this critical dialogue, and fostering continued collaboration in CV research.

A PARADIGM SHIFT FROM HIGH RATES TO HIGH RISK OF HEART DISEASE IN INDIANS

The UK Biobank study (nearly 500,000 participants) showed South Asians have double the CV event rate of Whites, even accounting for diabetes. Critically, standard atherosclerotic cardiovascular disease (ASCVD) risk tools *underestimated* this risk, with South Asians experiencing double the predicted events. This highlighted the need to recognize South Asians' inherently higher *risk*, not just *rates*, of heart disease, demanding deeper investigation beyond traditional risk factors and equations. "South Asians" here refers to those of Indian subcontinent origin (India, Pakistan, Bangladesh, Nepal, Bhutan, Sri Lanka), with Indians comprising 70–75%.

PERSISTING HIGH INCIDENCE OF HEART DISEASE IN YOUNG INDIANS

Despite decades of research, heart disease incidence remains alarmingly high in young Indians. Balarajan's 1991 work showed a 313% higher heart disease mortality rate in Indians under 30 years compared to Whites, a trend confirmed by the recent LOLIPOP study (2024). This 20-year study of 17,606 South Asians and 7,766 White Europeans (35–75 years old) found: (1) South Asian women's CAD incidence was much higher than White women's and nearly equal to White men's; (2) South Asian men had the highest heart attack risk across all ages; and (3) the highest relative risk was in South Asians under 45 years (88% higher), decreasing to 67% higher in those over 65 years. Professor Bhopal's 50-year analysis further supports this, finding no single explanation for the elevated risk, disproving many existing hypotheses.

MY EUREKA MOMENT IN CADI RESEARCH

In May 1990, I encountered a patient that would dramatically alter the course of my research. Dr X, the principal of a major medical school in South India, suffered a severe heart attack while visiting Chicago. Despite adhering to a strict vegetarian diet and maintaining a healthy lifestyle, he presented with no discernible risk factors. However, his coronary angiogram revealed extensive and severe heart disease **(Fig. 1)**, necessitating emergency quadruple coronary bypass surgery.

Witnessing the surgeon extract an enormous, 6 cm long plaque **(Fig. 2)** from Dr X's totally occluded right coronary artery, at my behest, proved to be a pivotal moment—a true "Eureka!" moment in my research career. This unexpected finding, unlike anything I had previously encountered, ignited a profound sense of curiosity and a

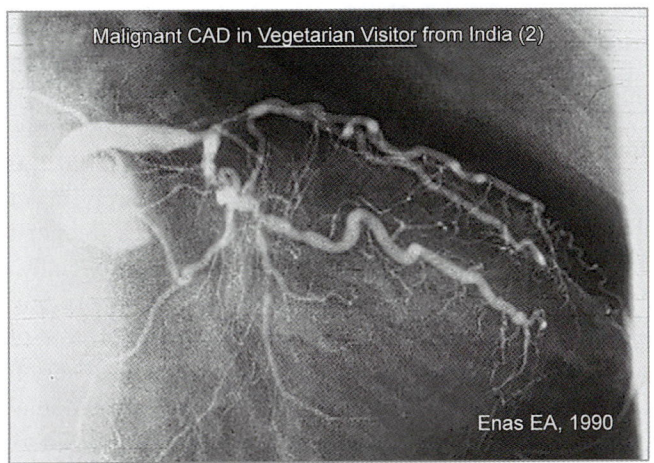

Fig. 1: Severe stenosis of the left main artery and subtotal blockage of left anterior descending artery and multiple stenosis of circumflex arteries.

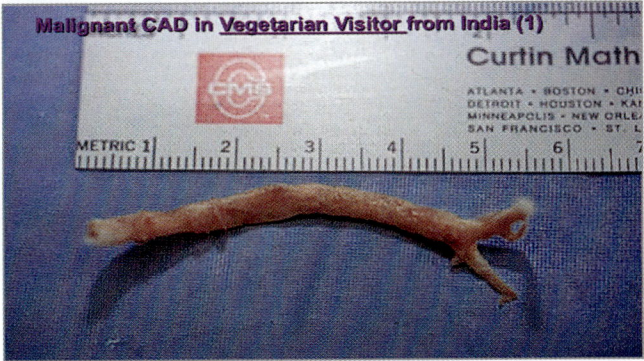

Fig. 2: An unusually large plaque that was removed from the right coronary artery.

determination to unravel the hidden forces driving heart disease, particularly in individuals like Dr X, who seemingly defied all the known risk factors. I meticulously documented the extracted plaque, capturing every intricate detail; even Dr X, a seasoned pathologist, was stunned by its size and unusual composition.

Dr X's inexplicable case, defying all known risk factors, solidified my conviction: "There's an unrecognized, more common and dangerous genetic risk factor in Indians". Feeling profound responsibility to my community, I vowed, "I won't rest until I find it". I confided in my wife. This wasn't just a medical mystery; it was a call to action, a solemn promise to unravel this hidden danger and challenge conventional wisdom.

A SERENDIPITOUS DISCOVERY: HIGH LIPOPROTEIN(a) AND MALIGNANT HEART DISEASE IN A YOUNG INDIAN PHYSICIAN

Dr Y's case—a heart attack of a 37-year-old physician—with no significant traditional CV risk factors but a strong family history of early heart attacks, became a turning point. Despite his heart attack, his initial workup, including a coronary angiogram and stress test, showed minimal disease **(Fig. 3)**. Nonetheless, his arterial plaque buildup progressed relentlessly, leading to severe heart failure within 10 years. A repeat angiogram revealed extensive blockages **(Fig. 4)**, prompting two surgeons to decline bypass surgery due to high risk and poor prognosis. A third surgeon reluctantly agreed, emphasizing the high mortality and poor long-term outlook. This case starkly illustrated the aggressive and unpredictable nature of heart disease in some young Indians.

A pivotal moment in my research occurred with the discovery of Dr Y's lipoprotein(a) [Lp(a)] level—a staggering 127 mg/dL—four times the normal limit. This pivotal discovery shifted my research trajectory. This missing piece revealed a deeper understanding of heart disease, especially in those defying traditional risk factors. Further confirmation came when his 14-year-old son was found to have an identical very high Lp(a) level of 127 mg/dL. This undeniable evidence of a powerful hereditary link—a genetic thread connecting father and son, both burdened

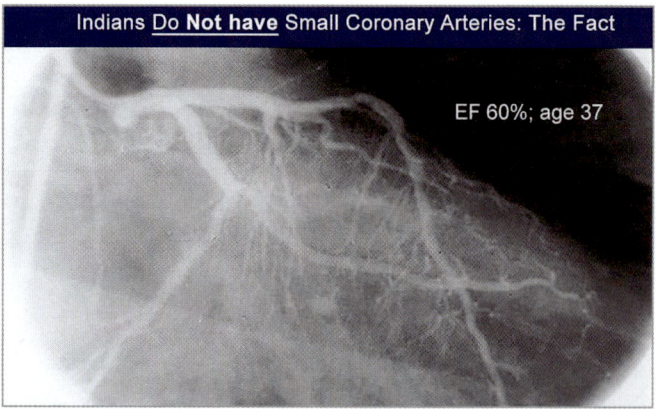

Fig. 3: Dr Y's first angiogram at age 37 years showing large coronary arteries. (EF: ejection fraction)

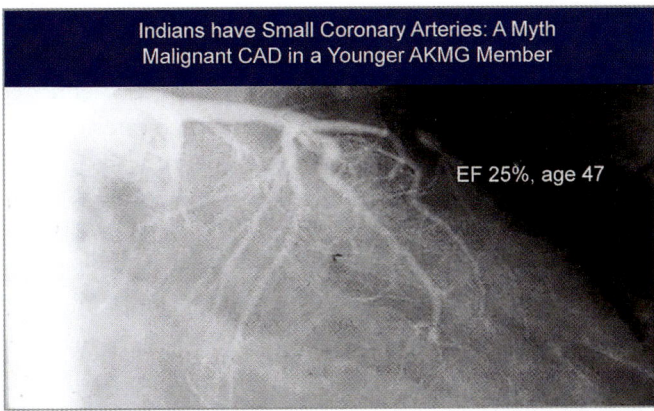

Fig. 4: Apparently small coronary arteries. Compare the size of the arteries of the same patient **(Fig. 3)** 10 years earlier.

with this hidden risk factor, served as a stark reminder that heart disease often defies predictable patterns.

■ THE "SMALL ARTERIES" MYTH

Dr Y's case challenged the misconception that Indians have inherently smaller coronary arteries. His initial angiograms showed healthy large arteries, but later images revealed seemingly "small arteries" due to extensive plaque buildup **(Figs. 3 and 4)**. This highlights the importance of considering factors beyond artery size, such as Lp(a), when assessing heart disease risk in Indians. Recognizing that extensive plaque can mimic small coronary arteries encourages a more nuanced understanding of heart disease risk in this population.

■ A BEACON OF HOPE

Dr Y's case, despite its grim initial prognosis, became a beacon of hope. Against all odds, he fought back with unwavering tenacity, defying the initial predictions of a shortened lifespan. Armed with cutting-edge medical therapies and aggressive lipid-lowering treatments, he was able to celebrate his 82nd birthday—a testament to the resilience of the human spirit and the power of medical innovation. We were able to gain 35 additional years of life for him, a far cry from the initial grim prognosis. Dr X's case, rather than a medical tragedy, became a beacon of hope, illuminating a new path in the fight against heart disease, a path I've dedicated my life to exploring.

This realization ignited a fire in me. I felt a renewed sense of urgency, a responsibility to delve deeper into the mysteries of Lp(a) and its role in premature heart disease. Dr Y's case, and the striking parallel with his young son, became a driving force in my research, pushing me to explore new avenues and challenge conventional wisdom.

Years later, Dr X's case provided a contrasting perspective. When he returned from India for a follow-up visit, his Lp(a) level was found to be modestly elevated at 48 mg/dL. This observation highlighted that cumulative lifetime exposure to Lp(a), rather than just a single measurement, significantly contributes to the development of heart disease.

This insight explained the delayed onset of his heart issues at 68 years in Dr X, compared to Dr Y's premature heart attack at 37 years. The contrasting cases of Dr X and Dr Y solidified my understanding of Lp(a)'s crucial role in malignant heart disease, particularly within the Indian population. Early aggressive lipid-lowering therapy in Dr Y's son, diagnosed with high Lp(a) at age 14 years, successfully prevented heart disease in the son as evidenced by consistently zeros scores, in later years including 2024.

Together these cases demonstrated that Lp(a) can be a primary driver of severe heart disease, even when other traditional risk factors are absent. Furthermore, Lp(a) emerged as a powerful predictor of familial risk, enabling early identification and management of individuals at high risk.

UNRAVELING THE INDIAN PARADOX AND HISPANIC PARADOX

In the early 1990s, awareness of Lp(a) was minimal, and research had seemingly stalled, until a landmark report, utilizing a more accurate assay, reignited interest by revealing a strong correlation between Lp(a) and severe heart disease. Individuals with very high Lp(a) exhibited a fourfold increased risk of severe CAD. This risk escalated to 12-fold in individuals with both very high Lp(a) and very high low-density lipoprotein cholesterol (LDL-C), highlighting the synergistic effects of these two risk factors. Leveraging Salim Yusuf's introduction, I collaborated with Thomas Pearson to analyze blood samples from the CADI study in his research laboratory, comparing Lp(a) levels across different ethnicities. Simultaneously, noting Steven Hafner's work on "Hispanic Paradox" (low heart disease rates, despite high traditional risk factors), I hypothesized that high Lp(a) might explain the Indian paradox (high rates of heart disease without high levels of traditional risk factors). This led to collaboration with Dr Steven Haffner's work suggesting that low Lp(a) levels might explain the "Hispanic Paradox". This sparked a question: Could high Lp(a) levels explain the "Indian Paradox"? We subsequently collaborated with Dr Haffner to compare Lp(a) levels in Indians and Hispanics.

HIGH LIPOPROTEIN(a) IN INDIANS

Our studies of nearly 500 individuals revealed that significantly elevated Lp(a) levels in Indians (25%) compared to Whites (17%) and Hispanics (10%) was a key factor in explaining the Indian Paradox. Subsequent US studies from the UK and Singapore have confirmed these findings with the UK Biobank showing 60% higher Lp(a) levels in Indians versus Whites. Similarly, Singaporean Indians, who have threefold higher heart disease rates than other ethnicities, also showed higher cord blood Lp(a) levels further supporting Lp(a)'s role in increased heart disease risk in Indians. The groundbreaking 2019 INTERHEART-Lp(a) study showed that South Asians had the second highest Lp(a) level (after Blacks) and the highest risk of heart attack associated with an elevated Lp(a). The evidence convincingly demonstrates that Lp(a) is a major independent risk factor for heart attacks, particularly in young individuals (<50 years) and very young individuals (<40 years), with approximately double the risk. This risk is further amplified to fourfold among those with other risk factors, particularly diabetes or elevated LDL-C.

THE GLOBAL BURDEN OF ELEVATED LIPOPROTEIN(a) IS THREE TIMES GREATER THAN DIABETES

According to the 2018 special report by the National Heart, Lung, and Blood Institute (NHLBI) elevated Lp(a) affects 1.43 billion individuals worldwide. For comparison, diabetes affects less than 500 million. Lp(a) levels vary by ethnicity: 25% of Indians have high Lp(a) levels, compared to 20% of Whites and 10% of Chinese. The report established the following Lp(a) classifications: <30 mg/dL is normal, 30–50 mg/dL is moderately high, and >50 mg/dL is high (Chapter 8).

LIPOPROTEIN(a), MALIGNANT HEART DISEASE AND RESEARCH PUBLICATIONS

Two striking features of elevated Lp(a) are its association with early heart disease and the severity of outcomes. Impressed by existing research and my own observations, I began routinely screening my patients for Lp(a). This revealed a strong correlation between Lp(a) levels and both the early onset and severity of heart disease in both Indian and White patients. In 1995, I collaborated with Jawahar Mehta on a review article highlighting the potential role of Lp(a) in aggressive heart disease in young Indians. My 2000 article, "Coronary Artery Disease Epidemic in Indians", emphasized the severe and early onset of heart disease in Indians both in India and within the diaspora. To address the misconception that Lp(a) screening should be limited to patients with unexplained heart disease, I authored a monograph in 2006 titled "Elevated Lipoprotein(a)—A Genetic Risk Factor for Premature Vascular Disease in People With and Without Standard Risk Factors: A Review".

Since my earlier work didn't have the intended impact on clinical practice, I wrote two comprehensive articles on Lp(a) for the Indian Heart Journal in 2019. The first focused on the general role of Lp(a) in CV disease, while the second specifically addressed its significance in young Indians with aggressive heart disease. I highly recommend these articles to readers interested in learning more about Lp(a).

AMERICAN GUIDELINES RECOGNIZE ELEVATED LP(a) AND INDIAN ETHNICITY AS ASCVD RISK-ENHANCING FACTORS

The 2018 American College of Cardiology/American Heart Association (ACC/AHA) Clinical Practice Guidelines marked a significant step forward by recognizing South Asian ethnicity and elevated Lp(a) as ASCVD risk-enhancing factors (Chapter 8). This recognition has important implications for treatment, warranting a more proactive approach to prevention, particularly with reference to statin therapy.

I have dedicated my career to raising the awareness about heart disease in Indians, delivering over 1,000 lectures and publishing more than 100 articles in major medical journals. I've strived to share the latest scientific progress with audiences in India and the US. My lecture series, "Heart Disease in Indians—A Global Perspective", presented at prestigious medical institutions in both countries, provided a valuable platform for engaging with leading cardiologists. My first book, "How to Beat the Heart Disease Epidemic Among South Asians", published in 2005, has helped countless individuals in India and the US. This 2025 edition synthesizes the latest scientific knowledge and treatment strategies in a clear and accessible style for

STRATEGIES TO ARREST AND REVERSE HEART DISEASE EPIDEMIC IN INDIANS

The rising heart disease epidemic in India is a complex issue fueled by lifestyle changes, dietary shifts, and the synergistic effects of various risk factors, notably the significant contribution of genetically elevated Lp(a). Urbanization and increased affluence have led to a sedentary lifestyle, a diet high in processed foods, and reduced physical activity, contributing to rising rates of obesity, metabolic syndrome, diabetes, and hypertension. High consumption of saturated and trans fats significantly increase LDL-C levels. Elevated Lp(a) significantly increases the risk of an early heart attack. An estimated 300 million Indians have elevated Lp(a), compared to 70 million with diabetes, highlighting the significant impact of this underappreciated risk factor. This risk is dramatically amplified when elevated Lp(a) coexists with other risk factors such as elevated LDL-C or diabetes, often increasing the risk of heart attack fourfold. Furthermore, the control of LDL-C and diabetes remains suboptimal in India, with only 10–20% of individuals achieving adequate control. This complex interplay of factors necessitates a multipronged approach to address the rising burden of heart disease in India. This approach must prioritize:

- Promoting healthy lifestyles through the early adoption of "Life's Essential 8" with specific targets tailored to the Indian population, including lower thresholds for waist circumference, cholesterol, and LDL-C (Chapter 17)
- Implementing strategies to effectively control LDL-C, diabetes, hypertension, and tobacco use (Chapters 4 to 7)
- Raising awareness about the significance of Lp(a) and developing strategies for universal screening and management of elevated Lp(a) (Chapter 8)
- Raising awareness that the American guidelines have lowered the desirable cholesterol level to 170 mg/dL, and our research suggests a target of 140 mg/dL for Indians (Chapters 7 and 17).
- Early identification of subclinical atherosclerosis, the foremost predictor of clinical heart disease and heart attacks, through coronary artery calcium scoring, also known as a heart scan (Chapter 2)

The PESA (Progression of Early Subclinical Atherosclerosis) study demonstrates that LDL-C levels below 60 mg/dL are needed to halt plaque progression, and levels below 30 mg/dL can induce significant regression. For Indians, achieving and maintaining an LDL-C level of 60–70 mg/dL should be a primary goal. The CV outcomes trial HORIZON, evaluating the Lp(a)-lowering agent pelacarsen, is expected to provide crucial data on the impact of significantly reducing Lp(a) levels on CV events.

By combining these efforts with personalized strategies, significant progress has been made in reducing heart disease rates among South Asians in Canada and the US, achieving near-parity with the dominant White population (personal communications with Salim Yusuf and Sonia Anand). This progress is attributed in part to awareness and educational initiatives championed by organizations like the CADI Research Foundation.

Inspired by these successes, this book provides practical tools to combat the disproportionately high rates of heart disease in young people. By implementing these strategies and fostering a proactive approach to CV health, we can significantly reduce the burden of heart disease and create a healthier future.

A LIFETIME OF GRATIFYING RESEARCH ON CARDIOVASCULAR DISEASE

It is incredibly rewarding to see the culmination of 50 years of research recognized in the growing understanding of the heightened heart disease risk in Indians and the crucial role of Lp(a). My professional idol, James Herrick, revolutionized our understanding of heart disease by being the first to describe myocardial infarction in living patients, challenging the prevailing belief that it was invariably fatal. Unlike Herrick, who may not have received widespread recognition during his lifetime, I am fortunate to witness my work gain widespread acceptance and be incorporated into national guidelines.

This legacy of knowledge, built upon the shoulders of giants like Jeremiah Stamler, Salim Yusuf, Jawahar Mehta, and Basil Varkey, whose guidance and mentorship were instrumental in my journey, will hopefully inspire continued research and innovation in heart disease prevention and treatment. Driven by a deep sense of compassion and a collaborative spirit, this journey has yielded discoveries with potentially global implications. To witness these findings, translating into improved lives for individuals and families fills me with immense gratitude.

The recognition of our work with the Most Distinguished Physician Award from AAPI and the AKMG Master Award has been a tremendous honor, acknowledging our contributions to the health and well-being of the Indian community. This 2025 book, along with the continued efforts of the CADI Research Foundation, will empower individuals to take control of their heart health by disseminating the latest data and promoting proactive lifestyle changes. I believe this work can serve as a testament to the power of dedicated research, the importance of collaboration, and the profound impact that scientific discovery can have on human health.

Index

Page numbers followed by *b* refer to box, *f* refer to figure, *fc* refer to flowchart, and *t* refer to table.

A

Acquired immunodeficiency syndrome 40
Acute coronary syndrome 22, 24, 26, 103, 118, 128, 138, 142*t*, 146, 183, 198
   diagnosis of 140
   management of 140
Acute interventional treatment, application of 147
Acute myocardial infarction 1, 2*t*, 24, 26, 27*t*, 34, 90, 100*t*, 103*t*, 138, 171, 174, 186, 187, 189
   prognosis of 144
   severity of 103
Adenosine triphosphate citrate lyase, inhibitor of 184
Adipokines 152*f*
   proinflammatory 227
Adiposity, central 152*f*
Adrenalectomy 58
Advanced glycation end products 36
Age-standardized death rate 12
Albuminuria 78
Alcohol use 37
Aldosterone, block effects of 160
Alpha-glucosidase inhibitors 75
Alpha-linolenic acid 210
American College of Cardiology 34*f*, 59, 173
   multisociety cholesterol clinical practice guidelines 40*b*
American Heart Association 134, 173, 222*f*
   multisociety cholesterol clinical practice guidelines 40*b*
Amiodarone 155
Anabolism 40
Anemia 27, 128, 143

Angina
   pectoris 128
   probability of 24
Angioplasty 141
Angiotensin-converting enzyme 146
   inhibitors 63, 78, 79, 119, 132, 145, 147, 201
Angiotensin-receptor
   blockers 63, 78, 79, 132, 145, 146, 201
   neprilysin inhibitor 160
Ankle brachial index 40, 41, 183
Anticoagulants 145
Antihypertensive medication 62, 63
Antiplatelet
   drugs 145
   therapy 119
Antisense oligonucleotides 107, 109
Aortic aneurysm 18
Aortic disease 50, 54
Apolipoprotein 19*f*, 41, 86, 94, 99, 101*f*, 116, 169, 188, 189
   high 72
   molecule of 19
   production of 108, 167
   test 91
Artery
   anterior descending 20, 21*f*, 29*f*
   posterior descending 21*f*
   small 239
Aspirin 132, 145, 147, 200
   role 202
   use 107
Asthma 50
Atherosclerosis 18, 19, 22, 24*f*, 30, 41, 50, 228*f*
   early detection of 30
   internal pudendal and penile 51
   multiethnic study of 41

   prevalence of 228*f*
   process of 138
   subclinical 228*f*, 242
Atherosclerotic cardiovascular disease 18, 33, 34*f*, 40, 42, 61, 87*f*, 89, 102, 102*f*, 105*f*, 117, 153, 167, 171-174, 186, 189, 226, 229
   high-risk 100, 145
   risk
      enhancing factors 40*b*
      management of 183*t*
Atorvastatin 145, 168, 169
Atrial fibrillation 50, 151-154, 154*fc*, 155*f*, 162
   adverse outcomes of 156
Atrioventricular nodes 20

B

Bangladesh Risk of Acute Vascular Events 8
Bare-metal stents 145
Basic pathogenetic mechanisms 72
Bempedoic acid 107, 183-185, 191
Beta-blocker 63, 132, 140, 160
Bile acid sequestrants 90, 185
Bisoprolol 145
Blood
   clot stemming 27
   flow 24*f*
   glucose levels 74*f*
   lipids 49, 222*f*, 227
   pressure 222*f*
      age-standardized prevalence of 61*t*
      category 59
      classification of 59*t*
      control of 61*t*, 64*t*, 198
      diastolic 59, 66
      high 28, 58, 71
      low 27
      lowering medications 201

Index

measurements 63t
systolic 59, 62f, 66, 174, 197
treatment of 61t
sugar 74f, 222f
high 76
low 75
tests 26
Bloodstream 213
Body mass index 38, 69, 70f, 71, 76, 151, 153, 197, 205, 225, 226, 226f, 226t
lowering 188
Brain 156
attack 156
Broken heart syndrome 118
Bronchitis, chronic 47, 50
B-type natriuretic peptide 159t
Buerger's disease 51

C

Calcific aortic valve stenosis 101
Calcium channel blocker 63, 132, 144
Calories 209
Cancer, types of 46
Cangrelor 145
Carbohydrates 35, 36, 36t, 74f, 205, 215f
complexity 74
Carbon monoxide 49, 51
Cardiac catheterization 128
Cardiac death, sudden 18, 24, 26, 27
Cardiac pulmonary resuscitation 26
Cardiomyopathy 118, 134
Cardioprotective medications, use of 79
Cardiovascular death 5f, 170f
Cardiovascular disease 1, 5f, 48, 49f, 50, 58, 59, 69, 71, 78, 101f, 117f, 145, 151, 195, 224f, 243
bedrock of 176
dominant cause of 18
large proportion of 224
lower incidence of 116
risk 49f, 90, 91, 106, 205
Cardiovascular events, incidence of 5f
Cardiovascular health 49, 221, 222f
scores 223, 224, 224f
study 41

Cardiovascular kidney metabolic syndrome 78, 151, 152f, 153t, 162
components of 152
Cardiovascular mortality 4, 213
Cardiovascular outcome trials 128, 182, 230
Cardiovascular phenotypic expression 100f
Cardiovascular risk factors 25, 33, 35f
development of 195
Cardiovascular system 86
Carotenoids 206
Carvedilol 145, 155
Case fatality rates 117f
Catheter ablation 155
Cerebrovascular disease 18, 50, 54, 69
Chest
discomfort 25f
pain 20, 26, 30
acute 30
diagnostic steps for 147
moderate-to-severe intensity midsternal 146
noncardiac 24
wall 24
Cholesterol 28, 48, 84, 85, 94, 99, 197, 213f
biosynthetic pathway 167
carrying atherogenic lipoproteins 94
clinical practical guidelines 42
era of 84b
high 8, 12, 38, 39, 43, 157, 199f
levels 93, 199, 213
reduction 198
screening 93
Chronic kidney disease 60, 78, 120, 153, 183
Chronic obstructive pulmonary disease 152
risk factor of 50
Chylomicrons 85
Circumflex artery 29f, 237f
Clopidogrel 132, 145
Colesevelam 75
Computed tomographic coronary angiography 8, 29, 130, 133, 153
Continuous glucose monitoring 75

Corneal arcus 89
Coronary angiography 29, 145
Coronary artery 21, 21f, 23f, 138, 237f, 239f
anatomy of 20, 20f
bypass graft 4, 183
surgery 21, 128, 134, 139, 167, 196
calcium 41, 42, 153, 174, 189
score 10, 24, 25b, 29, 37, 41, 42, 106, 106f, 172, 173
disease 1, 2t, 3f, 6f, 11t, 18, 25, 30, 35t, 50, 69, 100f, 103t, 120t, 130t, 138, 154, 155f, 162, 167, 171, 182, 195f, 196, 197t, 234
classic symptom of 128
cumulative incidence of 3t, 115
divergent management of 132
expression of 33
impact of 10
increased risk of 47
management of 24
premature onset of 7t
risk of 54, 212
severity of 8, 121
symptoms of 24
large 238f
layers of 140f
left main 20, 21f, 29f
remodeling 23
revascularization procedures 128, 130t, 134, 139, 167
limitations of 129
risk development 87, 87f
segment 139f
stent 167
surgery study registry 8
Coronary atherosclerosis
distribution of 21f
progression of 21, 23f
Coronary disease, chronic 134
Coronary heart disease 229f
Coronary interventions, trends of 129t
Coronary revascularization procedures 104, 134
Coronary stenosis 28
C-reactive protein, high-sensitivity 41

Index   247

D

Dairy products
 full-fat 211
 lower fat 64
Dapagliflozin 76
Deaths 11*t*
Depression 39, 157
Diabetes 38, 39, 48, 69, 69*t*, 71, 78, 120, 123, 199*f*
 control 77
 diagnosis of 73
 gestational 71, 73, 118
 mellitus 40, 69, 76, 78
 prevalence of 70*f*
 risk of 226
Diet
 high carbohydrate 34
 mediterranean 205
 unhealthy 34, 157
Dietary cholesterol inhibits 167
Dietary plant sterols, excretion of 90
Digoxin 155, 160
Diltiazem 155
Diospyros melanoxylon 52
Dipeptidyl peptidase-4 inhibitors 75
Disability-adjusted life years 10, 11*t*, 37, 52, 61, 228
Disopyramide 155
Docosahexaenoic acid 210
Dofetilide 155
Drug
 category 146
 classes of 183
Drug-drug interactions 175
Dual antiplatelet therapy 145
Dulaglutide 161
Dysbetalipoproteinemia 89
Dysglycemia 38, 39
Dyslipidemia 40, 71, 77
 atherogenic 87
 epidemiology of 92
 prevalence of 92*t*
 stems 89

E

Early subclinical atherosclerosis, progression of 223
e-cigarette
 associated lung injury 52
 use 52
Efferocytosis 19*f*

Eicosapentaenoic acid 210
Ejection fraction 238*f*
Electrical cardioversion 155
Electrocardiogram 27
 abnormal 140
Electronic cigarette use 52
Elevated lipoprotein 241
 global burden of 241
 management of 242
 striking features of 241
Emergency
 medical system 26
 quadruple coronary bypass surgery 237
Empagliflozin 76
Emphysema 50
Endothelial damage 20
Energy, replacement of 215
Epidemiology 1, 92
Epilogue 234
Eplerenone 160
Estimated glomerular filtration rate 78, 183
European Cardiology Society Guideline 140
Evinacumab 187, 185
Exenatide 161
Ezetimibe 90, 107, 183, 190

F

Fats 85
Fatty liver disease, nonalcoholic 175
Fertility treatments 118
Fibrates 190
Fibrinogen 23
Fibrinolytic therapy 141
Fibrosis 19*f*
Finerenone 78
Flecainide 155
Fluoroquinolones 185
Fluvastatin 168
Food Safety and Standards Authority of India 215
Food, types of 205
Framingham Heart Study 33, 48, 54, 197
Framingham Offspring Study 235

G

Genome-wide polygenic score 42
Glagov phenomenon 28
Gliptins 75

Global coronary artery disease deaths 11
Glomerular filtration rate 151, 152*f*
Glomeruli 151
Glucagon-like peptide-1 140
 agonists 76, 78, 161
 receptor agonists 76, 78, 132
 use of 76*t*
Glucagon-like polypeptide 1 receptor antagonist 153
Glycemic index 74, 74*f*
Glycemic load 74
Good blood sugar control 73
Groundbreaking cardiovascular outcome trials 139
Guideline-directed medical therapy 59, 128, 160
 treatment 131*t*, 134, 139

H

Health
 behaviors 221, 222
 evaluation 5
 factors 221, 222
 metrics 5
 social determinants of 23, 42, 65, 221
Healthy diet 205, 223
 prime importance of 205
Healthy eating index score 222
Healthy fats, classification of 210*fc*
Healthy sleep 221
Heart
 attack 26, 27, 40, 102, 131, 138, 145, 189, 196
 types of 27, 30
 bypass surgery scars, high prevalence of 234
 disease 20, 60, 84, 99, 102, 115, 158*t*, 182, 236, 242
 clinical manifestations of 24*t*
 death rate 4, 158, 198*f*
 diagnostic tests for 28
 high risk of 236
 impact of 195
 low risk factors for 202
 malignant 238, 240, 241
 natural history of 18
 overview of 1
 premature 8, 119

prevention of 167, 195, 199, 200t
rates, high 235
risk factor of 33, 42, 234
severe 237
treatment of 119, 167
electrical activity 28
failure 5f, 24, 50, 54, 60, 69, 117f, 151, 153, 158, 159, 162
severe 238
stages of 159t
with preserved ejection fraction 159, 161, 163
with reduced ejection fraction 159, 160, 160t
function 134
health issues 122
healthy diet 172
muscle 28, 134
rhythms, abnormal 27
scan 25b
transplantation 161
Heavy calcium deposition 29f
Hemoglobin 153
glycated 73
glycosylated 222
Hemorrhage
cerebral 60
subarachnoid 156
Hemorrhagic stroke 156, 157
management of 157t
Hepatocyte 108
High non-high-density lipoprotein 4
cholesterol 72
High-density lipoprotein 92-94
cholesterol 40, 41, 89f, 91, 169, 205
High-intensity statin 145
therapy 167, 189
Household air pollution 37
Human immunodeficiency virus 40, 175
Hydralazine 63
Hydrochlorothiazide 63
Hypercholesterolemia 38, 77, 84
familial 89, 184, 186
heterozygous familial 90
homozygous familial 89
Hyperglycemia
affects 69
promotes 72
Hyperkalemia 78
Hyperlipoproteinemia 89

Hypertension 8, 12, 38-40, 42, 43, 48, 58-62, 62f, 63, 64t, 65, 66, 77, 120, 123, 157, 226
adverse health effects of 59
control 65, 66
essential part of 63
global
impact of 60
prevalence of 60
prevention of 59
progress, control of 65
treatment of 199f
uncontrolled 66
Hyperthyroidism 152
Hypertriglyceridemia 187, 188t, 216
management of 189t
Hypertrophy, left ventricular 49
Hypoglycemia 75

I

Icosa pentyl ether 190
Icosapent ethyl 189
Immune cells 72
Inclisiran 186, 191
Indian Council of Medical Research 92
Inflammation 103, 152f
systemic 151
Institute for Health Metrics and Evaluation 115, 200
Insulin 75
resistance 3
Interleukin 6 207
Intermediate-density lipoprotein 19, 19f, 86
International Diabetes Federation 69t
Intraluminal thrombus 140f
Intravascular ultrasound 22
Invasive coronary angiography 30
Ischemia 25f, 141
recurrent 141
study 131
Ischemic stroke 27, 101, 156, 157
acute phase of 60
management of 157t
Ivabradine 132

J

Joint Association of Lipoprotein 106f

K

Kerala Diabetes Prevention Program 71, 71t
Keralite, daily diet of 212
Kidney
complications 77
disease 50, 60
chronic 60, 78, 120, 153, 183
diabetic 69, 77, 78t
failure 58
Kidney Disease Improving Global Outcomes 153

L

Lauric acid 212
Left ventricular
diastolic dysfunction 49
ejection fraction 134, 159
Lepodisiran 108
Leukocytes accumulate 72
Life's essential 8 221, 221t, 222f, 223
Lipids 85, 120
atherogenic 48
central role of 19
classification 85t
lowering therapy 23, 174t
profile 93f
terminology 85t
testing 93
Lipoproteins 10, 19f, 40, 41, 85, 86, 93, 94, 99, 101f, 103t, 106, 107, 174, 241
apheresis 107, 108
atherogenic 18, 86, 86fc, 167
cholesterol
low-density 19, 38, 40, 41, 71, 72, 86, 87f-89f, 92-94, 121, 167-169, 170f, 171, 174, 183t, 184, 185t, 186, 189, 205, 215, 222, 227, 228f, 229
lower low-density lipoprotein 182, 210, 215
non-high density 34, 90, 94, 121, 169, 222, 227
classification 85t
distribution 100t
gene 99
high 103t, 240
non-high-density 4

high-density 92-94
intermediate-density 19, 19*f*, 86
levels 94*t*
low high-density 72
low-density 19*f*
measurement 104
prevalence of 99
terminology 85*t*
very low-density 19, 19*f*, 86, 188, 189
Liraglutide 161
Lixisenatide 161
Lomitapide 187
London Life Sciences Prospective Population Study 3, 115
Loop diuretics 160
Lovastatin 84, 168
Low high-density lipoprotein 72
Low-density lipoprotein 19*f*
  apheresis 187
  cholesterol 19, 38, 40, 41, 71, 72, 86, 87*f*-89*f*, 92-94, 121, 167-169, 170*f*, 171, 174, 183*t*, 184, 185, 185*t*, 186, 189, 205, 215, 222, 227, 228*f*, 229
  era of 84
  high 39
  over life time, benefits of 169
  score 87, 88*f*, 88*t*
Lower low-density lipoprotein cholesterol 182, 210, 215
Lung
  cancer, increased risk of 47
  carcinoma of 46

M

Macronutrients 205
Main coronary artery 20
Major adverse cardiovascular events 41, 103*t*, 116, 144, 153, 167, 170*f*, 171, 182, 184, 186, 189, 196, 205, 229
  high risk for 27
  prevention 132
Major public health issue 71
Medium-chain fatty acid 212
Menopausal hormone therapy 118

Menopause 123
Metabolic disease,
  heterogeneous 69
Metabolic disturbances 3
Metabolic syndrome 40, 43
  feature of 43
  prevalence of 226, 226*t*
Metformin 75
Metoprolol 155
  succinate 145
Micronutrients 206
  trace amounts of 205
Microvascular complications 73
Million Death Study 4
Mineralocorticoid receptor antagonist 78, 160
Minerals 205
Miscarriage 50
  recurrent 118
Monoclonal antibodies 185
Monounsaturated fat 36, 210
  acid 209, 209*t*, 210, 211, 211*t*
Multiple end-organ damage 69
Multivessel disease 103
Muvalaplin 108
Myocardial infarction 4, 5*f*, 25, 40, 73, 88*f*, 117*f*, 143, 183
  increased risk of 39
  premature 103
  recurrence of 103
  types of 27*t*
Myocardial ischemia, silent 24, 28
Myocardial perfusion imaging 129*f*

N

National Family Health Surveys 51*f*
National Health and Nutrition Examination Survey 224
National High Blood Pressure Education Program 59
National Institute of Health 128
National Lipid Association Guidelines 93
Natriuretic peptides 159
Nebivolol 145
Necrosis 19*f*
Nephropathy, diabetic 77
Neuropathy
  autonomic 69
  peripheral 69

Niacin 107
Nicotine 49
  use 37
Nitrates 132
Noncardiovascular death 49*f*
Noncommunicable diseases 11
  burden of 39*t*
Nonobstructive disease 8
Non-ST-elevation myocardial infarction 27, 121
Non-ST-segment elevation myocardial infarction 138, 142, 142*f*
N-terminal pro-B-type natriuretic peptide 153, 159
Nuclear stress tests 28
Nurses' Health Study 48, 54
Nutrients, catabolism of 40
Nutrition intervention 215

O

Obesity 38*t*, 43, 71, 226*f*
  abdominal 34, 38, 38*t*, 39, 43, 71, 151, 157, 227
  central 226*f*
  generalized 39
Obstructive coronary artery
  absence of 143
  disease 143
Olpasiran 108
Omega-3 189, 210
  supplements 190
Omega-6 210
Oophorectomy, bilateral 118
Oscillometric devices 63
Overnutrition 40
Overweight 38, 71, 225, 226*f*
Oxidative stress 50

P

Pain, crushing 128
Palliative care 161
Pelacarsen 108
Percutaneous coronary intervention 4, 21, 27, 120, 128, 139, 183, 196
  indications for 141
Peripheral artery disease 4, 18, 50, 54, 69, 183
Peripheral vascular disease 195*f*
Periprocedural myocardial infarction 27

Phospholipids 99
  oxidized 101f
Physical
  activity 64, 223
  inactivity 37, 157
Phytochemicals 206
Phytosterols 90, 206
Pitavastatin 168
Plant
  protein 215
  sterols 90, 216
Plaque 22
  atherosclerotic 72, 139, 185
  formation 138
    process of 12
  hypothesis 139
  nonobstructive 30
  progression 23
  rupture 19f, 22, 23f
  stable 22, 22t, 30
  types of 22
  vulnerable 12, 22, 22t, 140f
Plasminogen gene 99
Polycyclic aromatic
    hydrocarbons 49
Polycystic ovary syndrome 118
Polygenic risk score, utility of 42
Polypharmacy 175
Polyphenols 206
Polypill 145, 147, 201
Polyunsaturated fat 36
  acid 209, 209t, 210, 211, 211t
Population attributable fraction
    34, 35f, 115
Potent atherogenic
    lipoprotein 121
Prasugrel 145
Pravastatin 168, 175
Prediabetes 73
Pre-eclampsia 118, 123
Pregnancy complications, risk
    of 50
Prehypertension 62f
Premature coronary artery
    disease 5
  severity of 9t
Premature vascular disease,
    genetic risk factor
    for 241
Prematurity 7, 8
Primary percutaneous coronary
    intervention 4, 119, 141
Primordial prevention 195, 201
Procainamide 155

Proinflammatory pathways 72
Propafenone 155
Proprotein convertase subtilisin-
    kexin type 9 184, 186
  inhibitor 107, 185, 191
    therapy 186t
Prospective Urban Rural
    Epidemiology Study 34,
    116, 206
Pyrogen injections 58

Q

Quadruple medical therapy 160t

R

Ramipril 147
Ranolazine 132
Remnant cholesterol 89f
Renal disease, end-stage 60, 175
Renal function 152f
Renal protection 76
Renin-angiotensin-aldosterone
    system 151, 152f, 154
Retinopathy 73
Revascularization procedures 4
Right coronary artery 20, 21f,
    29f, 237
Rosuvastatin 168, 169

S

Saturated fat 36, 36t, 196, 210, 215
  acid 205, 209, 211, 211t
  high consumption of 242
  major dietary sources
    of 211, 211t
Scandinavian Simvastatin
    Survival Study 167
Semaglutide 161
Seminal studies 46, 54
Septal perforator 21
Silent ischemia, sign of 28
Simvastatin 168
  low-dose 168
Single nucleotide
    polymorphisms 100f
Single photon computed
    tomography 129f
Single vessel disease 8
Sitosterolemia 90
Sleep apnea 152
Smokeless tobacco use 52

Sodium 63
  restriction 64
Sodium-glucose cotransporter-2
    76, 78, 140, 153
  inhibitors 76, 78, 132, 159, 160
Sotalol 155
Southall and Brent Revisited
    Study 2
Sphygmomanometer,
    cuff-based 58
Spironolactone 160
Spontaneous coronary artery
    dissection 118
Stable angina 24, 128, 131
  management of 131
Standard lipid profile test 104
Statin 107, 132, 140, 145, 147, 167,
    173, 190, 200, 228
  associated muscle
    symptoms 184
  lower cholesterol 167
  moderate intensity 168, 175
  target 167
  therapy 71, 168, 168t, 172,
    173t, 174, 175
    impact of 169
  treatment 41
  use of 198
ST-elevation myocardial
    infarction 26, 27,
    27t, 121
Stenosis
  degree of 21f
  severity of 129
Stress 157
  echocardiography 28
  psychosocial 39
  tests 28, 133
Stressor, physical 118
Stroke 60, 69, 86, 115, 117f, 151,
    156, 158t, 196
  death rate 158
  early detection of 156
  hemorrhagic 156, 157
  ischemic 27, 101, 156, 157
  rehabilitation 157
ST-segment elevation myocardial
    infarction 119, 141, 142f
Sulfonylureas 75
Sympathectomy 58

T

Tachyarrhythmias 118
Takotsubo syndrome 118, 123

Thiazolidinediones 75
Thrombin 22
Thrombolytic therapy 26, 141
Thrombosis 156
Thrombus burden 103
Ticagrelor 145
Ticlopidine 145
Tobacco
   deaths 37
   smoking 46, 50
   use 36, 51, 197
Total cholesterol 84, 85, 92, 93, 121, 174, 189, 213*f*, 222
Total daily calories 189, 215
Toxic effects 49
Trans fat
   acids 206
   high consumption of 242
Transient ischemic attack 156
Triglycerides 23, 85, 92-94, 99, 169, 187, 189, 215
   high 72, 90, 216
   lower mean concentrations of 116
   rich lipoprotein 189
Troponin 26
   high-sensitivity 28
   normal 143
Tumor necrosis factor-alpha 207

U

Ulcers, diabetic ischemic 69
Unhealthy fats, classification of 210*fc*
Unsaturated fat 188, 210, 215
Unstable angina 24, 26, 143

V

Vascular endothelium 49
Vasospastic angina 143
Ventricular arrhythmia, risk of 23
Verapamil 155
Very low-density lipoprotein 19, 19*f*, 86, 188, 189
   cholesterol 9
      benefits of 229*t*
Viscous fiber 215
Vitamins 205

W

Waist circumference 38, 225, 226*f*
Warfarin 155
Weight 38
World Health Organization 37

Z

Zerlasiran 108
Zipper club 234